HEALTH CARE IN RURAL CHINA

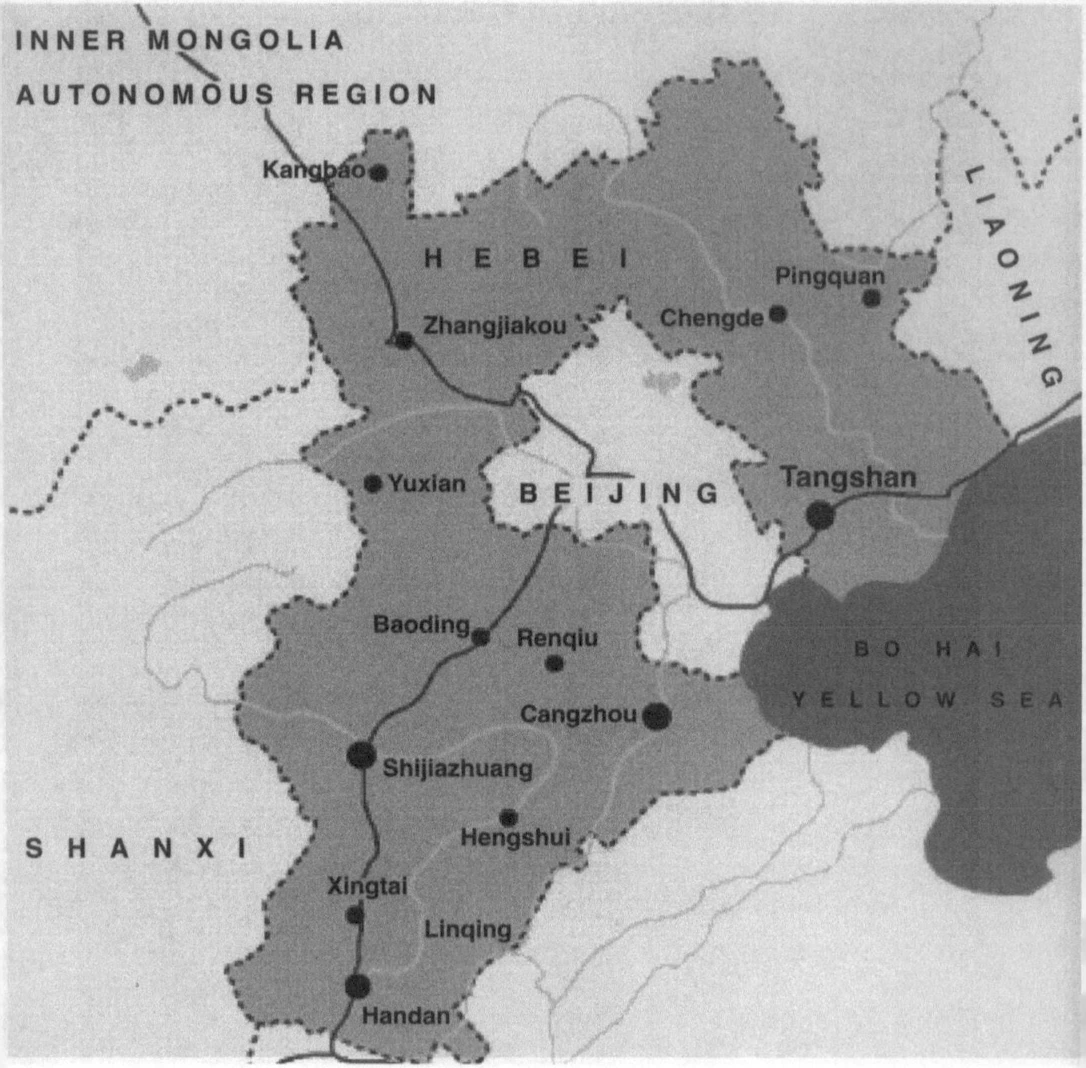
INNER MONGOLIA
AUTONOMOUS REGION
Kangbao
HEBEI
LIAONING
Pingquan
Zhangjiakou
Chengde
Tangshan
Yuxian
BEIJING
Baoding
Renqiu
BO HAI
YELLOW SEA
Cangzhou
Shijiazhuang
Hengshui
SHANXI
Xingtai
Linqing
Handan

Health Care in Rural China

Lessons from HeBei Province

OFRA ANSON
Ben-Gurion University of the Negev, Israel

SHIFANG SUN
HeBei Academy of Social Sciences,
The People's Republic of China

Routledge
Taylor & Francis Group
LONDON AND NEW YORK

First published 2005 by Ashgate Publishing

Reissued 2018 by Routledge
2 Park Square, Milton Park, Abingdon, Oxon OX14 4RN
711 Third Avenue, New York, NY 10017, USA

Routledge is an imprint of the Taylor & Francis Group, an informa business

A Library of Congress record exists under LC control number: 2004056938

ISBN 13: 978-0-815-38944-6 (hbk)
ISBN 13: 978-1-351-15664-6 (ebk)

Contents

List of Figures

List of Tables

Acknowledgments

We would like to thank the many organizations and people who have supported the project that made this book possible. We are grateful to the Netherlands--Israel Development Research Program (NIRP), which financed our study in HeBei Province and the preliminary editing of this volume. Recently, the government of the Netherlands has decided to terminate the funding of this program, which supported more than 60 collaboration efforts between scientists in Holland, Israel, and the developed countries of Africa and Asia. Valuable information was collected by these projects and presented to policy makers. Beyond the importance of supplying decision makers with missing data, the program has made it possible to train countless junior scientists. These were then able to participate in scientific work and experiments in their own countries, acquiring research experience in their respective fields and increasing their methodological knowledge and skills. We were fortunate to have had the opportunity to complete our own research and offer the hope that the program will be rehabilitated in the near future.

We haven't enough words to thank our friends and colleagues at the HeBei Academy of Social Sciences. Many of them were not directly involved in the research itself, and some were not even members of the Institute for Rural Development. We cannot name all of these kind, good-willed, hard-working people, and can only thank them for making themselves available when needed.

In particular, we are obliged to President Amaranthus Yan Lanshen and his successor President Li Zhoghua. Their support was invaluable and their advocacy opened all doors for us. We are deeply indebted to Mr. Zhang Xiaoping, the director of the Foreign and Public Affairs of the Academy, who coordinated all contacts with the authorities of the provinces, counties, and villages that we visited during the collection of the data. We admire his patience, dedication, and persistence. It is hard to imagine how he found the time to pursue his regular work during the four years of our collaboration.

Two other persons must be named: Dr. Yoav Sarig, the former Agricultural and Science attaché in the Israeli Embassy in Beijing, who skillfully managed the initial difficulties we encountered and actually saved the project. Without him, we would have stopped the project after studying two of the nine counties. Last, but by no means least, Dr. Frits W. Haanappel, our counterpart from the Netherlands, who kept the books in order.

Finally, this book was written while I spent a sabbatical leave at the Department of Interface Demography of the Vrije Universiteit Brussels. I would like to thank the VUB, the department, and Professor Ron Lesthaeghe in particular for making me so welcome and for the support they provided me.

Introduction

Periodic social, political, and economic transformations sweeping through mainland China have attracted worldwide attention for over five decades, ever since the Chinese Communist Party assumed power in 1949. But the world's absorbing interest in the People's Republic of China (PRC) cannot be attributed solely to its political and economic systems. China is home to one-fifth of the world's population (1,248,100,000 people in 1998). Almost 70 percent of the population lives in rural communities spread over 2,126 counties throughout the 9,600,000 km^2 mainland area and along its 18,000 kilometer long coastline. China has an area almost equivalent to that of the continental United States, but houses a population roughly five times the size. Providing adequate shelter, food, education, and health for a population of this size is an enormous challenge.

By international standards, China was a low income country until recently (World Bank, 2000, 2004). In 1998, the per-capita Gross National Product of the PRC was 750 US dollars a year, or $3,051 in terms of the international standard of Purchasing Power Parity rates (PPP). The average per-capita GNP in the world that year was 6.5 times higher ($4,890), and the world's average per-capita PPP was $6,300, twice that of the PRC. These figures ranked the People's Republic of China 145th and 132d, respectively, among the 206 countries listed by the World Bank. Nonetheless, China has made remarkable progress and recorded admirable achievements in providing health care for its population. By all accepted indicators, the PRC has reached mid-point in its 'epidemiological transition' within less than 50 years, a feat that took Western Europe at least twice that much time to accomplish (Omran, 1971).

As was the case in many countries, the PRC's health care system underwent important reforms during the 1980s (Chernichovsky, 1995; Twaddle, 2002). These reforms resulted largely from the dismantling of the rural collectives as part of the transition from centrally planned to free market economy and were thus more profoundly felt in the rural areas, where they affected the majority of the population. Two aspects of these reforms, the collapse of the collective medical insurance scheme and the introduction of private medical practice, raised concerns regarding equity in the distribution of health services, access to health care and treatment, and cost containment that are shared by other developing and industrially developed societies. It is these features that make the study of the PRC's rural sector interesting to students of the various disciplines of health care, and that have motivated us to write this book, which presents an analysis of the current health conditions of rural China, in their broadest definition, within their social and historical context. It endeavors to explore current social health patterns, behavior, and care, together with the processes leading to their development.

Health, however, is closely associated with cultural attitudes and beliefs, with the social structure and the distribution of goods, ideology and values, political and economical processes and patterns of behavior, in addition to the distribution and utilization of resources for coping with health problems. The book, therefore, seeks to examine the picture of health and health care in rural China by focusing on some of the primary issues studied by health specialists from various social science disciplines, as seen in the specific context of rural China. By exploring universal questions in the unique social, historical, and political context of the PRC we hope to advance understanding of the social processes which shape the social distribution of health care everywhere and to reveal implications of health care policy that are relevant to the PRC as well as to post-industrial and developing societies. Taking this approach, we set out to explore three main questions in this book:

1. What is the role of ideology, politics, and economic processes in shaping the rural population's access to health care? What are the unique ways in which the PRC copes with the tension between economic constraints and ideological commitments?

When the Chinese Communist Party came to power in 1949, the health status of the population was extremely poor. Poverty, inadequate living and sanitation conditions, and illiteracy, wars, and exploitation all contributed to the generally poor health status. Health services were scarce and inaccessible to the great majority of the population, who could not in any case have afforded them. Within 30 years (except for the period of the 'Great Leap Forward' and the famine of 1960–61), the health status of the rural population was dramatically improved, mainly as a result of an improved standard of living, raised levels of education, and effective public health programs. A three-tier health care system was built up in most parts of the country, in which more than 90 percent of the farmers were covered by cooperative medical insurance schemes. Health services became accessible and affordable to almost all.

The economic reforms of 1979 raised the rural standard of living, but also brought with them major, largely unforeseen, changes in the rural health care delivery system. Much of this change was a result of de-collectivization, which undermined the financial basis of the village as a unit. The village administration could no longer support the training of health personnel and the maintenance of the village clinic, nor could it retain the welfare safety net, including cooperative medical insurance. Within a few years, more than half of the rural health services were operating on a fee-for-service basis.

The first aim of the book is, therefore, to explore the ways in which the political, economic, and social transitions and processes experienced by the PRC since the establishment of the Republic have affected the health and the access to health care services for the rural population. Our analysis focuses on the most recent economic developments, that is, the transition from a centrally planned to a free market economy since 1979.

The health status of any population is closely related to health behavior, socioeconomic status, social support, and access to therapeutic and preventive health services. These issues will be dealt with in the book on three levels: the village, the household, and the individual. The second purpose of the book is, then

2. To explore behavior patterns among lay persons and health professionals. To what degree are different aspects of health behavior and professional practice shaped by the specific social context in which they take place?

The behavior of the rural population in sickness and health will be portrayed, including the assumption of health risks such as smoking and drinking alcohol, and patterns in seeking medical help. Like all other types of behavior, these patterns are largely non-random, tending to be shaped by structural factors, health values and attitudes, and the social characteristics of individuals and groups. The social patterns of health and illness behavior and the degree to which these follow the patterns observed in other societies will be presented and discussed.

The professional training of most village doctors in the PRC is very different from the medical education of their counterparts in industrial societies. Moreover, it has been argued that the economic reforms and the privatization of a large portion of the primary care services have increased profit-generating care on the one hand, and decreased the provision of preventive care and participation in continuing professional education on the other. The interactions among professional training, employment status, structural constraints and professional practice will be examined in the book.

Finally,

3. The book strives to examine inequalities in health, in the provision of health care and to evaluate the equity of health service distribution. Are health resources available to all in the post-collective economy of rural China today, and particularly to groups that in other societies are often disadvantaged (women, the elderly)?

The fee-for-service health delivery system often creates inequities in the distribution of health resources and unequal access to health and health care. In light of the mass privatization of primary care in rural China, we will look into the question of equity, that is, the quantity and the quality of health services available to those with greater need. The degree to which the availability of health care service is related to the social, economic, and geographical characteristics of a village will also be discussed.

The question of inequalities in health will also be addressed with respect to the individual. We will explore the well-documented relationship between the socioeconomic attributes of individuals and households, health and access to health care in rural China, with special consideration given to disadvantaged social groups, such as the poor, the elderly, and women.

Theory and Methodology

Our approach to the study of health and health care in rural China is commensurate with current trends in the sociological study of health. As a sub-discipline, medical sociology has not yet developed a comprehensive theoretical approach (Turner, 1997; Cockerham, 2001). It draws on the main theories of sociology, its mother discipline, in its effort to understand the social processes that bring about the observed distribution of health status, health behavior, and health resources in a given society. Thus, medical sociologists, or sociologists of health and illness as some prefer to call themselves, base their discussion on hypotheses submitted by structural-functionalists, symbolic interaction, and theories that place social conflict at the center of their understanding of social life in a rather eclectic manner.

This volume draws particularly on three traditions: the Weberian approach by which we seek to understand the individual actor, the structural/functionalist view of the interrelationships between social units, and the Neo-Marxist conflict theories, which guide us in our exploration of the conflicting interests within the health sector and in the doctor-patient dyad. Within the Weberian tradition, we search for the meaning attributed by the actors to their social actions, whether the actions concern their own health or the health of others. The two concepts, life chances and life style, are most useful for our discussion of health differentials, social distribution of health behavior and cultural meanings attributed to these types of behavior. The notion of a sense of 'calling' provides us with a helpful framework for analyses of the behavior patterns of care providers.

During the 1950s and 1960s, it was widely accepted that one basic characteristic of a service profession is a 'calling' orientation. Structural functionalists argued that this 'calling' orientation dictates professional behavior, which places service before personal interests. This school of thought, however, rarely dealt with the arguably paradoxical interpretation of the primacy of service that stems from the Weberian concern with bureaucracy and bureaucratic organization. The question of whose interests are to be served, those of the organization, of the professional group, or of the client, were not raised until the 1970s (Freidson, 1970).

Neo-Marxist analysis, conflict theory, and political economy have prevailed in the sociology of health and illness since the 1970's (Turner, 1997). Our book draws heavily on this tradition, particularly on current sociological critiques of the health reforms that have gained currency in Western countries during the past two decades. Central to these critiques is the withdrawal of the welfare state and the increasing privatization of social services, including medical care. These critiques suggest that vested interests of powerful social groups, that is, their efforts to retain power and economic privilege, have motivated the changes in the magnitude and the mode of the provision of welfare services and their ideological basis. These processes have led to increased emphasis on cost containment and profit generation. Competent management and competition between providers became magic means for achieving financial efficiency, quality of services, and patient satisfaction. Freedom of choice, autonomy, and individual responsibility for one's health and welfare have become central themes in the emerging ideology that underlies the new policies of many welfare states.

Current critiques posit that hidden motives behind the transitions in health and welfare policy of the state have legitimized increasing focus on the rewards of power and financial gain among both health organizations and individual practitioners. Consequently, equity in the distribution of health services has declined, while health differentials and inequalities in access to health care have increased. These theoretical propositions will guide our analyses of the health processes adopted by the PRC after the economic reforms of 1979 and the consequent reforms in the rural health care system during the early 1980s.

Given the size of the PRC in terms of area and population, and the enormous variability in its topography, resources, and economic development, a thoroughgoing and comprehensive analysis of health in rural China as a whole is not possible. The health consequences of the social, political, and economical processes discussed in this volume will therefore be demonstrated by focusing on just one of the 31 provinces, municipalities, and autonomous regions, HeBei Province in Northern China. Our analysis will concentrate on data collected by the authors as part of a joint Chinese-Israeli-Dutch research project. A random sampling of 288 villages in 9 counties was chosen to represent the geographical and economic development variability of rural HeBei. Between 1996 and 1999, information was collected by native interviewers from 14,895 persons of all ages belonging to 4,319 households. In addition, 416 doctors were interviewed and 1,262 patient records were collected. This data base will be supported and placed in focus by reference to published secondary sources. In so doing, we furnish the reader with a comprehensive review of the literature and a summary of the accumulated body of knowledge related to the transitions in health status and health delivery in rural PRC, in addition to extensive empirical evidence recently gathered in a specific province.

We wish, however, to call the attention of the reader to two limitations of the data presented in this book. First, we followed Riley and Gardner (1997), relying almost exclusively on the scientific literature published in the English language international scientific journals. There were two reasons for this choice, both related to the quality of the material. The articles published in scientific journals deal with universal questions and debates that are relevant to the international scientific community. Because our aim is to examine health issues which are universal, the body of knowledge seemed more relevant than studies published in Chinese alone, which usually reported data with limited, local relevance reflecting a more specific, narrower interest.

Moreover, in the past few years China's health and population policies seem to have lost their appeal to social scientists, and the number of publications appear to have declined particularly after 1997, the year of the IUSSP General Population Congress in Beijing. The reader will note that the bulk of the relevant literature was published during the 1980s and early 1990s.

The second limitation is our use of formal secondary data and statistics, which are also available to international organizations. The quality of these data is not always clear, because the PRC depends on the competence and understanding of local administrations with respect to the importance of accurate data. It is generally accepted that vital statistics and other data concerning the PRC before the 1980s is of relatively poor quality (Banister, 1998; Riley and Gardner, 1997). Because evaluations of corrections necessary to improve their accuracy vary considerably, we chose to use the data published by the PRC related to long term trends in population health and the general resistance resources available to it.

The Structure of the Book

The concept of health, as broadly defined by social scientists, is multifaceted. Each aspect reflects and interacts with other social aspects of life, such as cultural values, health attitudes, behavioral patterns, and access to social goods. In order to fulfill the three main goals of this volume, we decided to examine in detail several selected health issues before drawing conclusions. Each of the first eight chapters considers a specific aspect of health; each presents a focused analysis of one facet of the current health status and the provision of health care and explores the processes leading to its current status. The final chapter builds on the findings presented throughout the book, in light of the three stated aims of our research.

The first chapter sets the scene in which access to health care has increased since the establishment of the PRC in 1949, briefly reviewing the development of the rural health service system and health-related social criteria, such as standard of living, education, and social support.

Chapter 2 looks at the consequent health status and examines the health-related resources involved in the social, political, and economic processes described in Chapter 1. It presents long-term trends in health status, social investment in health, and health resources allocated to the rural population. Special emphasis is placed on the health reforms initiated as part of the transition to a market economy. Current health indicators and health resources in the PRC are compared with those of eight other Asian societies.

Chapter 3 presents the unique and innovative ways in which the PRC has achieved the remarkable improvement in the health of the rural population. The applicability of the PRC's experience in coping with extreme health difficulties as well as public health problems currently faced by China and other developing and post-industrial societies are also discussed in this chapter.

Chapters 4 and 5 focus on patterns of health behavior and their social context. Chapter 4 examines patterns of health care delivery as shaped by professional training on the one hand and the social setting of the practice on the other. Chapter 5 concentrates on the social patterns of lay health behavior, from confronting health risks to consumption of health services.

Chapter 6 addresses the most debated consequence of the economic and health reforms instituted in the rural sector of the PRC since the early 1980s: equality of access to health and health care and equity of health service distribution. These issues are discussed on two levels, that of the individual and that of the village as a social unit. Social class health gradients and gender health differences are considered on the individual level. On the village level, the interaction among economic development, geopolitical location, health and the availability of health services is presented.

Chapters 7 and 8 focus on two different, often disadvantaged, social groups. Chapter 7 is devoted to issues of women's health, with particular focus on the policies for population limitation implemented during the history of the PRC and their effect on reproductive health. Chapter 8 focuses on the special health needs of the elderly and on the formal and informal social support available to rural seniors.

Chapter 9 summarizes the discussion and highlights the information provided throughout the volume in light of the three main goals of the book. The discussion draws on current debates and theoretical developments in the medical social sciences and suggests possible lessons for health policy makers in China as well as in developing and industrial societies in general.

Chapter 1

Setting the Scene: Health, Health Services, Ideology and the Economy

Patterns of health and the specific form of health services in any society are largely the product of social, economic, and political processes unique to that society. The first goal of this chapter is to introduce the development of the rural health services and general coping resources in the People's Republic of China (PRC). The major political and economic events that occurred in the PRC during the first three decades of Communist regime left their mark on the health status, health care system, standard of living, level of education, and social support available to the population. This historical presentation sets the scene for detailed analyses of the different features of health and health services in the rural PRC.

The degree to which HeBei province represents rural China as a whole will also be discussed in this chapter. Such a comparison is valuable because the analysis of patterns of health and health services to be presented in the following chapters is largely based on research conducted in HeBei Province during 1996–1999. Such an evaluation will help to assess the extent to which our findings may be applicable to other parts of rural China as well.

The Development of Rural Health Services

The processes which led to the current health status and health care system in contemporary China can be divided into four major periods: the first three five-year plans, from the establishment of Communist China until 1958; the period of the 'Great Leap Forward'; the decade of the 'Cultural Revolution'; and the political change after the 'Cultural Revolution', which brought about economic reforms, starting in 1979. This section contains a brief presentation of the effect of these processes on the development of health and the health care system.

From Liberation to the 'Great Leap Forward': 1949–1958

The People's Republic of China (PRC) was established in 1949, after centuries of exploiting feudalism, colonialism, war with Japan, and civil war during the period of the communist revolution. In the rural areas, which is the focus of this volume, poverty prevailed, housing and sanitation conditions were inadequate, the majority of the population was illiterate. As a result, the health status of the population was extremely poor. Although vital statistics were rarely collected systematically, it is commonly accepted that life expectancy at birth was about 37 years, infant mortality about 250 per 1,000 live births, and maternal mortality was estimated at 150/100,000 (Young, 1989; Ministry of Public Health, 1993; Chen, 2001).

Health services were very scarce, especially in the rural areas. The few available services were concentrated in the cities and were privately owned. It is estimated that in 1949 there were 0.67 doctors per 1,000 population and only 3,600 health institutions in the whole of China. Of these, 2,600 were located in the cities, where only a minority of the population lived. Because of the paucity of roads and vehicular transportation, these services were almost inaccessible to the majority of the Chinese population, most of whom lived in the rural areas (Ministry of Public Health, 1984; China Year Book, 1998). The rural population had to rely on traditional healers and persons applying traditional Chinese medicine with little or no formal education and vocational training (Liu et al, 1994).

Poor health status and lack of health services were incompatible with CCP ideology and goals. Chinese socialism sought to establish a perfect publicly owned society, where the distribution of resources, goods, and products is based on and designed to meet the needs of all members of the society (Wong and Chiu, 1998). Indeed, in the 1954 constitution, adopted shortly after the Chinese Communist Party (PRC) rose to power, the PRC stated its commitment to provide each citizen with 'five guarantees' – the right of all to food, health care, education, shelter, and a funeral.

This ideology was the basis of the first five-year plan (1950–1954), when the health and welfare policy, aimed at establishing the foundations for a nationwide improvement of health and health services, was first declared. It was clear from the experience of the Soviet Union that the key to rapid improvement in the health status of the population lay in public health, particularly in light of the limited available resources that could not provide curative treatment for all who needed it. The 'Four Principles' were formulated at the First National Health Conference in August 1950 and measures were initiated to implement them. According to this policy (Dezhi, 1992; Liu et al, 1995; Wong and Chiu, 1998): (i) health care should be provided to workers, farmers, and soldiers by publicly owned and financed health services; (ii) health services should 'walk on two legs', that is, combine traditional Chinese medicine with Western medicine; (iii) give priority to public health, with emphasis on the prevention of communicable and infectious diseases and mother and child care; (iv) combine health care with mass health campaigns in order to break epidemiological triangles and educate the public on personal hygiene and healthy nutrition.

Actualization of these principles began during the second and third five year plans, together with the implementation of other goals of the CCP (Chen et al, 1995). From 1949 on, all types of private enterprise were gradually nationalized. Private capital and land were confiscated by the government and private industries were bought by the government at low prices. By 1956, land was redistributed to rural collectives and the share of private production, more than 60 percent of GNP in 1949, was reduced to less than one percent (Liu et al, 1995). Similar actions were taken in the health sector.

Table 1.1 Morbidity and mortality from infectious diseases, China 1952–1979 (per 100,000 population)

	Morbidity % change		Mortality % change	
	1952–65	65–79	52–65	.965–79
Animal control				
Anthrax	na	5.13	na	-50.00
Brucellosis	na	-84.85	na	na
Kala-azar	-94.11	-99.00	-86.67	-97.50
Leptospirosis	na	-85.55	na	0.00
Malaria	65.12	-71.55	-95.89	-66.67
Scrub typhus	na	-56.25	na	na
Environmental and personal hygiene				
Dysentery	203.82	38.99	-56.95	-18.75
Typhoid and Paratyphoid fever	9.77	-33.94	-86.36	-55.56
Typhus fever	73.21	-71.13	-84.62	-50.00
Immunization				
Diphtheria	100.44	-87.22	107.69	-90.37
Epidemic encephalitis	2,493.84	-60.80	621.67	-75.06
Measles	568.15	-85.96	21.40	-91.40
Pertussis	837.85	-59.64	155.00	-82.35
Poliomyelitis	Na	-85.96	na	-87.50
Scarlet fever	189.47	11.49	-92.31	-50.00

Source: Adapted from Dezhi, 1992.

From the 'Great Leap Forward' to the 'Cultural Revolution': 1958–1965

Health institutions were transferred from private or foreign ownership to the ministry of health or to the health departments of local governments. Doctors in private practice were gradually recruited by the developing public sector. Basic training programs were developed to prepare health workers to carry out public health policies and health campaigns.

The 'Great Leap Forward', launched in 1958, was aimed at achieving an agricultural and industrial revolution as quickly as possible (Peng, 1987). To meet these goals, collectivization of production, begun in 1956, was accelerated, new cultivation methods were implemented and rural manpower directed to industrial activity. By the end of 1958, virtually all of the rural population had been organized in communes. Villages became production brigades; large villages were sometimes divided into several production teams. Community dining rooms or public mess halls were established to liberate women from housework and enable them to fully participate in political, social, and economic activities. The most important objective of the Great Leap Forward was expeditious industrialization, with emphasis on heavy steel industry and boosting agricultural production.

The allocation of most social resources and rural manpower to industrialization and the implementation of unsuitable agricultural methods, such as over-farming, however, drained the soil, forestry, and food resources. A long period of drought and floods brought about a sharp decline in agriculture production, which together with a change in patterns of food consumption, misjudgment, and mismanagement of the available grains caused serious famine in many parts of rural China (Peng, 1987). Estimates of the human cost of the Great Leap Forward and the consequent famine vary between 20 and 50 million lives (Hesketh and Zhu, 1997). Nonetheless, several important developments took place in the rural health sector during this period.

With accelerated collectivization of the rural population, the recruitment of care providers also quickened. Data from Shanghai suggest that by 1962 only 3 percent of all health personnel were engaged in private practice, compared with 56.5 percent in 1950. Many of these practitioners were assigned to township health centers, which started to expand after 1959, enabling local training of health personnel (Liu et al, 1996). The well-known 'barefoot-doctors', farmers chosen by their fellow members of the working team and trained in three-month apprenticeship programs in township health centers, were introduced. Trained locally, the 'barefoot-doctors' remained in their home-villages, where their contribution to the rural health sector was considerable Chapter 2).

It was during this period that health insurance first appeared in rural China. This process can be seen in light of the CCP ideology, which regarded meeting the health needs of the population as a basic right, but also in light of the active involvement of the population in health issues and the spirit of collectivization sweeping the country at that time. The three insurance schemes available in the PRC are described in the next chapter; we need only note here that rural cooperative medical coverage started as a local initiative in several collectives before it was formally adopted as a national policy in 1960. It is difficult to imagine such mass mobilization in a voluntary mutual aid scheme without ideological commitment to the socialist value system and a sense of social responsibility, at least on the part of local leaders.

The Great Leap Forward and the famine of 1959–61 had other consequences, with positive health-related effects in the years to come. A system of grain transfer and distribution was developed that guaranteed each commune at least a minimum per capita grain supply ensuring survival in the event of flood, drought or other natural disasters (Tang et al, 1994). The supply of water, necessary for the industrialization effort, had been extended to remote parts of rural China. Water made more accessible to the population and the newly-created infrastructure enabled the development of rural industry in a later period. With the economic reforms of 1979, rural industry became an important source of income for both individuals and the local administrations.

The Cultural Revolution: 1966–1976

The era of the Cultural Revolution was a period of severe social and economic turbulence. Ideologically, the 'Great Proletarian Cultural Revolution' was consistent with Mao Ze Dong's perception of the Communist philosophy of perpetual social change and reexamination of values, attitudes, and structure. The objectives of the Cultural Revolution were to eradicate the remains of so-called bourgeois ideas, capitalist and Western orientations, old customs, and to recapture the revolutionary enthusiasm of early Chinese Communism. Mao also wanted to weaken the party bureaucracy, now entrenched in privilege, stagnation and nepotism brought about by the relative social stability of the post-revolutionary period, and to restructure the educational system to benefit farmers and manual workers. During the Cultural Revolution, the residual private economic enterprises that survived nationalization and collectivization had been banned, and self employment production prohibited. Many intellectuals, in particular those with Western training or specialization and persons with foreign relations, were publicly criticized, many of them losing their positions. Scholars, students, administrators, and others suspected of revisionist convictions or relaxed attitudes toward Marxist ideology were 'sent down' to be reeducated by farmers.

This period of turmoil deeply affected the health sector as well. The few doctors who still practiced privately either stopped practicing medicine altogether or joined publicly owned facilities. Like university education in general, higher medical education largely ceased, research projects were abandoned and many hospitals were closed. The number of practicing doctors declined from 1.05 per 1,000 inhabitants to 0.85, the number of health facilities declined by 33 per cent. Some health campaigns that had successfully decreased mortality from infectious diseases during the first 15 years of the PRC were discontinued (China Yearbook, 1998; Dezhi, 1992; Liu et al, 1994).

The Cultural Revolution, however, affected mainly urban health care institutions and personnel. Mao criticized the elitism of the members of the medical profession, the priority given by them to science, and their preference for urban hospitals. The administration of the Ministry of Public Health was criticized for having an urban bias and for the excessively slow development of primary medical services in the countryside. In a directive released in June 1965, on the verge of the Cultural Revolution, Mao wrote "Tell the Ministry of Public Health that it only works for 15 percent of the entire population. . . . It should be called the Urban Public Health Ministry, or the Ministry of Public Health for Urban Overlords." (Wilenski, 1976).

Indeed, rural health services flourished and expanded during this turbulent period. Private practices were replaced by public services and relocation of university trained physicians brought highly competent medical personnel to the rural areas. The population movement that destroyed the urban health services simultaneously fostered development and expansion of county hospitals, township health centers, and the training and updating of rural health workers, barefoot-doctors, and midwives. While the total number of health care personnel decreased by 5 percent between 1965 and 1970, the number of nurses and midwives increased by 25 percent. The spread of the three-tier health delivery network was also completed during this period. The number of village clinics and health centers increased dramatically, and by the end of the Cultural Revolution almost all villages had a clinic in which 2–4 barefoot doctors served populations of 1,000 to 3,000. The few exceptions were remote small villages, mainly located in the mountains. Barefoot doctors could consult with and refer patients to the nearest township health center that served some 25 villages, or between 15,000 and 50,000 people. By the early 1970s, most health centers were equipped with in-patient facilities and the range of their services expanded. If these were still insufficient, patients could be referred to the county hospital, which was responsible for about 14 township health centers.

The rural cooperative insurance scheme was also expanded during this period. Consequently, by 1976 health services were affordable and accessible to most of the population. The majority of the urban and rural populations were entitled to treatment under one of the three health insurance schemes, which covered a large proportion of their medical expenses. Hospital registration fees, the price of medications, medical treatment and procedures were centrally controlled at a low level. The three-tier grassroots facilities were well dispersed, though the variety and quality of care provided remained uneven. In general, village clinics provided services for the population within a radius of 1.5–2.5 kilometers, making them highly accessible. Moreover, rural health care providers were highly motivated to serve the population to the best of their ability (Chen et al, 1993; Dezhi, 1992; Kan, 1990; Liu et al, 1994).

At the same time, the 'Cultural Revolution' had serious negative health consequences. Some 17 million urban residents, the majority of whom were youngsters from high-school to college age, were mobilized and 'sent down' to agricultural work (Zhou and Hou, 1999). For many, this experience was rather traumatic. Urbanites were unfamiliar with the comparatively poor living conditions of the countryside and inexperienced in the manual labor they had to engage in for long hours, seven days a week. Above and beyond the physical difficulties, the relocated persons were disconnected from family, friends, and social support networks. In the cities most services and government agencies, including health, welfare, and job allocation, almost stopped functioning. The urban economy was largely paralyzed and unemployment rates increased dramatically. The negative health consequences of such processes have been documented in other developed and developing communist societies. Although, according to some estimates (Banister, 1997), there was no detectable increase in mortality during the Cultural Revolution, the social unrest, unemployment, and dislocation were bound to adversely affect the health of millions. The magnitude of these health consequences is still unclear.

The Economic Reforms, from 1979 Onwards

The upheaval of the Cultural Revolution severely damaged China's economy. The major challenge in the first years after this revolution was to revitalize the economy. During the period of 1977–1979, a transition from central planning, collective production and consumption toward a 'socialist market economy' was planned and gradually implemented. Development of the rural economy, which embraced 82 percent of the population at that time and was crucial for the guarantee of food supplies, became a top priority. Indeed, one of the first measures introduced was 'the responsibility system of household production' in rural China. Collective agriculture had been disbanded over a two-year period and land had been redistributed to families according to household size. Generally, households receive their portion of the brigade's land on a 15 year lease. Planned agriculture production had been gradually reduced and farmers increasingly enjoyed the freedom to cultivate products not stipulated by the state. A specified amount of produce per unit land was paid to the government in tax; the rest could be sold on the free market. This two-track approach enabled the government to maintain a supply of basic foodstuffs at relatively low prices, while gradually increasing the price of state supplies to market level (Sachs and Woo, 1996).

In contrast to the effect of the Cultural Revolution on the health sector, the new economic reforms left the urban health care system basically intact. However, they had profound consequences for the rural health services (Chen et al, 1993; Gian, 1991; Liu et al, 1994; Kan, 1990; Shi, 1993; Sun, 1992; Young, 1989; Hsiao, 1995). 'The responsibility system of household production' initiated a number of interrelated processes that led to the collapse of practically all cooperative medical schemes and to the privatization of almost half of the rural clinics within six years, leaving most of the rural population with no insurance coverage. By 1989, health services at reduced fees or other mechanisms for the reimbursement of medical expenses were available only in 4.8 percent of the villages in the whole of China. One of the most important factors underlying these process was the collapse of the financial base of the village brigade as a consequence of the dissolution of the collective structure.

Prior to the economic reforms, the cooperative medical scheme was financed by contributions of the members, the brigade's welfare fund, and the county or provincial government (Wong and Chiu, 1998). Accounts were kept by the village administration, which distributed cash in exchange for work points. In many places, the village administration had first deducted the premium, 0.5 percent of household income, distributing cash remainders only. Now, with the transition to household economy, the village no longer controlled its inhabitants' income, and was unable to maintain and finance the medical cooperative.

Mobilizing the population to participate voluntarily in an insurance scheme after the transition to market economy presented several problems. First, farmers had no concept of 'insurance', and those who did not anticipate medical expenses were not willing to join. Second, for many farmers, administrators, and politicians, the cooperative scheme, which developed rapidly and became compulsory during the Cultural Revolution, was associated with turmoil and was therefore dismantled along with other aspects of this period, already discredited by the People's Congress. Moreover, the disposable income of rural family increased dramatically within a short time, quickly followed by growing demand for high quality health care. Wealthier farmers preferred to seek medical help at county or city hospitals, despite the inconvenience and additional costs involved (Liu et al, 1996; Yip et al, 1998). The degree to which this preference was maintained in the long run and the social patterns of such preferences will be further discussed on the basis of our study in HeBei Province in Chapter 5.

At the same time, the income generated from practicing medicine in the village cooperative clinic was relatively low. Barefoot doctors, who had formerly enjoyed higher income than the farmers, now ran the risk of lagging behind their neighbors in per capita income. The demand for higher quality health services forced them to improve the equipment they used, store a wider range of medications, and upgrade their professional skills. With the fall of the cooperative medical system and its replacement by the individual responsibility system they had to bear all of the costs themselves. Some had exchanged the practice of medicine for a different economic activity or enterprise, such as agriculture, business, or the developing rural industry. Others combined business and/or agriculture with medical practice, a solution that seems to prevail today since, like their fellow farmers, village doctors received their share of redistributed collective land (see Chapter 4). The brigade clinic, no longer supported by the village administration, was frequently leased to one or more of the doctors who had operated it under the cooperative system. Others established group practices or opened clinics in their own homes or places of business. Most of the village doctors earned their living on a fee-for-service basis, whether the fees were paid entirely by the patients or partly covered by the newly emerging rural medical insurance schemes. In some cases, agreements were signed with village doctors for the continued provision of preventive health care in return for a fixed annual income financed by public resources.

The reforms deeply affected the entire three-tier rural health provision system. Township health centers, formerly financed by the public resources, were now increasingly dependent on patient fees and on the operation of non-medical economic enterprises (Wong and Chiu, 1998). Many township hospitals could not cope with the economic reforms in the health sector, such as the increase in material costs while patient fees remained under government control, or decrease in the government's share of financing their running costs, and had to close down or reduce the number of staff and beds. Between 1980 and 1987 the number of township hospitals decreased by 15 percent and the number of township level beds by 17 percent. Similarly, public funding no longer covered the costs of running the county hospitals (Hsiao, 1995). While facilities on both levels enjoyed more freedom in generating income and the use of surplus income, the pressure to increase income and cut expenses affected medical practice, equity and equality. The links among the three tiers of care weakened; health centers and hospitals were increasingly reluctant to invest in rural primary care and village doctors became solo practitioners, relatively free of collegial supervision.

At the same time, some hospitals opened branches in rural areas after 1979. This trend was motivated by a combination of three factors already discussed: (a) the collapse of the collective, which left some villages, especially remote and poorer ones, without any health care services at all, forced the government intervene in order to provide the health care needed by the population; (b) the opening of branches of upper level hospitals in the rural areas, staffed by graduates from colleges or universities, was one measure taken to improve the quality of rural health care (see Chapter 2); and (c) the creation of outpatient fee-for-service facilities enabled hospitals to better cope with growing pressure to generate a growing share of their own resources. The government continued to bear most of the expenses of public health, but due to the reforms of the health sector these services were administrated independently of the curative care services. It also became increasingly difficult to mobilize farmers for health campaigns, partially because they were not paid for the time spent on these activities (see Chapter 3).

The rise in standard of living, presented in the next section, together with the continuation of free public health and preventive medicine services, brought about a significant improvement in the health of the population since 1979. In 1987, some ten years after initiation of the transition from central planning and controlled market to a 'socialist market economy', life expectancy at birth was 71.5 in the cities and 67.3 in the countryside (Ministry of Public Health, 1993); infant mortality in the cities was 20.0 per 1,000 live births and 46.5 in the villages (Dezhi, 1992); maternal mortality in 1989 was 50 and 115 in the cities and villages, respectively (Lawson and Lin, 1994). Mortality rates for 23 infectious diseases declined from 18.71 per 100,000 populations in 1965 to 4.40 in 1979 and 1.49 in 1988; the respective morbidity rates were 35.0, 20.8, and 4.7 per 1,000 populations. Nonetheless, there were some indications that the improvements in health indicators leveled out during the 1990s, that the health consequences of economic prosperity in rural China since the economic reforms are far from satisfactory, and that the general improvement masks considerable national and regional variation (Liu et al, 1999). In other words, while some social groups have enjoyed dramatic improvement in health status, the health of other groups has stagnated, while that of still others seems to have deteriorated.

Open Questions

The changes that took place in the rural health care system raise several questions, some of which we will attempt to answer in later chapters. Most of these questions stem from the combination of fee-for-service health care provision system, in which an individual village doctor, working in professional isolation, and enjoys a great deal of professional freedom provides the primary care services. How does this situation affect medical practice? Are village doctors in such settings more inclined to concentrate on income-generating medical practices than are salaried village doctors? It has often been argued that fee-for-service may lead to focus on the income-generating curative care, with consequent neglect of the less profitable preventive medicine and health education (Cao and Zhong, 1990; Kan, 1990; Li, 1993; Zhou, 1992; Zhu et al, 1993; Hillier and Shen, 1996). Indeed, Gautam (1993) reported that since the extension of fee-for service health care, immunization coverage has declined from close to full coverage to 60 percent among urban children ans 33 percent among rural children. There is some evidence that the reduction in the incidence and prevalence of some diseases has slowed and even been reversed in some parts of the PRC (A World Bank Country Study, 1992; Zhu et al, 1989). Others have found that this was a short-term trend during the transition period alone (Chen et al, 1993; Haung, 1988). However, the health transition and the aging of the population present new challenges as the incidence and prevalence of chronic conditions such as cancer and cardiovascular diseases increase (Gautam, 1993; Tao et al, 1989). These health conditions are mostly incurable but somewhat preventable and can largely be delayed through risk control, health education, and health behavior intervention programs. Are village doctors in fee-for-service practices providing less preventive care than doctors whose income is not completely dependent on patient fees?

Except for narcotics and heavy tranquilizers, village doctors enjoy the freedom to prescribe all medications they find appropriate. The sale of drugs and medical procedures, such as injections and infusions, are the main sources of income for private practitioners, health centers and hospitals in the PRC (Gu et al, 1993; Umland et al, 1992; Dong, et al, 1999c). Indeed, according to several sources (McGreevey, 1995a, 1995b; Tang et al, 1994), medications account for some half of the total health expenditures in China (A World Bank Country Study, 1992). Do village doctors in private practice over-prescribe and perform medical procedures more often than village doctors whose income is not directly related to service?

Many of the village doctors practicing today started their careers as barefoot doctors and have limited professional training. In recent years, the Chinese Ministry of Health have made several attempts to improve their professional competence (see Chapter 2). Local governments have initiated continuing education programs in township health centers and county hospitals for village doctors (Chen, 1995). Yet without formal means of enforcement and coverage of their expenses, village doctors have little incentive to take part in these programs, save their professional commitment and consumer demand. What are the social patterns of such participation?

The transition from the rural cooperative medical scheme to a fee-for-service system raises the issue of equity and equality between regions, villages, households within the same village, and individuals within the same household (Bledsoe et al, 1988; MacCormack, 1988; Liu et al, 1994; Hillier and Shen, 1996; Chen, 2001). Both financial pressures and profit motive could lead to the establishment of clinics and medical practices in better off regions and villages, those that allow a private village doctor to achieve a comfortable standard of living, and a hospital to generate more resources. Yet, the well-documented positive association between standard of living and health indicates that it is the poor regions and villages that have the greater health needs. Are the rural health services distributed according to the needs of the population?

Before the economic reforms, health services were accessible and affordable for all. More than 90 percent of the rural population was covered by the cooperative medical scheme and a similar percentage of the villages had local clinics. The state provided a welfare safety net on the village level and the village administration provided such a safety net for individual households coping with crises that brought about heavy expenses and long periods of loss of work-points (Tang et al, 1994). With these no longer available, inequality between households, families and individuals is likely to emerge, despite the continuous government efforts to maintain affordability by controlling the price of medication. To what extent, then, is the economic standing of a household related to access to health services? Is the status of an individual within a household related to his/her access to health care? And if so, how is it related to household income?

The Development of General Coping Resources

Past research in medical sociology and social epidemiology has consistently shown that socioeconomic status and social support are strongly related to health and mortality (Link and Phelan, 1995; Uchino, et al, 1996). In the following section, the process of changes in the standard of living, education and social support are presented briefly. Rural China is the focus of the presentation, though much of the data, especially those published by international organizations, do not separate the indicators provided by rural and urban residents. Whenever possible, the processes which took place in HeBei Province will be compared with those that took place in China as a whole.

Standard of Living

Net income in rural China increased dramatically after the introduction of economic reforms. By the end of the land redistribution process, which lasted for some two years, the annual national average per-capita income in the rural areas increased by 39 percent in real terms. Ten years after the implementation of the 'system of household responsibility' was completed, the average annual per-capita income was three times higher than in 1978 (Table 1.2).

In HeBei Province, the rural population's income increased even faster, although until 1996 the average per-capita net income in rural HeBei was 31 percent less than the national average (Table 1.3). Within ten years of the dissolution of the collectives, average per-capita income was four times greater than that prior to the economic reforms, and by 1998 real net income per villager was more than seven times higher than in 1978 and 11 percent higher than the national average in that year. In our survey of 4,319 rural households in HeBei, the average annual per-capita income observed was 2,183.8 Yuan, but varied considerably among households (standard deviation = 3,805.0). Thus, the mode annual per-capita income was 1,000.0 Yuan, and the annual per-capita income of half of the households was more than 1,666.7 Yuan. The degree to which these income differentials are reflected in the access to health and health care will be explored in the following chapters (Chapters 5 and 6 in particular).

Table 1.2 Changes in standard of living, rural China 1978–1998

	1978	1985	1990	1995	1998
Per-Capita average nominal	133.6	397.6	686.3	1221.0	2162.0
Per-capita annual income	100.0	268.9	311.2	383.7	456.8
Per-capita expenditures for	116.1	317.4	584.6	1310.	1590.3
Per-capita expenditure for	78.6	183.4	343.8	768.2	849.6
Per-capita living space (m^2)	8.1	14.7	17.8	21.0	23.7
Durable goods per 100 households					
number of TV sets	–	11.7	44.4	80.7	96.2
number of refrigerators	–	0.1	1.2	5.2	9.3
number of motorcycles	–	–	0.9	4.9	13.5

Source: China Year Book, 1999.

In HeBei Province, the rural population's income increased even faster, although until 1996 the average per-capita net income in rural HeBei was 31 percent less than the national average (Table 1.3). Within ten years of the dissolution of the collectives, average per-capita income was four times greater than that prior to the economic reforms, and by 1998 real net income per villager was more than seven times higher than in 1978 and 11 percent higher than the national average in that year. In our survey of 4,319 rural households in HeBei, the average annual per-capita income observed was 2,183.8 Yuan, but varied considerably among households (standard deviation = 3,805.0). Thus, the mode annual per-capita income was 1,000.0 Yuan, and the annual per-capita income of half of the households was more than 1,666.7 Yuan. The degree to which these income differentials are reflected in the access to health and health care will be explored in the following chapters (Chapters 5 and 6 in particular).

Table 1.3 Changes in standard of living, rural HeBei, 1978–1998

	1978	1985	1990	1998
Per-Capita average nominal annual income	91.5	385.2	622	2405
Per-capita annual net income index*	100.0	380.3	412	741.9
Expenditures for consumption (yuan)	137.0	319.0	605	1299
Per-capita expenditure for food (yuan)				616.9
Per-capita living space (m^2)	7.8	14.0	17.3	22.5
Durable goods per 100 households				
number of TV sets	–	17.0	41.8	114.5
number of refrigerators	–	0.02	0.6	16.8
number of motorcycles	–	0.6	1.0	23.2

Source: China Year Book, 1997, 1999; HeBei Year Book, 1998.
* Adjusted for inflation.

The increase in net per-capita income enabled the rural population of the PRC to increase its standard of living significantly. If in 1955 per-capita consumption of the average rural household *exceeded* the average per-capita income by7.3 percent, the share of per-capita consumption *declined* to 73 percent of the net income of the average household in 1998. Moreover, the proportion of income spent on food declined steadily in relation to other expenses as income increased. In 1978, food comprised close to 60 percent of the per-capita household expenditures; in 1998 the share of food in total per-capita consumption declined to less than 40 percent.

With more spendable income, the rural population of the PRC was able to purchase durable goods and to improve its living conditions. Table 1.2 presents two examples of this process. Two decades after the implementation of 'the system of household responsibility', the number of rooms per household increased from 4.1 in 1980 to 5.6 in 1990, and to 4.9 in 1998. Considering the decline in fertility, the per-capita living space in 1998 was nearly three times the space available in 1978. Practically all rural households had a television set, and the number of households which owned a motorcycle and a refrigerator increased steadily.

The processes in HeBei Province resembled those observed throughout rural China. In 1978 per-capita net income in rural HeBei was lower than the national average and average per-capita consumption exceeded the net per-capita income by close to 50 percent. In 1998, however, as the net per-capita income in rural HeBei reached a higher level than the national average, only 25.6 percent of it was spent for consumption of goods, food, and services. Unfortunately, data concerning the proportion of money spent on food to total consumption are not available before 1995. In 1995, the share of food in total per-capita consumption was 65.9 percent, close to the national average of 62.9 percent; but in 1998, as net income surpassed the national average, food accounted for just 25.6 percent of total per-capita expenditures.

As in other rural parts of China, increasing disposable income in rural HeBei was translated into life style and living comfort. Villagers invested in increasing their living space and purchased consumer goods. In 1998, the number of durable consumer goods per 100 rural households in HeBei was above the national average, parallel to the increase in net per-capita income. Of the 4,319 households visited during our study in rural HeBei, a typical rural household had 1.3 room per-capita. While one quarter of the households had less than one room per person, a similar number had more than two rooms per person. The great majority of the houses were made of bricks (89 percent), 87 percent had running water in their yard, and 19 percent had an indoor bathroom. One quarter of the sampled households owned a motorcycle, 23 percent had a refrigerator, and less than 6 percent of the households had no television set.

Economic growth, industrial development, and prosperity, however, do not by themselves bring greater access to health and health care (Szreter, 1999). A market economy, if it follows the pure laissez-faire model promoted by the World Bank, involves the risk of social disruption and unequal access to health resources, increasing deprivation, poor health, and premature death for some social groups. These issues will be discussed in Chapter 6.

Education

The level of education is widely accepted as a crucial component in the economic and social development of any society (Schumacher, 1973; Lutz and Cao, 2000). For the individual, education is one of the most important general resistance resources, consistently associated with good health and general well-being (Antonovsky, 1979). Education has always been highly valued in the Chinese tradition and has determined socioeconomic class position for hundreds of years before the Communist revolution. Since the Tang dynasty (618–905), familiarity with the writings of Confucius and with Confucian literature had been a prerequisite for entry into state administration and enjoyment of the wealth and power of the ruling class. For the Chinese Communist Party, therefore, access to education was another mechanism to abolish the old, feudal, stratification system and a pathway to a classless society as well as an important agency for enhanced economic development and improved quality of life. The history of the rural education system and the ideology behind its development in the PRC thus resemble those of the rural health care system.

In 1949, there was, effectively, no school system in rural China, and some 70 per cent of the Chinese population had no formal schooling at all (China All-Women Federation, 1993). Enrollments were about 24 million in primary schools and 1,250,000 in secondary schools, or 2 percent of the corresponding age group. The eradication of illiteracy was another important goal of the newly independent government, seeking to reduce the social distinctions between manual and intellectual labor, between rural and urban dwellers, and between industrial workers and farmers. The right to primary education for all was established immediately after liberation and a mass movement to eradicate illiteracy was initiated. In the first two years of the communist regime (1949–1951), more than 60 million peasants enrolled in 'winter schools', established to take advantage of the slack season in agriculture. The reduction of the number of Chinese characters and the simplification of those left was another measure taken to provide all with literacy, a resource accessible only to a few before the revolution. Efforts were made to mobilize and increase school enrollment and by 1952 half of all children aged 6–12 attended a primary school, though there was still a considerable urban/rural discrepancy (Lutz and Cao, 2000).

The expansion of the education system and school enrollment was seriously interrupted during the Cultural Revolution. The 131 million youths who had been enrolled in primary and secondary schools, albeit mainly urban students, stopped studying; many became involved in the Red Guards, active in Mao's efforts to shake up the new, bureaucratic, elite of China. Primary and secondary schools began to reopen in 1968 and 1969, but all institutions of higher education remained closed until the early 1970s. Educational policy also changed dramatically during the Cultural Revolution. The traditional 13 years of education, from kindergarten to 12th grade, were reduced to a mandatory six years of primary education and three or four years of middle school for select groups of students. A two-year period of manual or agriculture labor became mandatory for secondary school graduates who wished to acquire higher education. The standardized college-entrance exams were abandoned and when the colleges reopened (1970–1972), political leanings, party activities and peer-group support became important criteria for admission and selection of candidates. Four and five year curricula were replaced by three-year programs, which included periods of productive labor in support of the school or the course of study being pursued, in line with Mao Ze-Dong's emphasis on being 'educated by farmers'.

A major review of these policies began with the political changes that took place after Mao's death in 1976. The need to revitalize and develop the economy called for a highly trained and educated labor force. In 1977, China launched a new campaign to achieve the 'four modernizations': it called for rapid modernization of agriculture, industry, defense, and science and technology. Gradually, pre-Cultural Revolution curricula were reinstated: primary and secondary schooling were slowly readjusted to encompass 12 years of study; the two years of labor in the countryside were no longer required as a prerequisite for college positions and the standardized college-entrance exams were reintroduced. Since 1986, the Chinese education system has taken a step forward, expanding compulsory education to include middle school, that is, from six to nine years.

Data regarding investment in education and the reduction of illiteracy are not available for the early years of the CCP regime, nor do the available data distinguish between the urban and the rural sectors. However, in 1965, just before the Cultural Revolution, expenditure per primary school student was 13 percent of the per-capita GNP, higher than the equivalent expenditure in Japan (World Development Indicators, 2000). Furthermore, despite the devastating effect of the Cultural Revolution on the educational system, the rate of increase in the number of teachers exceeded that of population growth between 1960 and 1980. Because the main victim of the Cultural Revolution was the urban school system, most of the increase in teaching staff took place in the rural sector. The transition to the 'socialist market economy' and the commitment to the 'four modernizations' were accompanied by a 10-fold increase in the government's per-capita investment in social, cultural and

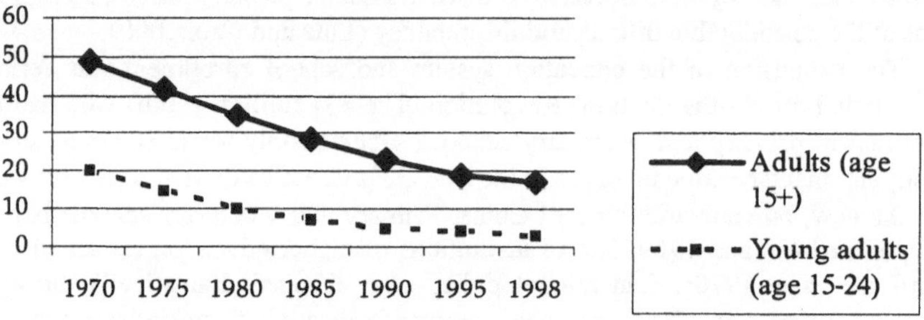

Figure 1.1 Illiteracy rates, China, 1970–1998 (percent)
Source: World Development Indicators, 2000.

educational development between 1980 and 1998 (China Yearbook, 1999). The increase in supply was followed by an increase in demand. The number of primary school students increased from 888 per 10,000 populations in 1952 to 1,602 in 1965, although as the population aged it declined to 1,118 in 1998 (China Yearbook, 1999). The number of secondary school students per 10,000 populations increased from 55 in 1952 to 588 in 1998. Primary school enrollment increased from 10 percent (gross) in 1960 to 12 percent in 1997, when the net enrolment reached 100 percent (World Development Indicators, 2000). During the same period, secondary school enrolment increased from 21 percent (gross) to 70 percent (gross and net).

Illiteracy rates declined steadily since the CCP came to power. Among adults over the mandatory education age (15 years and older), illiteracy rates decreased from 49 percent in 1970 to 17 percent in 1998 (Figure 1.1). Among young adults between 15 and 24 years of age, the social investment in education was already apparent in 1970. The oldest persons in this age group had been born during the civil war and turned school age upon the establishment of the PRC. Yet the number of illiterates in this age group had already reached half that of all Chinese adults in that year. By 1998, illiteracy rates of young adults declined to 3 percent, compared with 29 percent in India, a similarly rural society with more than one million citizens.

The development of the education system in HeBei Province took on a very similar pattern. In 1998, there were 49,495 rural schools; many of the village primary schools had been built following the economic reforms of 1979 (HeBei Rural Yearbook, 1998). The majority (88.6 percent) of the 288 villages in the nine counties sampled for our study had a primary school. The rest were small villages whose children attended school in a near-by village. On the average, the educational level in HeBei Province is somewhat higher than the national average. For the province as a whole and among its rural population in particular, illiteracy is less common and the proportion of persons with junior-high (middle) school education is greater than the national average. In 1998, when 13.7 percent of the Chinese population over 6 years of age was illiterate and 33.0 percent completed middle school, the respective figures for urban HeBei were 10.5 percent and 38.8 percent, and 11.0 percent and 36.2 percent among the rural population of HeBei Province (China Yearbook, 1999; HeBei Yearbook, 1998). An urban/rural educational discrepancy is apparent in the proportion of those who obtained a senior high school and college education in HeBei: 13.9 percent of the urbanites compared with 5.8 percent among their rural counterparts.

Our study in rural HeBei did not include a reading test, but the recorded the formal education attainment of the participants. These do not necessarily overlap, since one can be a semi-illiterate or even illiterate graduate from elementary school and reading skills can be acquired out of school. It does, however, indicate the degree to which the PRC had succeeded in carrying out its educational policy of providing universal access to an elementary school education. In our sample, 11.6 percent of the participants over 15 years of age had never attended school, while another 6.1 percent did not have a full primary school education. The relationship between age and education is most interesting: not only was the duration of formal school attendance highly and negatively correlated with age ($r = -0.498$), but half of the participants who never attended school were above the age of 56. In other words, they were born some ten years before the Communist revolution. Figure 1.2 illustrates the association between age and years of schooling. Note that the 20–24 year olds have attained higher education levels than the 15–19 year olds, many of whom will probably continue studying and ultimately reach at least the same level.

Social Support

Social support is another general resistance resource which affects health in different ways, providing tangible assistance and aid, emotional reassurance and comfort, knowledge and information. Nevertheless, data on social support are not easily collected and are rarely included in official publications for a society at large. China is no exception, so we will discuss the transition in the Chinese family as a proxy for social support. The discussion will follow Katz and Peres (1995), and look at patterns of marriage, divorce, living arrangements, and fertility.

Family and kin have traditionally been the most important source of social support in China (Zhou, 2000). Patrilocal living arrangements ensured provision for the elderly with a male descendant, while parents of daughters could only sometimes enjoy the support of their son(s)-in-law (Pearson, 1995; Wang, 1995). As a result of these preferred living arrangements, paternal kin have been a particularly important for the provision of emotional support, financial aid, and assistance with physical labor in times of need.

During the Communist regime, the formation of the brigades and the working teams during 'the great leap forward' further strengthened kin commitment, as most often an extended family sharing a household formed such a working team (Anson and Haanappel, 1999; Pearson, 1996). Patrilocality and economic bonds enabled local cadres and community leaders to enforce the traditional obligation of filial

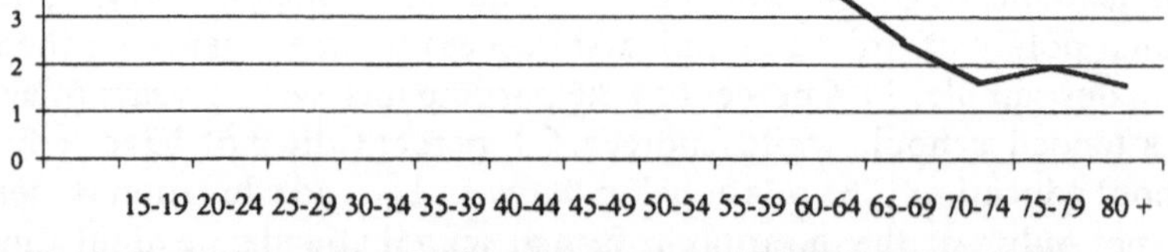

Figure 1.2 Mean years of schooling by age, HeBei, 1996–1999

responsibility, ensuring support for elderly and needy family members (Tang et al, 1994; Zhao, 2000).

In many other societies, modernization, have improved levels of education, and economic systems of individual responsibility have resulted in the attenuation of the traditional strength of the family. The Chinese family, so far, has remained very stable (Table 1.4). Despite exposure to Western culture, divorce rates remain extremely low and the proportion of married couples among the adult population is even increasing.

The extent to which the economic reforms and the dissolution of the working brigade affected living arrangements in rural China is not fully clear. Household composition was first monitored in the 1982 census and published without differentiating between urban and rural households. Nevertheless, according to the 1990 census and the annual 1.01 $^{0}/_{00}$ Survey Sample of Population Change, non-family households are extremely rare and their proportion has remained stable at 0.5 percent to 0.6 percent since 1982 (China year Book, 1999). In 1998, the average family size was 3.63 persons in the PRC as a whole and 3.64 in HeBei Province. Rural households in HeBei Province were considerably larger, with 4.18 members. The size of rural households in HeBei has decrease gradually, from 5.44 in 1978 to 4.92 in 1985 and 4.18 in 1998 (HeBei Year Book, 1998). This process seems not to be related to the 'system of household responsibility' but rather to the decline in fertility.

Table 1.4 Marital status of adults (over 15 years of age), China, 1982–1998

	Never married	Married	Divorced	Widowed
China,1982	28.6	63.7	0.6	7.2
China,1990	25.1	68.5	0.6	6.1
China, 1998	19.3	73.7	0.9	6.1
HeBei, 1998	18.9	75.2	0.6	5.3

Source: China Yearbook, 1999.

The decline in fertility in rural China will be discussed in detail in Chapter 7, which is devoted to the health of women. A brief description, however, will be presented in this chapter, as it has bearing on the current and future availability of social support. Fertility started to decline in China soon after the establishment of the independent state (Riley and Gardner, 1997). During the first two decades, the decline was rather moderate, from 37.0 births per 1,000 populations in 1952 to 33.4 in 1970. One goal of the fourth five-year plan (1971–1975) was to reduce the rate of natural population growth by close to 50 percent, in order to eradicate poverty, prevent the exploitation of resources and make faster economic development possible. This goal was to be achieved through increasing the age of marriage and a propaganda campaign aimed at promoting greater birth spacing and fewer children per family.

The age of marriage was specified as 23 years for women and 25 years for men in 1971. By 1975, birth rates had declined to 23.0 births per 1,000 populations and continued to decline to 18.2 in 1980. Birth rates started to increase during the 1980s, as the large number of women whose marriages had been delayed by the new regulations reached the age of 23 and relaxation of the marriage regulations enabled younger women to start childbearing at the same time (Zeng, 1996). The birth rate reported for 1987 was 23.3 per 1,000 populations.

Regulations regarding the number of children were issued in 1979. A one-child policy was implemented and is still in effect, albeit with some modifications. The one-child policy was fairly successful in the urban sector but encountered many difficulties in rural China (for a detailed discussion, see Chapter 7). Differences in socioeconomic factors, cultural preferences, and social control agencies between urban and rural populations brought about a slower decline in the fertility of rural women compared with their urban counterparts. The One-Child Policy was relaxed in 1984, allowing a second birth to daughter-only rural families. Fertility rates, however, declined steadily, from 23.3 births per 1,000 populations in 1987 to 16.0 per 1,000 in 1998. As in many other societies, the fertility rates in rural China remained higher than those of the cities. The patterns of rise and fall in rural and urban fertility rates, however, paralleled each other (Table 1.5).

The decline in fertility raises important questions regarding the availability of social support in the future. The first question has to do with caring for the elderly (for a detailed discussion see Chapter 8). The second relates to the disappearance of traditionally important supporting kin (Zhou, 2000). The number of seniors who have no son will increase and these elderly will be forced to rely on their daughter(s). Although the Chinese law only requires children to care for their own elderly parents, tradition obliges daughters to care for their husbands' parents and grandparents as well. Moreover, the current policy, which allows for more daughters than sons in a rural family, may in the future result in fewer paternal kin and a larger maternal extended family. Traditionally, paternal relatives are the important source of social support. The decline in fertility and the fertility regulations will probably bring about changes in the familial patterns of exchange. Families will have to rely on maternal kin, non-kin aid, and hired labor in order to obtain the support traditionally and currently provided by the family.

Familial support will be further challenged by migration to urban centers. Despite the lower fertility rates in the cities, the urban population has grown consistently since 1980 due to increasing migration. During the 1970s, the urban population accounted for 17.3 percent to 18.0 percent of of the total population. Its proportion increased to 30.4 percent of the Chinese population in 1998. Such migration interferes with the traditional kin support patterns, although there is some evidence that sons tend to bring their elderly parents to the cities with them.

Table 1.5 Urban and rural crude fertility rates, China, 1965–1998 (births per 1,000 population)

	Urban	Rural
1965	26.6	39.5
1975	14.7	24.2
1980	14.2	18.8
1990	16.1	22.8
1995	14.8	18.1
1998	13.7	17.5

Source: China Year Book, 1999.

Summary

This chapter presents a brief overview of the major historical processes that have shaped access to health, health care, and general coping resources, such as education and social support systems, in the People's Republic of China. We have focused as much as possible on rural China and on HeBei Province as a model.

Before the Communist revolution, the rural population of China suffered from poor health and its access to health care was extremely limited. Nor had the rural population access to such necessary health resources as adequate living conditions, nutrition, and education. This, of course, was incompatible with the ideology of the new regime and the Chinese Communist Party (CCP) made a major effort to change it. The economic resources available at the time did not allow for provision of curative care at the individual level. Relying on the Soviet model, the CCP focused on preventive health, health education, and public involvement. A massive effort was undertaken to establish a three-tier health care system in the rural areas. These efforts involved a large investment in health care personnel and facilities, and the system did not reach full development until the Cultural Revolution. By the mid-1970s, health services were available to almost all of the rural population and price control and the 'cooperative medical scheme' made these services affordable to the great majority of the population.

Similarly, elementary education became accessible to all. Levels of illiteracy among men and women declined dramatically. Schools were spread over the countryside and elementary school enrollment became almost universal. Mortality-based health indicators showed a remarkably rapid improvement in the health status of the population. We also present the changes in the health care system brought about by the economic reforms of 1979.

The factors that led to the fall of the cooperative health scheme and to the privatization of over half of the rural clinics are discussed. These processes leave several open questions related to the combination of a fee-for-service health care system, where services are provided by a professionally isolated village doctor, and the pressure experienced by hospitals to generate income. Of course, this combination is not unique to rural China, though it takes different forms in other societies. Its specific consequences for rural China will be explored in the following chapters. Nevertheless, the economic reforms increased the access to one of the most important health resources, disposable income and an elevated standard of living. Data on the increasing accessibility of a satisfactory income and the increase in the level of education are also briefly presented in this chapter.

The family, a traditional resource for social support in all societies, preserved its stability despite the political and economical changes, modernization, and the improving standard of education. This is evident from data indicating universal marriage, relative stagnation of divorce rates, and a slow decline in the size of rural households. The decline in fertility and increasing rural-urban migration, however, present new challenges to the traditional familial support, particularly in the absence of a welfare benefit system.

Chapter 2

Health and Health Resources

This chapter describes the health and health resources available to the Chinese population. Health statistics bears limited meaning when deprived of a context; its significance stems from an examination of the changes that have occurred over time in the society under study and from cross-cultural comparisons. We have striven to present long term trends in the PRC after the PPC came to power in 1949, and to compare these data with health statistics available for eight other Asian societies.

Unfortunately, this approach presents two major problems. First, it is limited to the data available from secondary, national and international sources, and the quality of health statistics available for the PRC varies from one period to another. Systematic data were not collected in the early years and good quality data are available only from the early 1970s on, when the first effort to map mortality, causes of death and, to a lesser degree morbidity, was made by the government (Banister et al, 1997, 2000). Thus, the Cancer Epidemiology Survey conducted in 1976 provides the first reliable data for mortality patterns in the period 1973–75. Several other data sets became available thereafter, such as national and sample censuses and mortality and fertility surveys.

The second limitation stems from the constraints of available international secondary sources. The international organizations which gather this information are dependent on the willingness of political leaders and policy makers in each society to share it with the world. As a result, the secondary sources available are inconsistent both in the health indicators published for each society and in years for which comparative data are available. Furthermore, differentiation between rural and the urban populations, crucial for our purposes, is rarely indicated.

In this chapter, therefore, the health and the health resources in the PRC are presented for the Chinese society as a whole, emphasizing in so far as possible those of the rural population. Long-term changes are examined, to the extent that the available data allow, with special emphasis on the economic reforms of 1979. Changes in the indicators for health and health resources in China are compared with those in the eight selected Far Eastern societies, again, to the extent our data permit.

Japan, India, Mongolia, the Republic of Korea, Singapore, Sri Lanka, and Viet Nam were chosen for comparison. All share some social characteristics with China, but differ from it with respect to others. Japan and Singapore are the two high-income countries of East Asia, in terms of per-capita GDP; India, on the other hand, is a poor country that, like China, has to provide for the world's second largest population, close to 70 percent of which is rural. Mongolia, the Republic of Korea and Viet Nam are geographically and ethnically closest to China. Viet Nam and Mongolia have lower income levels than China, and the Republic of Korea is considerably better off, being defined by the World Bank as an upper middle income society. Sri Lanka shares China's level of economic development in terms of annual per-capita GDP and demographic processes, such as its annual population growth and dependency ratio. Moreover, like China, Sri Lanka's health policy emphasizes public health and accessible primary care for the rural population. Thailand represents the lower middle income countries of the region.

Health Status

The health status of a society is not easily measured. Most commonly, mortality-based indicators are used for assessing health status, while morbidity, which better reflects quality of life, is largely neglected. In some countries only a few health conditions, such as preventable infectious, communicable, diseases and malignant neoplasms are officially monitored on a regular base. In others, data are available for health conditions treated in hospitals, though these represent just the top of the morbidity iceberg. Most health conditions treated by ambulatory health care, by the lay referral system, and/or by self care are monitored only by countries that regularly conduct health surveys. This costly path, however, is taken by very few countries.

In the following section the health status of the PRC is examined using mortality-based indicators: life expectancy, overall and adults' mortality rate, infant, child and maternal mortality, and the leading causes of death are discussed both vertically and in comparison to the eight societies mentioned above.

Life Expectancy

In 1998, life expectancy at birth in China was 68 years for men and 72 years for women. Most of the increase in life expectancy since the establishment of the PRC, 26 years for men and 25 years for women, took place before 1970. The increased life expectancy may be attributed mainly to the improvement in standard of living, implementation of public health programs, and development of rural health services as described in Chapter 1. No other country in the region has recorded a similar achievement, which cannot be explained simply on the basis of the extremely low life expectancy in China at the beginning of the period (Figure 2.1).

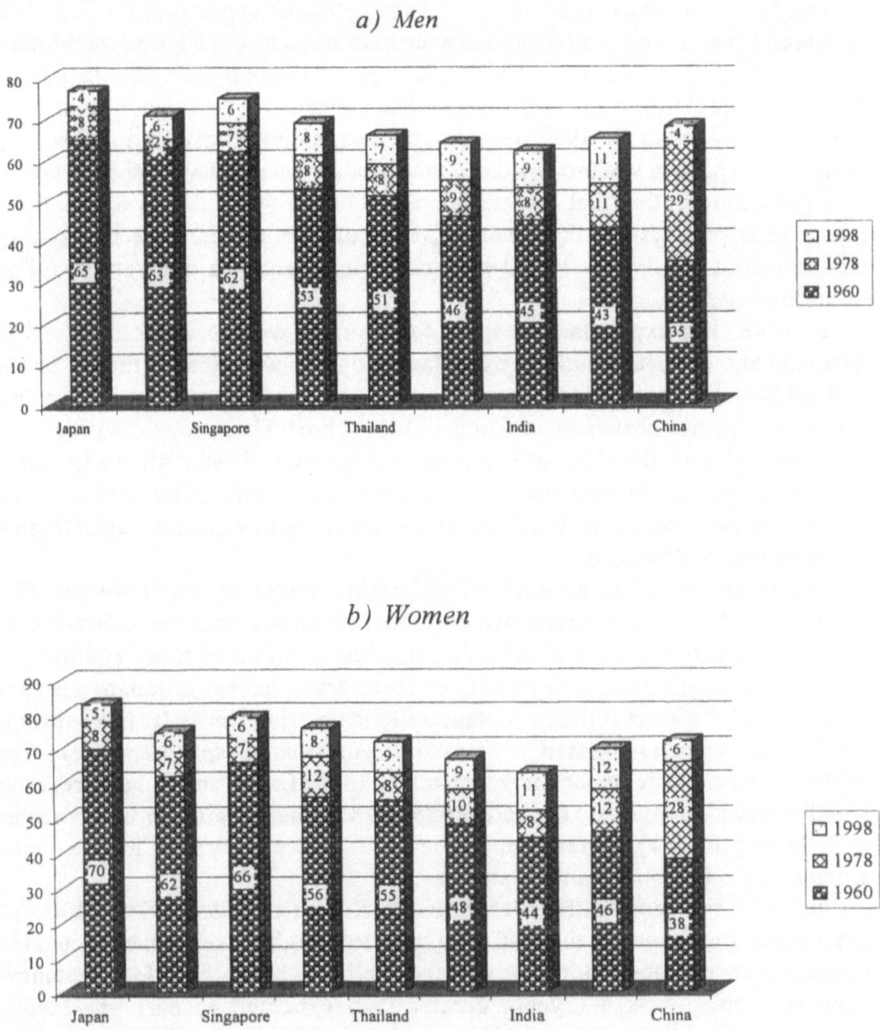

Figure 2.1 The increase in life expectancy 1960–1998, selected countries

* *Source:* The World Health Report, 1999; World Development Indicators, 2000.

During the two decades between 1978 and 1998, life expectancy for Chinese men increased from 64 years to 68 and for women from 66 to 72 (Figure 2.1). Moreover, the rate of acceleration seemed to be faster in the countryside than in the cities. Banister et al (2000), who compared the data collected in the Cancer Epidemiology Survey of 1976 with the 1993 mortality survey, calculated that during this 17 year period life expectancy of urban women increased by 4.6 years while that of women in the richest third of the rural counties increased by 5.1 years, and by 8.9 years in the poorer rural counties. During the same period of time, the life expectancy of urban men increased by 3.1 years, by 3.9 years in the richest rural counties, and by 6.1 years in the poorest rural counties.

In 1998, life expectancy at birth for Chinese women was close to that of Thailand and Sri Lanka and life expectancy for men was close to that of Thailand and the Republic of Korea, countries that enjoyed a higher standard of living and greater economic growth than China. The GDP of Thailand, for example, was over twice that of the GDP of China during the early 1990s, after adjusting for purchasing power. Furthermore, during the twenty years under study, Thailand enjoyed an average annual GDP growth of 6.0 percent, while annual GDP growth in China was 4.5 percent.

The increase in life expectancy for both Chinese men and women during 1978–1998, however, seems relatively moderate when compared with the changes that occurred in the eight other countries chosen. In all of these countries, life expectancy for men increased by six or more years, except in Japan, where men enjoy one of the longest life expectancies in the world. Similarly, life expectancy for Chinese women increased by one year beyond that of Japanese women, similar to the increase in life expectancy for women in Sri Lanka and Singapore, both of which enjoyed greater life expectancy in 1978. Thus, judging by life expectancy in 1978 (Figure 2.1), a greater increase in life expectancy for Chinese men and women could have been anticipated.

Indeed, according to the World Health Report of 1999 (WHO, 2000), life expectancy for women in the PRC is longer than might have been expected based on income level alone, but this advantage declined gradually. Life expectancy for Chinese women was 4.2 years greater than expected as early as 1962, an advantage that increased to 12.9 years in 1972. By 1982, however, life expectancy for Chinese women was 11.4 years greater than expected on the basis of economic development, and by 1992 it was 10.1. While this is a major achievement, it raises an important question: why did the trend reverse itself, particularly in light of the dramatic increase in standard of living after the economic reforms?

It is worth noting that no such reversal of trend has been observed in India, Sri Lanka, and Thailand. In India and Thailand life expectancy for women relative to income level increased steadily from 1952 to 1992. In Sri Lanka the increase in women's life expectancy stabilized at 12.2 years longer than expected since 1972. The steady increase in women's life expectancy in India can be explained by the fact that in 1952 it was 4.9 years lower than expected on the basis of income level. Yet the steady increase in Thailand and the stabilization in Sri Lanka cannot be explained by past decrease. Unfortunately, no comparable figures are provided for men or for women in high income countries.

General Mortality

The crude all-causes mortality rate in China decreased steadily after the revolution, but this trend seems to have ended during the late 1970s (China Year Book, 1999). After 1978, crude mortality rate increased from 6.25 per 1,000 population to 7.51 in 1998. Throughout this period, the rural mortality rate exceeded the urban rate and the gap has not closed since then. In 1978, mortality in the villages was 25 percent higher than that in the cities; in 1998 the corresponding proportion was 24 percent.

Increase in mortality rate is often attributed to a decline in fertility and the consequent aging of the population. Yet this explanation seems unsatisfactory when the crude death rate of the PRC is compared with those of Singapore, Sri Lanka, and the Republic of Korea (The World Bank, 2000). The proportion of elderly people in these societies is close to that of China and has accelerated during the past two decades, yet crude overall mortality rate in these societies has not increased.

Most relevant to this discussion is a comparison between China and Singapore, where the dynamics of population take on a comparable pattern. For example, in 1998 the elderly accounted for 6.6 percent of the population of Singapore, compared with 6.7 percent of the Chinese population. On the average, the elderly population of Singapore grew by 3.6 percent each year and that of China grew by 3.2 percent. Moreover, the decline in fertility in Singapore was very similar to that of China, starting with a crude birth rate of 17 and 18 per 1,000 population, respectively, in 1980 and reaching the rate of 13 and 16 per 1,000 population, respectively, in 1998. Yet, in Singapore the crude death rate continued to decline during the same years.

Judging by the crude death rate, then, the health of the Chinese population seems to fall somewhat behind that of seven of the eight societies selected for comparison. But the crude death rate reflects only part of the dynamics of mortality and its social distribution. A fuller picture of this dynamic may be obtained by looking at specific age groups that represent different stages in the life cycle and differentials in risk and vulnerability. The available data for adults of working age (15–59 years old), for example, show that the recent increase in mortality rate in the PRC is a result of a rise in the mortality rate of men of working age and of stagnation in the mortality rate of women of that age (Table 2.1). A similar pattern was found in Viet Nam, which is poorer than China and copes with a higher dependency ratio (0.9 vs. 0.7).

Table 2.1 Mortality of adults (age 15–59), by sex, selected countries, 1980–1998 (per 1,000 population)

	Men			Women		
Country	1980	1990	1998	1980	1990	1998
China	**185**	**160**	**171**	**148**	**135**	**135**
India	261	236	215	279	241	204
Japan	129	108	98	70	53	45
Mongolia	320	251	201	273	211	165
Republic of Korea	270	239	204	156	117	94
Singapore	199	138	131	115	80	75
Sri Lanka	210	184	153	152	120	97
Thailand	280	207	206	210	123	116
Viet Nam	262	215	225	204	153	153

* *Source*: The World Development Indicators, 2000.

Banister et al (1997) showed that despite the urban/rural mortality differences, the increase in the mortality rate of persons of working age was higher among urbanites than among farmers. In the cities, the central death rate for men aged 15–19 increased by 56 percent between 1981 and 1995, compared with 5 percent in rural China; during the same period, the central death rate for urban men aged 20–24 increased by 48 percent, and that for rural men by 22 percent. These urban/rural differences remind us that mortality is not determined by income level only. Social support, sanitation, health behavior and life style are other important determinants. The pattern of mortality in China could very well be explained by health risk behavior, such as consumption of alcohol and smoking, as presented in Chapter 5, and road and work safety, discussed in Chapter 3.

Infant and Child Mortality

Infant mortality is believed to reflect the general health of the population, because it is closely related to the health of women of reproductive age, to health resources such as nutrition, and to health services available to women in general, pregnant women in particular, and newborn infants. In addition, the increase in life expectancy has been largely due to decline in infant mortality during the first year of life in many societies.

Infant mortality in China decreased dramatically following the establishment of the independent PRC: from 132 per 1,000 live births in 1960 to 52:1,000 in 1978 and 41:1,000 in 1998. In other words, infant mortality in China decreased by 60.2 percent between 1960 and 1978 and by an additional 21.1 percent between 1978 and 1998. The decline in infant mortality during the period 1960–1978 exceeded the decline in all countries in the region, with the exception of the Republic of Korea (63.4 percent) and Singapore (62.9 percent).

There is some evidence, however, that the decline in infant mortality stagnated after the economic reforms, as did the rural/urban discrepancy (Carrin et al, 1996; Horsburgh, 1996), and that rural/urban differences even increased (Liu et al, 1999). The stagnation in the decline in infant mortality occurred mainly with respect to rural and female infants (Banister et al, 1997). From 1981 to 1995, the central death rate (mx) of urban male infants decreased by 47 percent, while that of rural male infants was only 24 percent. The 28 percent decline in the central death rate of urban female infants was slightly higher that of rural male infants, but the central death rate of rural female infants increased by 10 percent. It has been argued that the sex differences in infant mortality that explain much of the stagnation are related to the population policy launched in 1979, rather than to the economic reforms and the privatization of rural health services that took place almost at the same time. These issues are discussed at greater length in Chapter 7.

From 1978 on, the decline in infant mortality in the PRC was slower than in the other countries selected for comparison (Figure 2.2). In all eight countries, infant mortality declined at a faster pace, ranging from 42–44 percent (Mongolia and India, respectively) to 62–67 percent (Singapore and the Republic of Korea, respectively). In Thailand, for example, which entered the 1980s with an infant mortality rate similar to that of the PRC, a decline of 48.2 percent was reported; in Sri Lanka, whose standard of living and economic development resemble those of China, infant mortality dropped by 56.1 percent.

The moderation of the decline in infant mortality in the PRC is also evident when the actual rate is compared with that predicted on the basis of China's income level. In 1962, infant mortality in China was 14 percent less than the rate expected in a society with a comparable income, an advantage that increased to 67 percent fewer infant deaths in the early 1970s, a rate similar to that of Sri Lanka. In 1998, however, the difference between the actual and the expected infant mortality rates in the PRC narrowed and was 33 percent lower than that predicted by the level of economic development. In Sri Lanka, by comparison, chances of infant survival continued to improve, and the mortality rate for infants in 1998 was 96 percent below that predicted.

Like infant mortality, child mortality before the fifth birthday reflects the general standard of living and accessibility of health care, but also patterns of child rearing and nutrition. Between 1980 and 1998, child mortality in China declined by 44.6 percent, from 6.5 percent to 3.6 percent of all children (The World Bank, 2000). Compared to the other selected societies, China remained fourth in the child mortality rate, after India (8.3 percent), Mongolia (6.0 percent), and Viet Nam (4.2 percent).

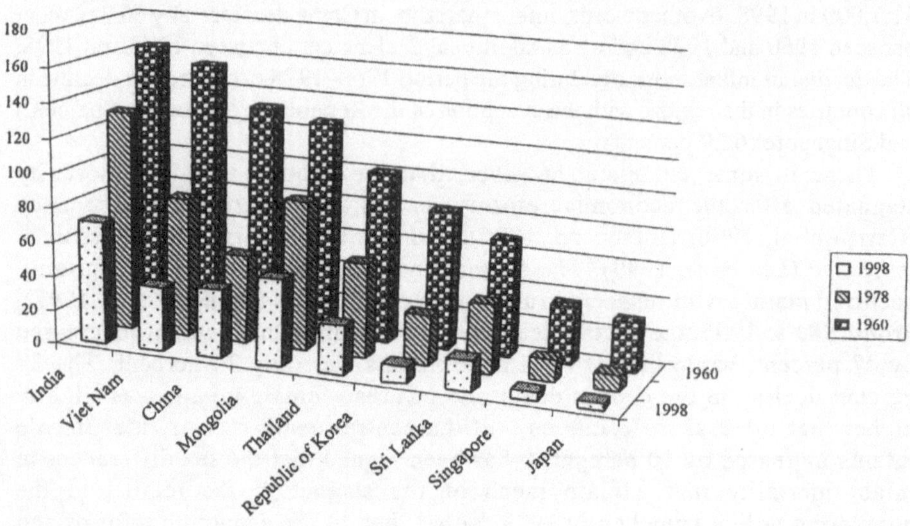

Figure 2.2 Infant mortality in selected countries, 1960–1998 (per 1,000 live births)

The rate of decline in mortality of children under five years of age was similar to that of Thailand (43.1 percent) and higher than that of Japan (38.5 percent). Both countries, however, entered the 1980s with lower childhood mortality than China (Figure 2.3). Considering the higher than expected child mortality observed in the PRC in 1973–1975, the mortality survey of 1993 and the 1.0 percent sample population survey of 1995 documented a sharp decline in child mortality for both sexes, in the cities as well as in the countryside (Banister et al, 1997, 2000). Rural and female children, relatively disadvantaged during their first year of life, benefitted particularly. From 1981 to 1995 the central death rate (mx) of rural females aged 1–4 declined by 62 percent and that of rural male children by 54 percent. This decline was achieved by the improved standard of living described in Chapter 1, as well as by increased investment in improved sanitation, a growing safe water supply (see below), and immunization programs launched in 1979 (Chapter 3).

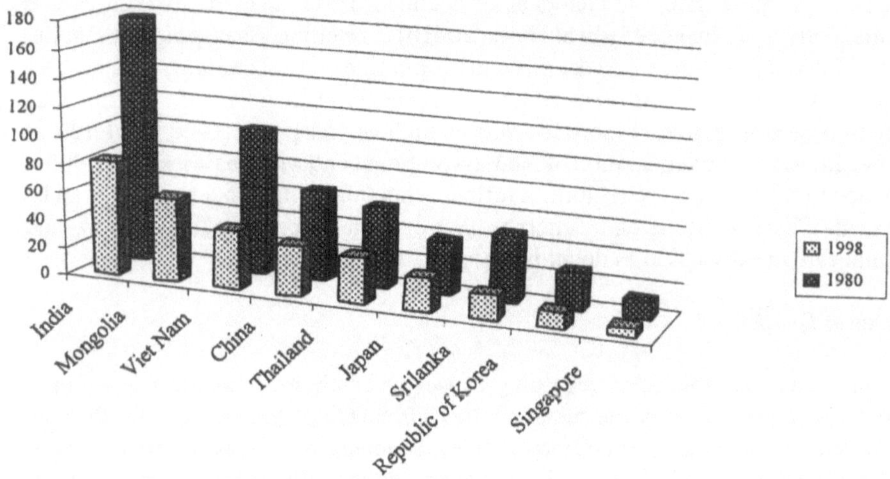

Figure 2.3 Mortality of children under five years of age, 1980–1998, selected countries (per 1,000)

**Source*: World Development Indicators, 2000.

Maternal Mortality

Maternal mortality, as reported by the WHO for 1990, was 95 per 100,000 live births. This figure was higher than the maternal mortality reported for Japan, Singapore and Mongolia, but lower than that of the other five societies selected for comparison that year. Previous reports suggested that maternal mortality was higher in the rural than in the urban areas, 114.5 per 100,000 live births in 1989 (Lawson and Lin, 1994). In the data collected by the authors from 288 villages in Hebei Province between 1996 and 1999, 49.2 maternal deaths per 100,000 live births were reported from three of the four standard causes of maternal mortality (deaths caused by induced abortions were not included in the data provided by the village authorities. It is difficult to imagine, however, that induced abortions would increase maternal mortality by a factor of almost 2.5).

According to recent reports from the PRC, maternal mortality continues to decline (Chinese Medical News, 2001b). During the last eight years of the 20th century, maternal mortality declined by 40 percent, though there is large regional variation both in the pace of the decline and in the rate reported. The urban rate, for example, dropped by 42.6 percent, while the rural rate fell by 35.5 percent. The leading cause of maternal mortality is obstetric bleeding, which counted for 54.2 percent of all maternal deaths in 2000.

One of the most important factors in the decline in maternal mortality in the PRC is hospital delivery (Chinese Medical News, 2001b). In Beijing, Shanghai, and Tianjin, where 97 percent of deliveries take place in hospitals, maternal mortality was 12.4 per 100,000 live births; in northwestern China, where fewer than half of all births take place in hospitals, maternal mortality was as high as 164 per 100,000 live births in some regions. As implementation of the Law on Infant and Maternal Health of 1995 is extended to more and more regions, a further reduction in maternal mortality can be expected. The law itself, and patterns of utilization of pre-natal, post-natal, and hospital care are discussed in detail in Chapter 7.

Causes of Death

The only data available to us regarding causes of death are crude data based on a survey of a sample of cities and rural counties. Urban China has clearly gone through the epidemiological transition (Omran, 1971); degenerative diseases were the major causes of deaths in 1997 (Table 2.2). However, while malignant neoplasms, cardio- and cerebrovascular diseases accounted for 62.1 percent of the deaths in the cities surveyed in 1997, these causes accounted for fewer than half of the deaths in rural China that year, when the leading cause of death was respiratory disease (22.9 percent of all deaths). Moreover, pulmonary tuberculosis and infectious diseases, absent from the list of the 10 main causes of death in urban China, were responsible for 2.8 percent of the rural deaths.

It is worth noting that death due to external causes such as trauma and intoxication were almost twice as frequent in rural areas as in urban areas. This trend may be the result of differential accessibility of emergency health services, crucial in the occurrence of trauma. This explanation is supported by the number of deaths caused by traffic accidents and fire, which are twice as high in rural China as in the cities (China Yearbook, 1998).

Unfortunately, it was impossible to compare the relative contribution of the major causes of deaths in China with those of the eight countries selected, both because of the different coding systems used and the lack of rural/urban differentiation in the available data. Nevertheless, some comparative insight can be drawn from the work of Murray and Lopez published in 1997. In their analysis of the patterns of mortality, China is in the midst of a demographic transition, still behind the established market and the former socialist economies but ahead of the developing world. This is evident from figures for the probability of dying from infectious communicable diseases, of which the PRC had the lowest probability in the developing world for all ages in 1990 (15.8 percent of all deaths in China, compared with 50.9 percent in India, 49.5 percent in the rest of the developing world, and 6.1 percent in the developed world). At the same year, noncommunicable diseases were responsible for 72.7 percent of the deaths in China, compared with 40.4 percent of deaths in India, 40.5 percent in the rest of the developing world, and 86.2 percent in the developed world.

Table 2.2 Ten leading causes of death in urban and rural China, 1997*

Cause	Urban[a]	Rural[b]
Malignant neoplasms	22.7	17.1
Cerebrovascular disease	22.6	17.8
Heart trouble	16.8	11.5
Respiratory disease	14.1	23.4
Trauma and intoxication	6.2	11.7
Digestive diseases	3.1	4.4
Internal system, nutrition, metabolic and immunity diseases	2.7	
Urinary disease	1.5	1.4
Mental disease	1.2	
Neuropathy	1.0	
Newborn baby disease		1.5
Pulmonary tuberculosis		1.4
Infectious disease (excluding TB)		1.4

**Source*: China Yearbook, 1998.
[a] Covers 91.8 percent of deaths occurred in 35 cities including Beijing, fully or partially.
[b] Covers 91.5 percent of deaths occurred in 79 counties, including counties in Beijing.

Health Resources

Social Investment in Health

In 1995, China's investment in health was 3.8 percent of its total GDP, according to the WHO. The figure provided by the World Bank for the 1990s was somewhat higher: 4.5 percent of the GDP. This investment was higher than the investment in health by Sri Lanka (1.9 percent of the GDP according to the

WHO and 2.6 percent according to the World Bank), whose per-capita GDP is comparable to that of the PRC, by Singapore (3.5 percent or 3.2 percent, respectively), whose per-capita GDP is much higher; and possibly by the much poorer Viet Nam (4.3 percent according to the World Bank, but 5.2 percent according to the WHO). In terms of purchasing power parity (PPP), the investment in each Chinese citizen reached 142 International Standardized Dollars that year. This sum was almost double the per-capita investment of Mongolia ($68) and India ($73), whose per-capita GDP is lower than that of the PRC, and Sri Lanka, which has developed economically to a similar degree ($72).

Public resources accounted for about half of China's social investment in health (Figure 2.4). Compared with the other eight countries selected for comparison, the public resources allocated to health by the PRC fall behind Mongolia, Sri Lanka, and Japan, where public resources comprise more than three-quarters of the investment in health. Yet the other five countries fall far behind China in public financing of health care, covering between 22 percent (India and Viet Nam) to 37 percent (Singapore) of the costs of health. Despite the relatively high share of the public resources invested in health by China, private expenditures on health could constrain access to medical care, especially for the rural population.

Although the per-capita annual income of the rural population increased faster than that of the urban population after the economic reforms, urban residents were economically better off throughout the Communist regime. In 1978, when the average per-capita income in the cities was 739.1 Yuan, that of rural residents was just 397.6 Yuan, almost half that sum (China Yearbook, 1998). In 1997, nearly twenty years after the economic reforms were introduced, the average per-capita income of urban dwellers reached 5,160.3 Yuan, while that of the rural population had still less than half that amount, 2,090.1 Yuan.

Out-of-pocket medical expenditures increased considerably between 1985, at the height of privatization of rural primary services and a year before co-payment was introduced to beneficiaries of government and labor insurance, and 1997. These expenditures increased, on the average, from 16.7 to 179.7 Yuan for urbanites and from 7.5 to 62.5 Yuan for rural households. In other words, urban per-capita out-of-pocket medical expenses were 10.8 times higher in 1997 than in 1985, and rural per-capita expenses were 8.2 times higher. The rise in per-capita income, however, increased at a much slower pace in both sectors. Between 1985 and 1997, the average per-capita income of an urban household increased by a factor of 7.0, that of a rural household by a factor of 5.3. The proportion of expenditures for health increased from 2.3 percent to 3.4 percent of total per-capita income in the cities, and from 1.9 percent to 3.0 percent in the countryside.

Data for HeBei Province are available only from 1996 on. The net per-capita income for a rural household was below the national average, 1,394.8 Yuan in 1997, 4 Yuan less than in 1996. Out-of-pocket per-capita expenditures for health, however, increased slightly, by 0.27 Yuan. Thus, in 1996 medical out-of-pocket expenses for a person living in the countryside accounted for 4.3 percent of the net income in HeBei; in 1997 it accounted for 4.4 percent of it.

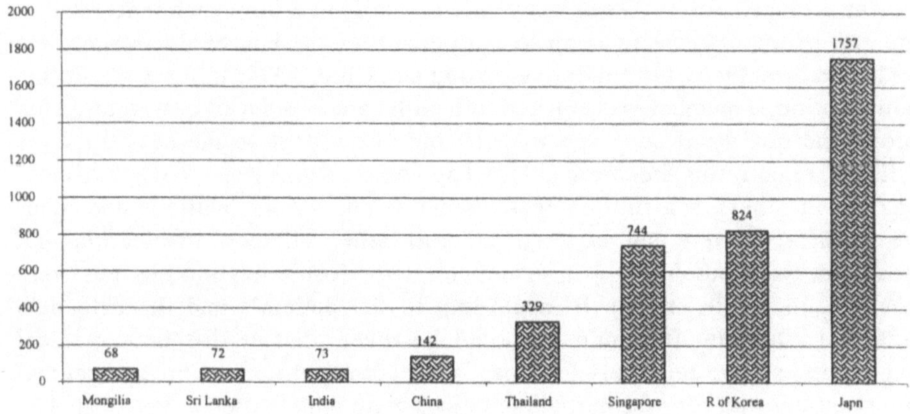

Figure 2.4 Per-capita investment in health, 1990–1998, selected countries (PPP in US dollars)

Source: World Development Indicators, 2000.

Out-of-pocket expenditures were closely related to the changes in the village collective economy after the economic reforms of 1979 and to implementation of the 'responsibility system of household production' (Chapter 1). During the 1950s, three insurance schemes were developed, covering 90 percent of the population by the middle of the Cultural Revolution. Free health care, financed by the state, was provided for government employees and their families for life. Employees of state-owned enterprises were entitled to a Labor Protection Scheme that covered all of their own health expenses and half of the expenses of their immediate families for life.

In the villages, cooperative medical care was established for members of the commune and the production brigades. This system relied heavily on the collective economy system and was based on voluntary collaboration by the residents of each village. Starting as a local initiative, the system was adopted by the Chinese Ministries of Health, Agriculture and Finance in 1960. Together these ministries established guidelines for regulation of the rural medical cooperative schemes. Shortly after publication of the 'Rural Medical Cooperation Rules (Tentative Draft)', over 90 percent of the villages (then, brigades) established medical cooperative schemes that drew on three sources for financing of the health services: contributions by the members of the brigades, the welfare funds of the brigades, and the public welfare funds of the commune (Lennart et al, 1996).

On average, 1.5–3.0 Yuan per year were collected from each individual at the end of the crop year, or up to 2.0 percent of the household income was deducted directly by the collective (Wong and Chiu, 19980). In return for this contribution, a member was entitled to health care at reduced cost, though the scope and quality of coverage varied from one village to the next. In some villages, registration fees were charged and medications were provided free of charge; in others, registration fees were waived, but medications and other treatment fees were not covered; in still other villages, medication and treatment were purchased at a discount price. Hospitalization charges were covered, in whole or in part, according to the patient's and the brigade's financial situation. It should be noted however, that at that time medical expenditures were relatively low, partly because traditional Chinese medical interventions and Chinese herbal medicines were widely used at low cost. The medical cooperation scheme was thus able to guarantee access to basic health care for almost the entire rural population.

The dissolution of village collective economy after the economic reforms of 1979 removed the financial basis for medical cooperative insurance. By 1989, coverage of health services was available only in 4.8 percent of all villages in China (Ho, 1995). Concurrently, the proportion of rural health services in the total of public resources allocated to health, that is, the government's expenditures for health, fell from 21.5 percent in 1978 to 18.1 percent in 1980, 12.1 percent in 1985, and 10.5 percent in 1990 (Wong and Chiu, 1998; Liu et al, 1999).

Currently, some 5 percent of the rural population is still covered by medical insurance and an additional 9 percent by government insurance or the labor protection plans (Dong, et al, 1999c). But 86 percent of all rural households have to pay for health services from their own pockets, incongruous with the CCP's commitment to health as a basic right of all the population. Indeed, as China prepared to carry out "The program of 'Health for all in 2000' in our rural areas", ways to revive and improve the cooperative medical scheme were sought. The result was document No.18, "Suggestions for Developing and Improving the Rural Cooperative Medical System", drafted by the Ministries of Health and Agriculture, the Treasury Planning Committee, and the Civil Administration Office, and issued by the Chinese State Department in 1997.

'Under the leadership of the government, regulated by the local people, and supported by the public', it was proposed that the main financial source for the new schemes be individual contributions. The extent of coverage, however, was to be decided at the county level. It was hoped that if the cooperative health insurance system was adapted to local economic conditions and health needs, farmers would be motivated to join it. Under this assumption, decisions regarding methods of fund raising, collection of premiums, and eligibility were to be made locally, so that universal insurance coverage would gradually be achieved. Within two years, over 350 counties developed cooperative medical insurance programs, though a definitive model of rural medical insurance has not yet developed and the proportion of the rural population covered is not yet clear.

A survey of 42 experimental townships showed that, on the average, the premium for cooperative medical insurance in 1996 was 17.7 Yuan. Most of the funds of the scheme (84.2 percent) were raised from the premium paid by individual members. An additional 8.9 percent of the funds was contributed by the village committee, 5.6 percent was paid by the township authorities, and 1.4 percent by the county government. The average reimbursement for outpatient services was 29.4 percent of the services provided in a village clinic, 20.8 percent of those provided in a township hospital, and 7.1 percent for outpatient services purchased in a county hospital (Yang, 1998).

Physical Health Resources

Very few physical health resources existed in China immediately after the revolution. In accordance with the stated goals of the CCP, a concentrated effort was made to increase the availability of health care to the population and the number of health institutions increased dramatically. By 1952, there were close to 37,000 health institutions, ten times as many as in 1948 (China Yearbook, 1999). The number of clinics established throughout the country increased from 769 in 1949 to more than 29,000 in 1952. The number of hospitals increased during these early years from 2,600 to 3,540 at county level and up. Township hospitals began to emerge during the early 1960s and their number grew almost steadily until 1992.

The economic reforms of 1979 brought about a radical change in the hospitalization system. First, the number of hospitals fluctuated considerably: from 65,450 in 1980 it declined to 59,614 in 1985 (China Yearbook, 1998) and then started to increase again from 1986 on, reaching a peak of 67,964 in 1996 before it started once again to decline slightly. Most of the decline took place on the township level: 14.5 percent of the township hospitals closed down between 1980 and 1985, with an additional 4.2 percent decline by 1993 (Liu et al, 1996). Throughout this period, however, the number of hospitals at county level and above increased. The pace of this increase, like the pace of the decline in township hospitals, changed from one year to the next, but never declined.

The crisis in township level hospitalization was directly related to the economic reforms. Under the 'socialist market economy', health institutions had to purchase an increasing portion of their materials on the free market, at steadily rising prices. For every 100 Yuan spent on medical materials in 1980, 155.7 Yuan had to be spent in

1985 (Liu et al, 1996). The salaries of health personnel increased, but the portion paid by the government decreased by over half. At the same time, patient fees were controlled at levels lower than the real cost of the health care, a measure taken by the government to assure access to health care for the majority of the population.

Because township health centers were an important component of the three-tier system and geographically located to facilitate access to health care for the rural population, several policy measures were taken to revive and strengthen the system. Much of the effort was aimed at increasing the scope and quality of the services provided and to make the township health centers more affordable to consumers. Between 1994 and 1995, the number of these facilities grew by 15 percent and the utilization rate, for both hospitalized and outpatients, was also on the increase.

A more accurate estimate of the physical health resources available to a population is the number of hospital beds. This number increased dramatically, from 0.1 per 1,000 population in 1949 to 12.7 per 1,000 in 1998. A massive development took place during the early years of the Communist regime, reaching 11.2 hospital beds per 1,000 population within ten years. The economic reforms of 1979 did not affect this process of development. The ratio of hospital beds to population continued to increase by an average of 1.03 percent until 1995. In 1998 there were 12.5 hospital beds per 1,000 population.

The equity of hospital bed distribution is not easily determined. Some insight may be gained, however, by looking at the development patterns of city, county and township level hospitals. Until the Cultural Revolution, which put more emphasis on the needs of the farmers, the number of hospital beds in the cities exceeded that of the counties. It was not until the late 1960s that hospital beds became more accessible to the rural population and the number of hospital beds in county hospitals surpassed the number in city hospitals. Yet the investment in county hospitals slowed down after the economic reforms and their number leveled out by 1988 (Figure 2.5). Thereafter, the process was reversed and the number of county hospital beds started to decrease, while the city hospitals continued to expand. Thus, in 1980 the city:county ratio of hospital beds was 0.6 and by 1998 it became three times higher – 1.8.

The number of inpatient beds on the township level followed a similar trend (Liu et al, 1996). From 30,224 beds in 1958, the number had increased more than fourfold by 1965, on the eve of the Cultural Revolution, during which the service expanded by a factor of five and reached 620,281 beds. But the decline in the number of institutions was followed by a decline in the number of beds, from 775,413 in 1980 to 730,828 by the end of the 1980s, a decline of close to 6 percent.

It is not unreasonable to argue that city hospitals were more successful in competing for the social resources allocated to health. It is possible that city hospitals, located closer to the power centers and the decision making social institutions had greater access to the funds allocated by the government. Some support for this explanation can be found in Yu's (1992) analysis of health expenditures during the 1980s. He reported that the government clearly favored city and upper level hospitals in its budget allocations.

Yet, it is also possible that city hospitals were more efficient in generating income, in developing services and increasing the demand for these services among the urban, generally more affluent, population. The pressure to generate income seems to have resulted in some neglect of preventive health services and to have increased inequality between rural and urban residents and between the poor and the rich, both individuals and regions (Yu, 1992; Liu et al, 1996).

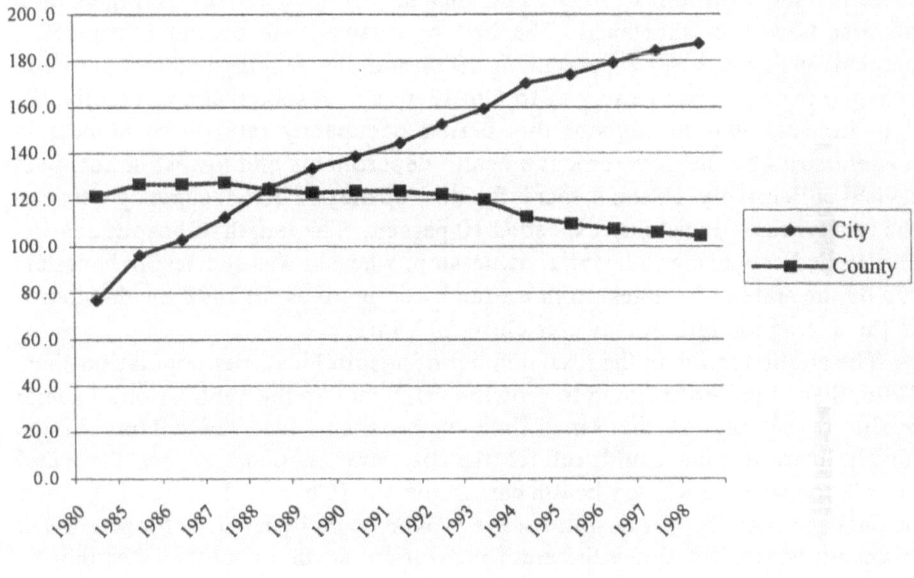

Figure 2.5 Number of hospital beds by location, 1980–1998 (in 10,000 units)

**Source:* China Yearbook, 1999.

Although each level of the three tier system is available to the rural population when needed and farmers are not restricted to township or county hospitals, past research has documented the negative relationship between utilization of health services and accessibility barriers. The cost of access to city hospitals for the rural population includes not only expenses for transportation in time and money, but also the social costs of the withdrawal of social networks and support. In our study of a sample of 288 villages in HeBei Province, the average distance of a village from a township hospital was 2.0 Km, ranging from 0.1 Km to 9.0 Km; the distance of a village from a county hospital ranged from 1.0 Km to 50 Km and averaged 15.6 Km; the average distance of a village from a city hospital, on the other hand, was 52.9 Km and the most remote village in the sample was located 200 Km away.

Although the increase in the number of hospital beds per population since the economic reforms was somewhat slower than the population growth (an annual average of 1.3 percent), there is evidence that the PRC does not experience a shortage in hospitalization beds. Similar to tendencies in industrial societies, the hospitalization rate in China has declined and the average length of hospitalization shortened. The bed occupancy rate declined from 82.7 percent in 1985 to 60.2 percent in 1998 and the length of hospitalization changed from an average stay of 15.8 to 13.1 days, respectively. Generally, the data indicate that throughout this period occupancy rates were highest in hospitals run by the government's health departments and lowest in hospitals owned collectively. In some years, the discrepancy in bed occupancy between the two types of ownership exceeded 10 percent. The length of hospitalization also varied according to hospital ownership, where it was shortest in hospitals run by the state and longest in those run by collectives. In 1998 the difference in the average length of stay was close to 3.5 days.

The slight decline in the total number of hospital beds per population since 1996, then, can be attributed to growing efficiency in the application of social health resources. At the same time, some argue that the decline in the hospitalization rate could reflect the barriers encountered by the rural population seeking tertiary health care in the city (Chen et al, 1997). However, no data are available for hospital usage broken down by level, or for patterns of township hospital and health center utilization, so this hypothesis cannot be explored.

International comparison of the number of hospital beds cannot be conclusive, because of inconsistency in the definitions of the unit(s) of analysis. The number of hospital beds published in the statistical abstracts of the PRC includes all types of beds, that is, acute, long term, and specialized. However, when all these types of hospital beds are considered, China has one of the highest beds per population ratio even in terms of the industrially developed world. Comparison with the other eight societies chosen indicates that the number of hospital beds in the PRC fell behind those available in Japan (16.2 beds for 1,000 population) and Mongolia (11.5 beds per 1,000 population). However, when only county and city acute hospital beds are taken into account, the number of hospital beds available per 1,000 population drops to 2.7 in 1998, similar to the number of beds available in Sri Lanka, but higher than the number of beds in the more affluent Thailand (2.0:1,000) and the poorer India (0.8:1,000).

Data regarding hospital beds in HeBei Province are not available. In 1998, however, 5.3 percent of the national hospital beds were located in HeBei Province, similar to the province's portion of the total population of the PRC. Occupancy rate declined below the national average, from 82.2 percent in 1985 to 58.9 percent in 1997, and the length of stay from the average of 15.0 days to 12.6 days (HeBei Yearbook, 1999). As with the national utilization patterns, bed occupancy rates were lowest in collectively owned hospitals (41.0 percent in 1997) and highest in the health department hospitals (62.6 percent), though hospitalization length was similar in the two types of facilities.

The dynamic of primary care clinic development, in general, follows that of hospitals. A massive investment in developing the grass-roots health services occurred during the early years, increasing the number of clinics from 769 in 1949 to 170,708 in 1965. The number of clinics continued to increase steadily from 1975 to 1990. Since then, a slight but steady decline in the number of clinics was reported. By 1997, however, 89.3 percent of the villages in rural PRC had a clinic, 44.6 percent of them owned by the village collective and 48.3 percent privately (Yearbook of Sanitarian Statistics, 1998). In HeBei Province, 96.2 percent of the villages sampled for our survey had at least one clinic, but the proportion of private clinics was much higher (77.0 percent).

Other kinds of physical resources are the supply of safe drinking water and sewage disposal systems. Long-term data regarding such facilities are not available for the PRC (WHO, 2000). Data available for 1989–1990 and 1990–1991 indicate that a safe water supply is becoming more readily available. In 1989–1990, 70.3 percent of the population enjoyed safe water and the proportion increased to 82.9 percent in 1990–1991. Yet, continued linear development cannot be assumed with certainty. The quality of water supply has to be consistently monitored. Recent growth of rural industry, for example, threatens the quality of water accessible to the population, as described in Chapter 3.

It has only been since the mid-1990s that policy makers have started to pay attention to environmental risks. The budget allocated for pollution treatment increased by 236 percent in four years and was more than 12 billion Yuan in 1998 (China Year Book, 1999). The number of sewage treatment projects increased sevenfold since 1995. The proportion of industrial water which reached the standards set for safe discharge increased from 55.4 percent in 1995 to 67.0 percent in 1998.

Developing a sewage disposal system for the rural population demands an enormous investment of resources. In 1997, 68.4 percent of the urban population and 15.8 percent of the rural population enjoyed adequate sewage disposal. This figure was almost five times higher than that for the rural population of India, with equivalent proportion of rural population, only 3.7 percent of whom have access to sewage disposal. In Viet Nam, whose population density is comparable to that of the PRC, adequate sewage disposal as available to 3.6 percent of the rural population.

In HeBei Province, 94.4 percent of the villages surveyed in 1996–1999 were connected to a piped water system, two-thirds were supplied with purified drinking water. Yet, regardless of its source, the water was considered to be of poor quality by 11.5 percent of the village doctors who participated in the study. All of the villages in the survey had an open sewage system, that is, ditches that run along the streets of the village. Only in 14.6 percent of them, however, were all households connected to the system. Of the village doctors we interviewed, 58.4 percent maintained that there is no sewage system at all in their village. An additional 19.9 percent felt that the system was not adequate.

Medical Professionals

Doctors

When the CCP came into power in 1949, it developed a multilevel medical education program to fit the planned three-tier health care delivery system. To date, four main programs prepare doctors to provide health services at different levels (Chen et al, 1995; Gong et al, 1997). A five-year university medical education program, which may be extended to seven years, prepares 'qualified' physicians for the third tier facilities or research institutions. These education programs resemble those of Western medical institutions, training persons who have completed 12 years of formal schooling to serve in county or urban hospitals offering either Western or traditional Chinese medical treatment. The first two years are devoted to basic science and the last three to clinical studies. Graduates of the five year program receive a Bachelor of Medicine degree and enter practice; those who continue for an additional two years acquire research skills and are granted a Master of Medicine degree usually turn to medical research.

Three years of college training are offered by many local governments, that is provinces, municipalities, and some counties. The curricula of these programs are oriented toward the preparation of medical personnel to run primary medical curative and preventive care facilities at the township or factory level. High school graduates (12 years of formal schooling) are accepted into these programs and obtain a Certificate of Medicine upon graduation. The graduates of these programs are often employed as qualified doctors.

The third major training program is offered in high schools to graduates of middle or junior high schools, who have completed nine years of formal schooling. The graduates of secondary medical schools are capable of providing primary curative care and carrying out public health programs with the support of qualified doctors of the township health centers, or county or city hospitals, for specialized and more complicated treatment.

Nonetheless, shortage of health personnel has led to a lack of differentiation between the functions performed by graduates of the different training programs. Further, most rural health care is delivered by village doctors who are not graduates of any of these formal vocational schools. Most grass roots level doctors have acquired their knowledge and skills by serving as apprentices in the army, or were formerly trained as 'bare foot doctors'. These grass roots primary care providers are of particular interest to this volume. Many of them were members of the working brigades, chosen by their comrades or the village administration. They were initially trained in township health centers or small hospitals in apprenticeship-like courses of three months, followed by regular refreshing and upgrading courses. The primary aim of these training programs was to produce large numbers of health personnel to implement public health campaigns and preventive health services along with the provision of simple curative treatment for their fellow farmers. Commonly known as 'bare foot doctors', these medical practitioners were highly motivated to serve the population to the best of their ability, for three reasons.

First, they were members of the community they served and felt responsible for the well being of their fellow brigade members, who expressed trust in them by choosing them for the job. Second, their training was paid for from the collective funds and they were accountable to the village committee. Finally, their employment conditions were comfortable compared with those of their counterparts in agricultural work and their earnings were higher, sometimes even in comparison with the income of the village leadership (Dezhi, 1992; Huang, 1988; Kan, 1990).

The result of the efforts of the CCP to effectuate its commitment to the health of the population was a dramatic increase in the number of medically trained personnel. During the period prior to the cultural revolution, the ratio of doctors per population increased by 50 percent, from 0.74:1,000 in 1952 to 1.05:1,000 in 1965 (China Year Book, 1999). The massive privatization of rural health care following the economic reforms of 1979 and the implementation of the 'responsibility system of household production' as described (Chapter 1) did not reverse this process. Most of the rural medical personnel continued to provide curative and preventive health services for the rural population despite these changes; during the 1980s, the number of rural care providers increased as graduates of secondary medical schools and army veterans trained as paramedics returned to their home villages and started local medical practices.

The economic reforms of 1979, however, had two consequences regarding the quality of the rural doctors. First, doctors gained more freedom in their career decisions. During the planned economy period, graduates of training programs were assigned to a workplace, which they could not leave without authorized permission. In the health sector, these restrictions on migration were used to assure the county and township health facilities of an adequate supply of trained doctors. With the relaxation of this policy and the onset of the financial crisis of township health centers, a considerable proportion of the qualified health personnel left the countryside to join urban hospitals, which offered higher income (Gong et al, 1997).

Second, the growing disposable income of the rural population created a growing demand for higher quality medical care (Liu et al, 1996). Most health personnel in the villages before the reforms had only basic training, with periodical refreshing courses. There was no licencing, since only persons chosen by their peers or village administration could engage in medical practice and be compensated by the village administration with work-points. With the dissolution of the collective, these control mechanisms also faded. It was necessary to develop a licensing procedure to ensure the competence of the practitioners.

As a result, after January 1985, rural health practitioners were required to take a qualification examination prepared by the Health Department of the province in which they practiced. Officially, no formal medical training was required as a prerequisite for these examinations. Those who demonstrated a knowledge equivalent to a secondary medical high-school level were qualified as 'village doctors', those who failed, about one-half of the applicants in 1985, were certified as 'medical persons'. Following the new licencing regulations, 'bare foot doctors' were no longer legally recognized by the Chinese Health Ministry as providers of health care.

Yet the mandatory examinations were not sufficient to assure quality health care and the professional knowledge and competence of many of the rural health care providers were far from satisfactory. 'The education plan for rural practitioners (1991–2000)' was launched by the Chinese Ministry of Health in order to provide the rural practitioners with a systematic secondary medical school education. This program increased the number of certified village doctors in the rural health care system and reduced the proportion of 'medical persons'. In 1997, 73.8 percent of all village doctors met the secondary medical education criteria, an increase of 51.2 percent from 1985 (Yearbook of Sanitarian Statistic, 1998).

A thorough description of the professional training received by village doctors today, based on our survey of 416 village doctors in HeBei Province, is presented in Chapter 4. In this chapter, however, let us note that 44.5 percent of the village doctors currently practicing started their professional careers as apprentices in township health centers or hospitals, but over two-fifths of them (62.2 percent) successfully completed upgrading programs.

In total, the effort to expand the knowledge and improve the competence of the village doctors since 1985 resulted in an increase in the number of doctors per 1,000 population from 1.3 in 1985 to 1.6 in 1995, a proportion which remained stable thereafter. In HeBei Province, however, the doctor:population ratio was lower than the national average, decreasing from 1.5 doctors per 1,000 population in 1995 to 1.3 in 1997 (HeBei Yearbook, 1998).

An international comparison of the number of doctors available for the population is not reliable, because societies differ from each other in the structure and the content of their medical education and the licensing procedures and prerequisites. Despite these reservations, however, it is worth noting that according to the World Bank report of 2000, by the end of the 20th century there were 2.0 doctors per 1,000 population in the PRC, a ratio lower only than that reported by Mongolia (2.4) and higher than that of the two developed and richest countries in the region – Japan (1.8) and Singapore (1.4).

Nurses, Midwives and Other Health Professionals

In practice, very few nurses provide primary care in rural China today. In general, nurses and other technical personnel, such as pharmacists, laboratory and image technicians, can rarely be found below the level of township hospital or health center, so that a thorough discussion of these health professions is beyond the scope of this book. Yet, a short description of development trends involving these health occupations is called for.

Data regarding the long-term trends in the expansion of the health professions in the PRC are only available from 1985 on. During this period, the number of registered nurses increased from 68,000 in 1985 to 745,000 in 1998, much faster than the growth of the population or the number of hospital beds (Figure 2.6). The number of practical nurses, however, decreased during the same period from 569,000 to 474,000 and that of assistant nurses from 259,000 in 1985 to 95,000 in 1998. In other words, the number of registered nurses increased eleven-fold, while the number of practical nurses declined by 17 percent and that of assistant nurses by 63 percent.

It seems that nursing started a process of professionalization and expansion similar to those that have taken place in developed societies. The total number of nursing personnel increased steadily over a period of 14 years, from 0.40 nurses per hospital bed and 0.8 nurses per 1,000 population in 1985 to 0.45 and 1.0, respectively, in 1998. Furthermore, this increase was accompanied by a consistent professional upgrading of nursing personnel, a transition from care provided by auxiliary nurses to care provided by better trained and more professionally competent registered nurses.

The number of midwives also declined during 1985–1998, from 76,000 to 49,000, a decline of 36 percent. This decline, however, seems to be part of the transition to professional nursing, as the vocational training for midwives is similar to that of practical nurses. The degree to which the decline in the number of midwives affected the reproductive health of Chinese women is not clear. As mentioned above, maternal mortality is on the decline, but the proportion of births attended by trained personnel also declined from 94.4 percent in the mid-1980s to 89.3 percent in the mid-1990s. Only 78.6 percent of all pregnant women received professional prenatal care, similar to the figures reported by Viet Nam but lower than those of the other countries selected for comparison. The reproductive experiences of the women interviewed during our research in HeBei Province are presented in detail in Chapter 7.

Other medical and technical personnel increased in number by 25.5 percent between 1985 and 1998, from 2,439,000 to 3,061,000. This increase is proportional both to the population growth and to the increase in the number of hospital beds (China Yearbook, 1999). Similarly, the number of managerial personnel increased by 21.5 percent and the number of logistics workers by 6.8

percent during that period. It seems that the PRC evaded development of the large bureaucracies that drain health related social resources in so many other industrial societies (Shuval, 1992).

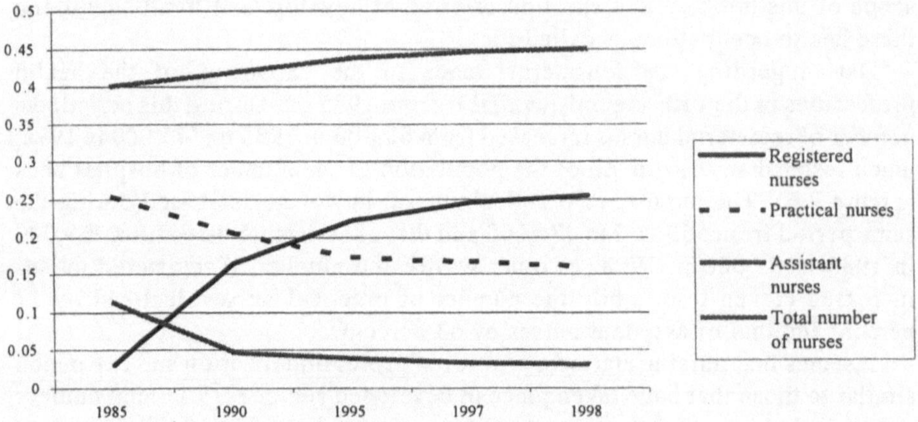

Figure 2.6 Number of nurses per hospital bed, 1985–1998

**Source:* China Yearbook, 1999.

The division of nurses, midwives and other medical and technical personnel between the urban and the rural populations cannot be accurately estimated on the basis of the data available. All we can do is to compare the proportion of health professionals who practice on the county level, that is, closer to the locations of the rural population, with that practicing in the cities. After 1957, the number of practical nurses working in county level health care institutions fell behind that o9f cities. By 1970, 39.2 percent of all registered and practical nurses were employed in county level health institutions, a proportion which declined further to 35.6 percent in 1980, just after the economic reforms, and to 28.6 percent in 1998.

Moreover, the number of nurses per hospital bed in the cities was higher than in the counties, although the gap has narrowed consistently since the late 1980s. Thus, while in 1980 there were 0.14 nurses per county bed, in the cities 0.39 nurses were available per hospital bed. In 1998, the number of nurses per hospital bed in the counties increased to 0.33, while the increase in the cities was much more modest, only up to 0.46.

The apportionment of other medical and technical personnel between county and city health facilities was more equitable, although the proportions of allied health occupations practicing on the county level had declined almost steadily since the early 1970s. In 1970, 61.5 percent of all medical and technical personnel were practicing in county level health institutions, while only 41.4 percent of these personnel had been practicing in the counties in 1998. Yet, the number of medical and technical personnel (other than doctors and nurses) per hospital bed in the counties was almost always higher than that in the cities, possibly compensating for the shortage in doctors and nurses. Nonetheless, none of these processes was associated with thc cconomic reforms of 1979, the focal point of the current analysis.

HeBei Province underwent processes similar to the national trends described above. From 1990 to 1997, the number of registered nurses increased by 67.1 percent, similar to the national average, though the number of practical nurses and midwives in HeBei Province declined more rapidly than the national average. The number of practical nurses declined by 23.4 percent in HeBei, compared with the national average of 20.7 percent. The number of midwives declined by 20.5 percent, compared with 15.5 percent for the whole of China. The number of assistant nurses in HeBei, however, increased by 13.6 percent, while on the national level their number declined by 18.9 percent. Thus, the expansion of the nursing profession and its professionalization appears to have been somewhat slower in HeBei Province. By 1997, the number of registered nurses per hospital bed in HeBei was 0.17, compared with the national average of 0.25. The respective figures for the total number of all nursing personnel was 0.33 in HeBei and 0.45 in China as a whole.

The shortage in nursing personnel reflects a general shortage in medical care providers of all categories in HeBei Province. By 1998, 4.8 percent of all Chinese medical and technical personnel (excluding doctors) were practicing in HeBei Province, less than the province's proportion of the total Chinese population (5.3 percent).

Summary

This chapter is devoted to the health status of the population, social investment in health, and available health resources, both facilities and personnel. To provide additional insight into the current state of health and health resources, long term tendencies are examined, with emphasis on the 1979 economic reforms, and the PRC data are compared with those available for eight other East Asian societies.

The health status of the Chinese population is described by exploring long-term trends of mortality-based indicators in the PRC and other eight East Asian societies. In 1998, life expectancy in China was similar to that in Thailand, a richer society whose members enjoy a higher standard of living, and Sri Lanka, whose economic development has been similar to that of the PRC. However, most of the increase in China took place in the first two decades following the revolution, after which the increase in life expectancy in China was moderate when compared with the increase observed in the other eight societies.

Crude mortality declined in China after the revolution, but increased again after 1978, a process that appeared not to be related to the aging of the population. Rather, it appeared to be the result of increasing mortality of men of working age and a relatively slow decline in infant and childhood mortality, as compared with the decline in the other eight East Asian societies.

The social resources invested in health are also described in this chapter. In 1995, China allocated 3.8 – 4.5 percent of its GDP to health, half of it from public resources. Although the public share in the financial resources allocated to health was higher than in most other countries selected for comparison, it raises concerns regarding the equality of access to care, especially in rural China, where income is lower than in the cities. The efforts to revive the rural health cooperative system, adapted to local economic conditions and health needs, raise similar concerns: unlike the pre-economic reforms era the financial basis of the new systems is the premiums contributed by the individual members, rather than state support (Carrin et al, 1996).

The economic reforms of 1979 did not have a long-term effect on the social investment in physical health resources, or their availability in general. This conclusion is based on long term fluctuations in the number of hospital beds, clinics, and health personnel per population. The transition to a market economy combined with the government's effort to control prices at affordable levels, however, brought about a decline in township hospital services. Policy measures taken to revive this important component of the rural health care system seem to have been effective. China is making a considerable effort to provide the population with the necessary physical health resources, such as health care institutions, safe water supply, and adequate sewage disposal, within the limits of its economic capability. Standards for licensing of rural doctors and the upgrading of professional nursing personnel are being improved in order to increase the number of available competent care providers.

Chapter 3

Public Health: Past Achievements and Future Challenges

Irvin K. Zola often relates to the story about a physician who was so busy saving individuals drowning in a river that he didn't have the time to look for the person persistently throwing them into the water (Mckinlay, 1974). The remarkable improvement in the status of health in the PRC, presented in Chapter 2, came about primarily by focusing on "up-river" causes.

The volume of health-related problems facing the Chinese Communist Party as it came into power in 1949 was so great that it was impossible to meet the health needs of each individual with the limited resources available to it at the time. It was clear that a significant improvement in the health status of the population could be achieved only by 'putting prevention first', rather than by treating and curing individuals.

China's public health policy after the revolution drew on the experience accumulated in the Soviet Union, but also contained several innovative and unique features, some of which will be presented in this chapter. Many of these features were abandoned after the economic reforms of 1979 and the dismantling of the collective. At the same time, new potential health hazards, related to increasing industrialization and urbanization, emerged. Yet the economic reforms were accompanied by a gradual relaxation of the isolation policy followed strictly during the Mao Ze Dong era. Its changing foreign policy enabled China to recruit international support and to join forces with other nations to preserve public health and cope with emerging challenges.

These are the issues that will be described in this chapter, which begins with a description of the innovative public health policy developed and pursued during the first three decades of the People's Republic of China, using one communicable endemic disease, schistosomiasis, as a case study. The courses of action taken within the context of social and political processes that followed the economic reforms will be represented by the way in which one non-communicable endemic disorder, iodine deficiency, was handled. We shall then turn to discuss some of the, new, emerging public health concerns.

Putting Prevention First

Above and beyond its commitment to the well being of the Chinese population, the CCP recognized the importance of good health to the economic development of modern China. In all societies, the health of the population is a key economic factor. In the newly established PRC, the rural population was the most readily available economic resource and its good health was essential for the effort to overcome long-standing shortages of food and hunger. The perception of public health as a cardinal asset in rural production was explicitly communicated to all levels of the public administration, social and political organizations, and the public at large. This explicit and publicized recognition was one of the components used to motivate the whole society to support and participate in programs to improve public health (Wilenski, 1997).

In keeping with this perception, public resources were increasingly allocated for public health programs soon after the revolution. Public health workers were trained and anti-epidemic stations were established, from national down to village level. For the first time in China's history, farmers enjoyed the benefit of public resources, although the share of city dwellers in the resources allotted to health was higher than that of their rural counterparts, up until the 'Cultural Revolution' (Chen, 2001).

A unique feature of the CCP's approach to public health was the effort to integrate public health with social life and political activity. Preventive medicine was not left in the hands of the Ministry of Public Health alone, but was treated as an all-party concern, and party resources were recruited to the public health effort. Multi-sectorial committees, named Leading Groups, were established at all administrative levels. These committees included health professionals, health workers and representatives of volunteer organizations such as the All Women's Federation and the Youth League as well as ordinary citizens. In the villages, public health committees were often chaired by the brigades' barefoot doctors' (Jamison et al, 1984). Farmers and city dwellers were consulted regarding their public health problems, informed about possible ways of coping with a given problem, and consulted regarding the design of a public health strategy suitable to their particular situation.

Another innovation was 'the patriotic health campaigns' conducted by means of 'mass line'. Local committees of 'the patriotic health movement' successfully mobilized a large number of citizens, including children and seniors, to take part in public health activities. News papers, posters, public meetings, discussions, evening classes, street propaganda and other means of publicity were used to educate the people about a given health problem and the reason particular means were chosen to cope with it, calling on everybody to participate actively in the health campaign. Health campaigns were conducted two to three times a year, carefully timed so as not to interfere with regular economic activity. In the countryside, campaigns were carried out during agriculture slack seasons. The involvement of the masses in public health work played a major role in improving the health of the general population (Wilenski, 1977).

Finally, the Chinese public health policy changed the power structure among health care providers, eliminating the monopoly of medical professionals in particular (Chen, 2001). The Western model of health care provision, which relies heavily on highly skilled personnel whose training is long, costly, cure-oriented and utilizes expensive technology, was not feasible in the young PRC. Skilled medical doctors were extremely scarce after the Communist revolution, as were health facilities and financial resources. The needs of the population, however, were many and called for immediate and efficient action to promote the health of all, not only of privileged individuals. As described in chapters 1 and 2, China chose to train large numbers of health workers capable of doing public health work, transmitting health education, and providing basic health care under the existing local conditions. Practitioners of traditional Chinese medicine were integrated with public health activities, increasing the number of trained personnel involved in preventive health work. Scientific research was carried out in the countryside with the help of the local population, demystifying and popularizing science (Wilenski, 1977).

As with many other aspects of the rural health care system prior to the economic reforms, once the 'system of household responsibility' was implemented new public health strategies were called for. While some aspects of the unique approach to public health, such as multi-level and multi-sectorial collaboration, could have been maintained, others, such as mobilizing 'mass line', became increasingly difficult to actualize. The privatization of primary health care encouraged care providers to focus on the curative, more profitable, aspects of health care. The government had to use its administrative authority and offer financial incentives to mobilize village doctors for public health work (Hsiao, 1995). The increasing demand for high quality medical care and the emerging need to ensure the providers' competence (see Chapter 2) gradually transferred the emphasis to professionalism and technical skill.

At the same time, the economic reforms of 1979 were accompanied by the relaxation of the policies of self-sufficiency and isolation. In keeping with the perception of health as an economic asset, foreign investments were not restricted to raising capital, knowledge, and technology. Rather, China opened its doors to collaborative efforts with other nations and with international organizations, with the aim of solving long-standing endemic health problems and attacking newly emerging problems. We now turn to examine in some detail the strategy taken to eradicate schistosomiasis and cope with iodine deficiency disorders before and immediately following the economic reforms of 1979.

Fighting Infectious Diseases – Schistosomiasis

Schistosomiasis is caused by blood flukes of the genus Schistosoma, which invade the human body and inhabit it. Schistosomiasis is endemic in 74 countries and territories and despite control efforts and the development of new treatment technologies, the number of infected persons throughout the world did not decline during the 20th century. Paradoxically, economic development, particularly the utilization of water for electricity and irrigation, seem to have increased transmission of the disease. It is estimated that some 200 million people throughout the world are infected with schistosomiasis, of whom 120 million are symptomatic and 20 million are severely ill (Chitsulo et al, 2000).

The Schistosoma blood flukes spend most of their life cycle in two hosts: the immature stages are spent in Oncamelania snails, while the adult stage is spent in a mammal, usually human. Eggs discharged from the mammal host hatch into larvae in fresh water before invading the snail, their intermediate host, where they partially mature. The mature larvae escape back into the water and later penetrate the skin of a mammal. In this host the mature larvae migrate through the blood vessels to specific organs, remain there, and lay eggs.

The schistosoma prevalent in China is Schistosoma Japonicum, which concentrates in the blood vessels of the large intestine and liver. Some are carried up the portal veins to the liver, where they cause inflammation and scarring, with enlargement of liver and spleen. Obstructing the blood flow through the liver, it may cause distension of veins, which often rupture, causing serious hemorrhage.

Untreated schistosomiasis often results in death. Effective chemotherapy free of severe side effects was not available until 1982, when oral praziquantel chemotherapy was introduced. Though effective, praziquantel is too expensive for many developing countries and prevention by means of adequate sanitation and extermination of snails remains the best option for these countries (Chitsulo et al, 2000).

China was one of the first countries to control schistosomiasis, though the goal of eradication has not yet been fully reached to date. Of the ten provinces, one autonomous region and one municipality along the Yangtze and the Pearl Rivers, five are still struggling with the parasite that Mao Ze-Dong named 'the god of plague'. Sleigh et al (1998a, 1998b, 1998c) described the fight against schistosomiasis in the Guagnxi Zhuang Autonomous Region, from the first five-year plan of the early 1950s to 1992, three years after the eradication of schistosomiasis in this region. This case study provides insight into the China's unique approach to curing and preventing further affliction with schistosomiasis.

As early as 1950, the Ministry of Public Health called on health specialists and rural administrators to prepare for a campaign to eradicate schistosomiasis. They were requested to form mobile teams of medical staff who, together with students of medical and nursing colleges on their summer vocations, were to detect schistosomiasis cases and Oncamelania snails and identify the regions in which they were endemic. From 1954 to 1956, the masses were also mobilized to locate such regions and assess the volume of the problem. Vignettes and descriptions of schistosomiasis symptoms and five Oncamelania snails were mailed to local leaders at all levels, directing them to report possible cases in their community, and to encourage villagers to collect suspect snails and send the information and suspicious snails to the public health authorities.

A national control effort was launched in 1955. The strategy chosen was to eradicate the disease by changing the snails' inhabitant and thus limiting their ability to transmit the disease. A massive health education effort was undertaken, using all available methods to teach farmers about the disease, the parasitic life cycle, transmission, and prevention. Health education took place at every opportunity in every possible way, in regular schools, in village meetings, and through the widespread use of street posters.

Multi-sectorial Leading Groups were established at all levels of administration; institutes for disease control and specialized hospitals were founded in large central cities. The role of the Leading Group at each level of administration was to specify the actions appropriate to its specific conditions and to adapt the strategy proposed by the upper administrative level to local situation. Representatives of the public health sector served as advisors on matters of health education, treatment, sanitation, and research; those of the agricultural sector were responsible for the control of schistosomiasis in livestock and reclaimed wasteland. Representatives of the water conservation authority coordinated the eradication of snails with other water engineering plans and facilities. The propaganda office was responsible for health education. The Women's Federation and the Youth League motivated their members to take part in the actual environmental work and to adhere with the recommended health behavior.

'Mass line' was regularly used in eradicating snails. Farmers, students and teachers, soldiers and office employees participated in the 'patriotic health campaign'. They scraped the earth and redirected water to change the snails' inhabitant, as well as actually destroying snails. While the pace of the work did slow down during the 'great leap forward' and difficult period that followed, it regained its initial momentum in 1970. Sleigh et al (1998b) estimated that between 1974 and 1980, 7,680,000 person-days were invested in environmental change aimed at eliminating the snail hosts.

The control program was designed to increase agriculture production. Mass mobilization overlapped slow agricultural seasons, hardly interfering with production. Draining swamps, building dams, and diverting water eliminated snails on the one hand, while creating and improving agriculture resources on the other. In Guangxi alone, for example, more than 6,600 sq km of wasteland were reclaimed and 360 sq km of fishing pools built between 1953 and 1991 (Sleigh et al, 1998a, 1998b). Freed from schistosomiasis infection, the productivity of livestock grew significantly.

With decollectivization and the abolishment of the work-point system, however, mass mobilization became increasingly difficult and slowly faded away. New strategies were designed, relying on specialized teams for the continuous monitoring of snails and infection in humans and animals. Consequently, wages now comprise half of the annual budget allocated to maintain control of schistosomiasis, and the costs of administration have almost doubled (Sleigh et al, 1998b).

At the same time, it is very possible that mass mobilization is no longer necessary and, despite the rise in individualistic and materialistic attitudes, the great majority of farmers are still willing to participate in collective schistosomiasis control efforts (79 per cent of those aware of the condition; Sleigh et al, 1998c). More alarming is the decline in knowledge regarding schistosomiasis and the prevalence of unsafe behavior. Sleigh et al, (1998c) reported that 33 per cent of the farmers who live in a county where schistosomiasis was previously endemic have never heard of the disease and over half of the population engage in unsafe fishing, swimming, and rice planting. This neglect in health education should concern the public health authorities of the PRC, who have been struggling with schistosoma for over five decades, with total success in five out of the ten provinces and autonomous regions where the disease was once endemic.

There are two additional obstacles to full eradication. One is the lack of a widespread safe sewage infrastructure, the other is the use of untreated human waste as agriculture fertilizer. The use of communal toilets, where human feces were disinfected before being used for agriculture, seems to be on the decline since decollectivization. As the human waste will be necessary for maintaining and increasing agriculture production for the foreseeable future, it is necessary to find simple and cheap ways to disinfect it (Lai and Hsi, 1996). Treating human waste will also serve to control intestinal nematode infections, which are also highly prevalent along the Yangtze River (Sun et al, 1998).

Coping with Non-communicative Disorders: The Case of Iodine Deficiency

Iodine, which is essential for the normal functioning of the thyroid gland, is one of the elements among the mineral nutrients which must be constantly supplied in the diet. A normal thyroid gland consists of cuboidal epithelial cells arranged to form small sacs known as vesicles, which are usually filled with a colloid substance containing the protein thyroglobulin in combination with the two thyroid hormones, triiodothyronine. Thyroglobulin is especially rich in iodine and the two thyroxin hormones are composed of multiple copies of the amino acid tyrosine, which contains either four or three iodine atoms. Iodine is thus essential for synthesis of thyroid gland hormones, which increase the cellular rate of carbohydrate metabolism and synthesis and the breakdown of protein. The two thyroxin hormones therefore play a vital role in the growth and development of children and the pace of metabolism in adults.

Iodine is a trace element found in small quantities in the soil, air, and seawater. The distribution of iodine in the environment depends on geographical distance from a sea as well as on past and present climate. Geographical regions far from a sea, rich in rainfall and snow, or prone to recurring floods, are generally poor in iodine. Furthermore, the glaciation that ended the last Ice Age some 10,000 years ago scraped the surface of the landscape, living behind insufficient iodine for mankind and animals. Currently, 130 countries in the world are affected by iodine deficiency (ICCIDD, 1999).

A daily dose of only 100–150 micrograms of iodine is required for normal functioning of the thyroid gland. Its absence, however, causes several health disorders. In humans, goiter and cretinism are visible in severe cases. Less obvious are different degrees of stunting of growth and mental retardation caused by prenatal iodine deficiency or deficiency in infancy and childhood. Lethargy is common among adults in iodine deficient environment, even if they were not deprived of iodine in infancy or childhood. The International Council for the Control of Iodine Deficiency Disorders estimates that 1.6 billion individuals worldwide are at risk for iodine deficiency disorders (IDD). Of these, 50 million are children (ICCIDD website, 2000). Of the population at risk, 1–10 per cent are Cretins, 5–30 per cent have some degree of brain damage, and 30–70 per cent suffer from lack of energy.

The rural economy in iodine deficient environments is doubly jeopardized, because livestock, like humans, also develop IDD. In such environments, still birth rates and calf mortality among domestic animals are twice as high as in environments with sufficient iodine. Production of wool, eggs, and meat is low and work animals are relatively weak (Pandav, 1994).

Most IDD cannot be fully cured. These disorders, however, are relatively easy to prevent by the administration of small doses of iodine to the population in iodine deficient areas. Prenatal treatment is strongly recommended, because postnatal intervention will prevent stunting of growth and mental retardation, but will not improve neurological conditions and will not necessarily prevent low intelligence levels (Xue et al, 1994). Furthermore, unlike infectious diseases, iodine deficiency cannot be eradicated. It needs to be constantly treated to ensure not only the adequate growth and development of children, but the well-being and productivity of adults as well.

The soil in a large part of China is iodine deficient, due to glaciation and repeated flooding. All provinces, autonomous regions, and municipalities, with the exception of Beijing and Shanghai, include number of cities and counties at risk for IDD (Wang, 1997). IDD has been known in China for more than 4,000 years. It is documented in Chinese medical scripts from the 3rd century BC on and was described by Marco Polo in the 13th century. A survey in Yunnan Province during the 1930s documented the scope of the problem, though persons who appear to be normal but have low intelligence were probably not included in the survey as IDD cases.

IDD was yet another endemic problem facing the CCP as it came into power in 1949. During the 1950s, public health research teams conducted epidemiological and applied research into the nature of IDD. It was specified as a priority health target in the third five-year plan (1959). Nevertheless, apart from some local initiatives to distribute iodized salt, a large scale national effort was not undertaken until the end of the 'great leap forward'.

The first multi-sectorial Leading Group on national level was established in 1960, followed by the subsequent formation of similar committees on the provincial level. Nationwide distribution of iodized salt was initiated in 23 provinces in 1964, but interrupted by the Cultural Revolution before the necessary infrastructure for production and distribution could be developed. With the end of the period of unrest, researchers from national and provincial institutes strongly advocated for prevention and control of IDD, bringing about serious attempts to cope with the problem in 1978.

During that year several policies were designated and operational steps taken for their implementation. Recognizing the importance of IDD control, the government took upon itself the full expense of iodization. Guidelines for the production, distribution, and quality of iodized products (mainly salt, but also oil) were set and a network of quality control laboratories was founded in iodine deficient areas. Because iodized salt is highly sensitive to environmental conditions during storage and transportation, the laboratories were responsible for quality control at both the production and consumption ends. A simple kit for field monitoring of the iodine content of salt was developed and is still widely used by health workers as well as by school teachers.

The large-scale efforts to prevent and control IDD, however, begun on the verge of the economic reforms, which brought about considerable social, economic, and political transitions. It may be argued that these processes were reflected in the way in which China coped with IDD: the Ministry of Health was in charge of coordinating and managing the strategies developed by national and provincial committees, in cooperation with the Chinese Medical Association (Wang, 1997). Now it was the Department of Endemic Disease Control, not the propaganda office, that was charged, in addition to its responsibility for epidemiological monitoring and surveillance of treatment, with organizing the health education and communication programs on the provincial and county levels. Most work was done by experts and professionals, the masses were not involved; community participation was minimal.

Nevertheless, the relaxation of the PRC's political isolation during the early 1980s enabled it to join forces with other nations and international organizations in the work of controlling IDD. Its first collaboration, begun in 1986, was undertaken with the Australian government and public health authorities. During the first stage of this joint effort, four experimental regions were chosen in which to develop and establish effective systems for the surveillance of iodine levels in water as well as in newborn infants and adults. The system of collecting and transporting specimens of water, blood, and urine developed during the pilot stage was later implemented throughout China. The collaboration with Australia began its work with IDD research on animals, and with training specialists in IDD-related fields such as psychology, neurology, and biochemistry.

In 1990 representatives from the PRC participated for the first time in the World Summit for Children held in New York. This summit started a cooperation between the PRC and the United Nations aimed at eliminating IDD by the year 2000, which yielded training programs for health professionals, scientists, public health educators, and technical support personnel. In 1995, the World Bank joined the UN–China collaboration, providing additional funding and technical assistance. This intervention was associated with changes in the distribution system, from planned central distribution to a more market-oriented pattern of production and supply. However, while the laboratories have been equipped and maintained by the World Bank, the monitoring of the quality of iodized salt and oil remained the responsibility of national and local governments.

Considerable progress has been made towards IDD control in the PRC since the beginning of collaboration with other nations and international agencies (Chen, 1998, 1999, 2000). Criteria for the diagnosis of IDD have been developed, manufacturing and quality control methods of iodized products (salt, oil, and tea) are constantly updated, their distribution is regulated, and health education in the schools and via the mass media continues unabated. The production of iodized salt increased from 3.7 million tons in 1993 to 7.53 million tons in 1999, far beyond population growth and close to the level of self-sufficiency.

The quality of iodized salt is also increasing: 94 per cent of the 1999 production met the national standard, compared with 50 per cent in 1993. Household use of iodized salt increased from 51 per cent in 1995 to an average of 89 per cent in 1999. However, the quality of the salt consumed varies significantly from one region to another. Only in one province (Hunan), did 90 per cent of the salt sold meet the national criteria of 20–60 mg iodine/kg salt in 1997, and the national average was 69 per cent. Moreover, non-iodized salt still compromised 10 per cent of the edible salt market and is considerably cheaper for the consumer. Given the variability of economic development in the PRC, the use of iodized salt is significantly less widespread in poor regions.

Health education is most important in controlling IDD. The rural population tends to respond mostly to acute conditions (see Chapter 5) and needs to be educated regarding the permanency of iodine deficiency. In 1994, May 5th was set as an 'IDD Control Day' and devoted to increasing awareness among the public of the importance of iodine supplements to brain development of fetuses and newborn infants, to the growth and development of children, to general adult well-being, and to livestock production. Special attention is given to women of childbearing age and IDD prevention and education are guaranteed by the 1995 Law for the Protection of Infants and Women (Chapter 7). A survey conducted after the fourth IDD Control Day, held in 1997 reported national coverage of 65 per cent, with the highest coverage of 82 per cent in Liaoning Province and the lowest coverage of 53 per cent in Jilin.

Research into new methods of iodization is continuing in China. In several pilot regions, iodized salt for domestic animals and iodized drinking and irrigation water have been used with promising results. The data collected seem to indicate a higher urinary iodine level in women of childbearing age, a decline in infant mortality, and an increase in lamb production by close to 50 per cent. Similar increases were observed in rice production and in the iodine content of rice grains and of the soil (Chen, 2000).

Table 3.1 China IDD control as compared with WHO standards*

Criterion	WHO standard	China[a]	
		1995	1999
Iodized salt (% of households)	> 90%	51.0%	88.9%
Urinary iodine			
(% median less than 100 ug/l)	< 50%	na	6.5%[a]
(% median less than 50 ug/l)	< 20%	na	3.3%
Goiter (% age 6–12 with thyroid size above 97th percentile)	< 5%	20.4%	8.8%
Neonatal TSH (% above 5 mU/l)	< 3%	33.3%	33.3%[a]

* *Source:* World Health Organization, 1994; Chen, 1999, 2000; Wang et al, 1997.
[a] Percent of the 31 provinces, municipalities, and autonomous regions.

Most alarming are the findings of an analysis of over 22,000 neonatal cord blood samples performed in 1997. Fully one third of the provinces did not meet the standard and the prevalence of higher than 5 mU/L thyroid-stimulating hormone (TSH) exceeded the WHO target of 3 per cent. A similar proportion was reported in 1995, indicating that a large number of newborn infants still ran a high risk of neurological disorder and mental retardation if not treated.

The multi-sectorial effort and multi-dimensional campaign has in fact improved IDD control in China and brought the country closer to the control standards set by the WHO (Table 3.1). In 1999, the median level of urinary iodine was 306 mcg per $1{,}000^3$, compared with 165 mcg per $1{,}000^3$ in 1995. The prevalence of goiter among children declined from 20.4 per cent in 1995 to 8.8 per cent in 1999. However, full control has not yet been reached. As with the consumption of iodized salt, the median level of urinary iodine masks a considerable regional variability. In 3.3 per cent of the urine samples iodine level was lower than the recommended safety level of 50 mcg per $1{,}000^3$. In one province the median was lower than 100 mcg per $1{,}000^3$.

Future Challenges

As described in the previous chapter, China is in the process of epidemiological transition. Infectious diseases have not been fully conquered yet, but the prevalence and incidence of chronic degenerative diseases and the proportion of deaths caused be these diseases are on the increase (Banister, 1998). Since the economic reforms of 1979, rural to urban migration has grown, as did the rural industry. These processes have introduced new public health challenges: risks caused by environmental pollution. Some of these old and new challenges will be briefly described in the following section.

Infectious Diseases

a) Parasitic infections

The unique public health approach taken by China to the eradication of endemic parasites that have impaired human health and inhibited agriculture production for generations has already been described. Despite these admirable achievements, parasites remain a significant public health problem in China. Cystic echinococcosis is endemic in 87 per cent of the country (Wen and Yang, 1997) and the prevalence of some nematode infections was close to 50 per cent in 1997, particularly among farmers in paddy agriculture in some areas (Sun et al, 1998; Lai and Shi, 1996).

Chemotherapy is not feasible, mainly because of its high cost. In line with the four principles determined by the CCP after liberation (see Chapter 1), priority was given to the treatment of these health conditions among children. Benzimidazole anthelminthic is administered annually to children from kindergarten until they graduate from school, and in 1997 a zero prevalence of Ascaris, Trichuris, and Hookworm was found among school-children along the Yangtze River. Nevertheless, those children who enter agriculture run a 15–50 per cent risk of being infected in the future.

Lessons learned from industrial countries indicate that the elimination of parasites is possible through a combination of four factors: environmental change, adequate sanitation, medical curative intervention, and behavioral change (Shuval and Anson, 2000). To date, most public health efforts have been concentrated on environmental change and health education. Health education alone, however, is not sufficient to bring about behavioral change. Structural and economic constraints, such as the lack of adequate sanitation and the use of human waste as fertilizer, limit the effectiveness of health behavior advocated by educators.

b) Malaria

Malaria is endemic in central China (at present, mainly in Henan and Yunnan provinces). Efforts to eradicate the disease started soon after the CCP came into power in 1949, when mosquitoes were one of the 'four pests' on which war was declared. 'Mass line' was recruited to spray standing water to eliminate the vector anopheles, and bed-nets were distributed. In later years, chemotherapy has been provided, treating acute conditions and preventing relapse in persons with a history of malaria.

Henan Province experienced three major outbreaks of malaria between 1950 and 1970, when the rate of incidence reached 16.9 per cent. Consistent eradication efforts have yielded considerable advancement toward malaria control: from 1989 to 1997, not even one case of malaria caused by plasmodium falciparum, the more severe form of the disease, was reported, and the incidence of plasmodium vivax malaria in 1994 was just 0.82 per 100,000 population (Li et al, 1999).

Nevertheless, malaria has not yet been fully conquered and several local outbreaks have been registered in Henan Province since 1994, including 14 sporadic cases of falciparum malaria. Two factors are probably responsible for the persistence of malaria in rural China (Li et al, 1999; Xu and Liu, 1997). One is related to the topography of some tropical regions of China, which restricts access to standing water for effective, regular, spraying. Some villages in these areas are equally hard to reach. There is some evidence that bed nets are not effective in these villages, either because of the poor quality of living conditions, or because of the reluctance of the local farmers to use pesticide-sprayed nets.

Internal and international migration, which increased with the transition to the socialist market economy, is another factor which inhibits malaria control. Migrants from malaria-free regions lack natural immunity as well as knowledge regarding protective measures. They are, thus, highly susceptible and easily infected. Many of these are seasonal working migrants. At the end of the season, they return to their home areas carrying malaria plasmodium, which may be transmitted to others by the anopheles vector. All 14 falciparum malaria cases diagnosed in Henan Province in 1977 were imported by seasonal workers returning home.

Yunnan Province shares over 4,000 kilometers of its border with three countries where malaria is endemic, Lao, Myanmar, and Viet Nam. All three have only limited anti-malaria programs. Refugees from Myanmar, for example, increased the incidence of malaria in Yunnan Province from 0.52 per 1,000 populations in 1987 to 4.57:1,000 in 1989. Coffee, tea, sugar cane, and fruit are cultivated in the south of the province, attracting seasonal workers from other parts of China as well as traders from across the border. Local residents, on the other hand, migrate to work in construction and mines on the other side of the border. It has been estimated that many of these workers return home bearing malaria plasmodium.

In the early 1990s, the persistence of malaria in China lead public health authorities to increase anti-malaria activity and tighten migration surveillance. All relevant departments, that is, customs, public security, border police, the bureau of industry and commerce, and the office of farm management, assist the Provincial Health Departments to identify national and international mobile populations. The purpose of this activity is rapid identification and treatment of imported malaria cases. In Yunnan Province, 34 surveillance centers were established along with 390 blood examination stations. Close to four-thousand primary health workers were trained to draw and analyze blood samples, provide treatment when necessary, and promote health education. The incidence of malaria in the province declined from 5.67 per 10,000 population in 1985 to 3.99:10,000 in 1995, and from 19.19:10,000 to 12.12:10,000 along the border areas (Xu and Liu, 1997).

c) Immunization

China started a large-scale child immunization program during the early 1960s. Public health workers and barefoot doctors were responsible for the inoculation of children and pregnant women with the vaccines available at the time. Since 1979, children are entitled to receive vaccination against tuberculosis, diphtheria, tetanus, measles, whooping cough, and poliomyelitis, while pregnant women are entitled to hepatitis screening and their children are entitled to vaccinations, if necessary. Reports on immunization before the mid-1980s are not available, but it is generally believed that the coverage reached over 90 per cent (MacCormack, 1988).

The transition to fee-for-service health care seriously hampered the immunization program. Although the government continued to fund the inoculation program, the early stages of the transition were characterized by uncertainty regarding the responsibility for all public health functions, including immunization. Immunization coverage declined to 60 per cent in the urban areas and to 33 per cent in the countryside (MacCormack, 1988). As a result, the rate of decline in the incidence and prevalence of some diseases decreased and the trend even reversed itself in many parts of China (Dezhi, 1992; Zhu et al, 1989).

The ambiguity regarding the division of public health work was soon resolved, however (Huang, 1988). In most villages served by private practitioners only, local village doctors were commissioned to perform public health tasks for a fixed annual fee, a program that has been supported by UNICEF since 1984 (Hsiao, 1995; Hillier and Shen, 1996). Wherever villages retained the collective medical scheme or were served by a branch of a public hospital, public health responsibility was assumed by these clinics. In the 1990s, charges for immunization and some limited health insurance coverage for preventive care were introduced, but apparently with no effect on immunization coverage. The proportion of children immunized against measles before their first birthday, for example, increased from 78 per cent in 1985 to 97 per cent in 1990 and, despite annual fluctuations, was stabilized at 95–96 per cent by the end of the 1990s (The World Bank, 2000).

The poliomyelitis outbreak of 1990 raised some doubts regarding the validity of the immunization coverage figures reported (Zhang, 1997, 1998), although limited outbreaks were observed in some Western societies with good immunization coverage during this period as well (Israel, for example). The figures reported by the 314 village doctors responsible for public health or mother and child care interviewed in rural HeBei indeed indicated that coverage varied by type of vaccine and that coverage in some villages was lower than the official 95 per cent (Table 3.2).

Table 3.2 Child immunization coverage, HeBei, 1996–1999 (percent immunized)

	Less than 95%	Mean percent
Poliomyelitis	5.9	98.5
Measles	13.4	97.1
Tetanus[a]	23.4	95.8
DPT[b]	20.1	96.0
Hepatitis Bc[3]	54.1	31.0

[a] Including booster, according to age.
[b] Diphtheria, tetanus, whooping cough.
[c] Immunized or screened (the child or his/her mother)

In 1990, 5,065 poliomyelitis cases were diagnosed, raising concern regarding the risk of a national epidemic (Zhang, 1997, 1998). In the winter of 1991–1992, six provinces conducted a 'National Immunization Day', in which 71 million doses of Oral Poliovirus Vaccine (OPV) were distributed to children under the age of four. Calling on the public health strategies developed during the 1950s, teams of health personnel and volunteers from the Women's Federation and the Youth League administered two doses of OPV, four weeks apart, in permanent health facilities and mobile units. In 1991, the number of diagnosed polio cases declined to 1,372, and the operation was extended to another 29 provinces, autonomous regions, and municipalities. A year later, 186 million doses of OPV were administered, bringing the number of poliomyelitis cases down to 653 cases in 1993. Another three 'National

Immunization Days', supported by WHO, UNICEF, CDC/Atlanta, Rotary International, and the Japanese International Cooperation Agency, were conducted between 1993 and 1996. Over 200 million children were vaccinated at that time and the number of cases dropped farther to 134 in 1995.

d) AIDS/HIV infection

The first AIDS case in China was diagnosed in 1985, two years after identification of the HIV retrovirus (Wu et al, 1999). However, while most post-industrial countries experienced an AIDS panic, the risk of epidemic had not been recognized in China until 1989. Relative isolation, restricted migration, and strict enforcement of anti-drugs and anti-prostitution laws were believed to protect China from a large scale spread of HIV/AIDS infection.

Indeed, an appreciable incidence of HIV infection was first documented in Yunnan Province (De Cock and Weiss, 2000), on the border of the Golden Triangle, where Thailand, Laos, and Myanmar meet. In both Thailand and Myanmar HIV infection is extremely high, around 70 per cent among injected drug users. Drug injection seems to be the main mode of transmission in China too, though in the early 1990s HIV infection started to spread among sex workers in the area. In other parts of the PRC, however, only sporadic cases were reported (Wu et al, 1999).

Yet, infected needles may become a more important mode of transmission in the future, particularly if the prevalence of HIV infection increases (Normile, 2000). Disposable syringes are not used in rural China, and many village doctors do not have adequate means for sterilization (see Chapter 4). Some refrain from sterilizing needles used for acupuncture, because sterilization reduces the flexibility of the spring located at the top of these needles. It is worth noting that the scarcity of autoclaves was suggested as one explanation for rural/urban differences in the incidence of Hepatitis B, the transmission of which resembles that of HIV infection (Shimbo et al, 1998).

By the end of 1999, there were 670 confirmed cases of AIDS and 18,143 confirmed HIV positive cases in the PRC. Like elsewhere around the globe, the reported cases were based on positive diagnosis of the small fraction of the population tested and the estimated figures are much higher. The China Center for AIDS Prevention and Control estimates the number of HIV positive cases at close to half a million, five times higher than estimated in 1996 (Normile, 2000).

Some HIV health education was introduced in 1989 and workshops were held for health professionals (Wu et al, 1999). Most of the workshops were organized by hospitals to educate their clinical and technical staff with respect to different aspects of HIV/AIDS infection and modes of transmission. These were local initiatives and varied considerably in content and structure. The number of such workshops and participants is not clear. However, a survey among 1,400 clinicians conducted by Wu et al (1999) in 1995 indicated that knowledge about HIV among health workers in China is inadequate, though most of the participants in this study (85 per cent) attended at least one HIV/AIDS workshop.

For example, only half of the respondents knew that the most efficient transmission agent is blood, or that the length of time after infection during which HIV infection cannot be detected by blood analysis. Furthermore, just 3 per cent of those questioned were aware of the meaning of universal precaution, that is, the need to treat the body liquids of all patients as if they were HIV positive. Though the association between awareness and behavior is generally weak, these findings raise serious concern regarding the preventive activities of the health care workers themselves, their own personal practice, and the health education they provide their patients.

In an effort to identify cases and control the spread of HIV infection, HIV was added to the list of sexually transmitted diseases (STD) that have to be reported to the anti-epidemic centers. The surveillance includes regular blood sampling from several groups: persons at high risk, such as employees of the entertainment industry, drug users, blood donors who could endanger others if infected, and two conveniently accessible groups – gynecological patients and persons applying for marriage license (Choi et al, 1999).

Two additional measures were taken in 1998. Commercial blood donation was banned and the National Center for AIDS Prevention and Control (NCAIDS) was established within the Academy of Preventive Medicine. NCAIDS's activity focuses on supporting AIDS-related epidemiological research and preparing for a nationwide health education campaign. Some health education activity for the public has already been started in the mass media, along with a specific program for drug users.

The relaxation of the isolation policy enabled the PRC to become the first to try the HIV/AIDS vaccine (Normile, 2000). Restricted migration has resulted in a stable population and prevented the different strains of HIV from commingling. These features, together with the infrastructure of widely dispersed anti-epidemic stations, make China an excellent location for testing the vaccines developed for specific subtypes of the virus. The first trial, funded by the European Union, started early in 2001 in Xinjiang Province, in collaboration with scientists from the University of Regensburg (Germany). Later in 2001, NCAIDS and Rockefeller University started a second clinical trial in Yunnan Province, funded by the International AIDS Vaccine Initiative. A third collaboration between NCAIDS and researchers from Johns Hopkins University is planned for 2002, funded by the US National Institute of AIDS Prevention.

Non-communicable Diseases

Non-communicable diseases are usually attributed to the health behavior of individuals and to health risks rooted in the physical environments in which they live (Berrios et al, 1997). Patterns of health behavior and their social distribution in rural HeBei are described in detail in Chapter 5. The purpose of the following section is to describe how the danger of non-communicable diseases was intensified in rural China by the social and economic changes introduced by the transition to a 'socialist market economy' after 1979.

Economic reforms were introduced in the industrial sector in 1981. One result of the transition from a planned, state-owned economy to a market economy was to provide individuals and local administrations with the autonomy to initiate and develop industrial enterprises. Much of the industrialization occurred in the rural areas, where the dominant mode of development was the creation of enterprises run jointly by townships or villages and farmers' organizations (Wu et al, 1999). This type of industry formed the base on which China's economy has grown rapidly during the past two decades. The share of township-village owned industry (TVE) in China's gross domestic product increased from 7.0 per cent in 1978 to 55.8 per cent in 1995.

The rapid development of rural industry took place despite a scarcity of managerial personnel, safety engineers and experts in environmental and occupational health (Guidotti and Levister, 1995). Furthermore, the new entrepreneurs and the managerial staff had little or no previous industrial experience or vocational training and were not always aware of the short- and long- term effects of production processes on health in general, nor the particular health risks in the specific enterprises they were developing. Similarly, they were unaware of possible measures they might take to prevent the risks involved. As in market economies in general, priority was given to production, competition and profit.

The combination of population growth and an uncompromising dedication to increasing national agricultural and industrial productivity led to increasing environmental pressure, in terms of both pollution and resources exploitation, following the establishment of the PRC (Banister, 1998). The 1978 revised constitution was the first to introduce some measure of environmental protection and the Environmental Protection Law was passed in 1989. The law was followed by the foundation of the Environmental Protection Office within the State Council and a National Institute of Environmental Protection, which monitors the use of chemicals, herbicides, and insecticides. Similar agencies were established on the provincial level to coordinate solutions to environmental problems. The Environmental Protection Offices, however, has little power over local and rural industries. Furthermore, natural catastrophes and recent environmental deterioration, which has severely damaged China's agricultural land in the past 40 years, have led China to focus its environmental protection activity on forestation, erosion control, and water conservation. Consequently, as a result of past neglect, environmental hygiene, together with work- and traffic-related injuries, are now emerging as urgent public health issues.

a) Air Pollution

In spite of the pastoral image of the countryside, the rapid development of rural industry during the past two decades has brought about a considerable air-pollution risk. The main sources of air-pollution in rural China, and to a large extent in urban areas as well, are industry and domestic cooking and heating (Xu et al, 1999; Xu et al, 2000). Currently, leaded fuel is used in industry, discharging large quantities of heavy metal particles, including lead, cadmium, and arsenic.

Exposure of young children to lead raises particular concern, since frequent exposure to even small quantities of lead interferes with normal physical growth and intellectual development. Although systematic data are not available, it has been estimated that at least half of the children in China have over 10 ug/dl, the internationally accepted safety level (Shen et al, 1996). Industrial plants, particularly those that use unleaded fuel, and developing rural cottage industries, such as recycling newsprint and lead-acid batteries, are considered to be primary sources of exposure.

Indoor air pollution is another common source of concern for the health of children and adults in rural China (Xu et al, 1999; Xu et al, 2000). Coal that produces intense smoke when burned and contains a higher concentration of toxic materials than smokeless coal is used extensively in rural areas for both cooking and heating and even more commonly by city dwellers. Along with the burning of bio-fuels, such as twigs, leaves, straw and wood, domestic air-pollution seems to impair the breathing of children and families.

Several air pollution control policies were implemented by the government since the 1980s. Data on the quality of outdoor air in rural China are not available, though some success in controlling air pollution has been measured in the urban areas (Banister, 1998). In order to overcome indoor air pollution, the Ministry of Agriculture has popularized more efficient stoves supplied with vents, which by 1992 were installed in over half of all rural households.

b) Water Pollution

As with air pollution, there is a paucity of available data related to the scope of water pollution in China. Nonetheless, the data we do have indicate that water pollution is becoming a serious public health problem and that the administrative organization for controlling water-related risks has enhanced the maintenance of safe drinking water.

From 1981, when the principles of the 'socialist market economy' were first applied to industrial production, until 1996, the quantity of industrial waste water increased by 27.8 per cent, or by an annual average of 1.7 per cent. In 1995, rural industries owned jointly by townships and villages (TVE) discharged 21 per cent of all industrial waste water in China, a total of 5.9 billion tons (Wu et al, 1999). Close to one-third (30.0 per cent) of this waste water was discharged by the paper industry, that is, the production, recycling, and printing industry. During the same year, the chemical industry was responsible for 5.9 per cent of all industrial waste water, and the textile dyeing industry discharged 4.6 per cent of the total. Yet, only 17.0 per cent of the industrial waste water was treated in compliance with national standards.

One result of large-scale rural industrialization was pollution of many of the sources of drinking and irrigation water for the rural population. Some studies showed that the levels of organic mater, heavy metals, acids, alkalis, nitrogen, phosphate, and other materials in drinking water from sources located close to industry far exceed the national standards for permissible amounts in drinking water (Wu et al, 1999). In some places, the water does not meet the national standard for agriculture use either.

Table 3.3 Investment in environmental control, China, 1996–1998*

	1996	1998	% Change
Industrial growth:			
Number of industrial enterprises (10,000 units)	798.65	797.46	- 0.2
Total number of employed persons (10,000 persons)	68850	69957	1.6
Environmental control:			
Number of agencies (unit)	8400	9937	18.3
Total number of staff & workers (person)	95562	112626	17.9
Of these:			
Scientific and technical personnel	45691	54873	20.1
Monitoring personnel	36586	37467	2.4
Supervising and administrative personnel	17312	23659	36.7

**Source:* China Yearbook, 1997, 1999.

Another source of water pollution in the countryside is the intensification of agriculture production (Wu et al, 1999; Cho et al, 1999). The implementation of the 'system of household responsibility' offered farmers incentives to intensify agriculture production, which in turn has gained momentum thanks to the increasing standard of living and demand for garden and livestock products. Modernization of agriculture introduced improved hybrids, along with extensive use of fertilizers and pesticides. The latter have a severe effect on the quality of drinking water. Moreover, as mentioned above, sewage systems are scarce in rural China. Raw domestic waste water as well as untreated human and livestock waste further serve to contaminate water supplies.

A number of studies have indicated that water pollution is already taking a heavy toll of health in rural China (Wu eta al, 1999; Cho et al, 1999). Cancer-related mortality, especially cancer of the liver, is on the increase; birth defects, and spontaneous abortion rates are significantly higher and directly related to poor quality water. At the same time, however, the incidence of infectious water-born diseases such as dysentery and typhoid is on the decline (Banister, 1998). These paradoxical reports may indicate the effectiveness of the efforts made to control infectious diseases, while the risks in water-born diseases caused by industrial waste were neglected until recently.

Since the mid 1990s, several new programs aimed at environmental protection, such as the prevention of air and noise pollution and further contamination of water sources, together with programs for cleaning up already polluted sources have been initiated. The number of agencies and administrative and professional personnel involved in the effort increased at a greater rate than that of industrial growth, though the number of persons engaged in monitoring remained rather stable (Table 3.3). One result of these efforts was the stabilization of the emission of industrial organic water at 0.14 Kg per worker per day (The World Bank, 2000). In 1998, 88.2 per cent of all industrial waste water was treated before being discharged, compared with 76.8 per cent in 1995 (China Yearbook, 1999). Of the treated industrial waste water, 23.4 per cent complied with the official standard in 1998, an increase of 1,464.9 million tons since 1995.

c) Work and Traffic Injuries

Once again, official statistics on the incidence of work and/or traffic injuries, deaths and long- and short-term disability are not available. However, there are indications that rapid industrialization and the development of transportation associated with it have increased work and traffic accidents to an alarming level (Guidotti and Levister, 1995; Roberts, 1995). According to estimates of the early 1990s, work and traffic accidents caused 300,000 deaths and 500,000 disabling injuries a year (Jiang et al, 1996). Traffic fatalities, for example, more than doubled within one decade, from 2.2 per 100,000 population in 1983 to 5.4 in 1993, despite the low level of motorization of the PRC compared to highly industrialized societies (5 vehicles per 1,000 population in 1993). Moreover, the increasing death rate among men of working age, while death rate of women and that of other age groups is declining steadily (Chapter 2), may be, at least partially, attributed to road and work accidents.

The challenge facing China today is to shift the emphasis from surveillance and the treatment of work-related health problems to the prevention of occupational hazards, and to develop efficient trauma care (Guidotti and Levister, 1995; Jiang et al, 1996). Since the revolution of 1949, the PRC followed the model of the Soviet Union, which focused on early detection and treatment of occupational diseases and work injuries. Its ideological commitment to the well being of laborers and the work force as its most valuable economic asset has led China to develop special services for industrial employees whose health has been impaired by their work.

A plethora of occupational health activities has been developed, yet so far it has focused more on cure than prevention. Medical units were established in large- industrial plants; smaller enterprises contracted with external health services to care for their employees. Specialized hospitals or wards within a general hospital provide hospitalization and outpatient care for specific work-induced health conditions, such as pulmonary diseases, to employees and persons afflicted by poor work-related health conditions in their immediate geographical vicinity. Generally, these curative services also include periodic screening and research related to prevalent occupational diseases. Rehabilitation services and financial support have been provided to workers who have been disabled or become chronically ill due to their occupations. Nonetheless, very little attention has been paid to regulating the work environment, controlling potential health hazards, or preventing workplace exposure to health hazards.

The degree to which the services described above hold true for rapidly developing rural industry is not clear. The nature of the rural three-tier health care system suggests that such occupational health services were more likely to be available to employees of industrial enterprises located close to cities and county administrative centers than for those employed by TVEs. Township health centers are not sufficiently provided with either the technology or health personnel needed to support curative care for work-related disease or injuries. Yet, these very enterprises have often been constructed without the consultation and support of safety engineers, occupational health experts, or environmental hygiene authorities.

While the occupational diseases and disabilities suffered by rural industrial laborers can be treated with the help of specialized services on the county or city level, injuries require immediate attention. Efficient trauma services and care have been shown to reduce both fatalities and disabilities resulting from work and traffic accidents (Shackford, 1995). As yet, however, this aspect of care delivery has not reached an adequate level in the PRC (Jiang, 1996; Roberts, 1995). First-aid services for on-site treatment are still largely local initiatives. When available, they are too limited to meet all needs. Specialized trauma centers are extremely rare and casualties are treated in the general emergency departments. In these departments, the available technology and personnel qualified for trauma care are often insufficient. Rural health centers are even less able to provide adequate trauma care. Indeed, the death to injury ratio in the countryside is some 50 per cent higher than in urban areas (China Yearbook, 1999).

The transition from treatment-oriented occupational health to a policy of prevention has taken place slowly (Guidotti and Levister, 1995). The Institute of Occupational Medicine, a branch of the Chinese Academy of Preventive Medicine, has been developing safety standards suitable to China's level of economic development. The implementation and enforcement of these standards depend on lower level, that is provincial and county, administrations. These, are faced with a conflict of interests related to the cost of safety versus the urgent needs of economic development.

Equally slow has been the introduction of road safety regulations. As yet, laws forbidding drinking and driving, mandatory use of helmets and safety seat belts remain local, mainly urban, initiatives (Jiang et al, 1996). Regulations, of course, are not sufficient to change behavior. Institutional measures, infrastructure, and health education are all required to promote road safety. None of the 149 bicyclists involved in traffic accidents and treated in three of the hospitals of Wuhan, the capital of Hubei Province, had been wearing a helmet at the time of the accident, and only 4 per cent believed they should have worn one (Li and Baker, 1997).

To limit injuries, fatalities, and disability resulting from work and traffic accidents, the old principle of 'putting prevention first' must be applied. Multi-sectorial collaboration, mass mobilization, and health education, so successful in overcoming the endemic infectious diseases that have plagued China's population for centuries, are well devised for management of the current and future public health challenges facing China.

Summary

In all societies, public health is the most important determinant of the current and future health status of the population. This chapter is devoted to the unique and innovative ways in which the PRC has coped with the enormous public health problems encountered upon its establishment, and its plans for confronting current and future challenges.

Unlike the regimes of some developing countries, the Chinese Communist Party has consistently emphasized public health as the key to rapid improvement in the health of its citizens. Access to health was central to the fulfillment of the CCP's commitment to ameliorate the quality of life of the population and, with manpower as its major resource, facilitate economic development and growth. Curative care on a massive scale was not feasible, so a policy of 'putting prevention first' was adopted.

The policy carried out had several unique and innovative characteristics. Public health was combined with political activity through the creation of multi-sectorial Leading Groups at all levels of administration. Policy decisions were taken at each of these levels and special funds were allocated to the rural sector. Public health work involved mass mobilization, carefully designed not to interfere with agricultural production and other economic activities. Public health was removed from the jurisdiction of the medical profession, which traditionally emphasizes the treatment of the individual by highly trained personnel using expensive technology. Rather, the efforts of professional health care personnel were directed toward research work related to public health and basic training was provided for a large number of cadres working in the preventive health field. A 'mass line' strategy was taken, involving the whole population in public health work. The control of schistosomiasis and iodine deficiency disorders are presented as illustrations of this unique approach to public health. The new opportunities opened up by the economic and political transitions of the late 1970s are also presented.

Despite past achievements, communicable diseases still present considerable challenges to the public health authorities. Infectious disease control requires permanent environmental monitoring, population surveillance, and behavioral change. Parasitic infections still prevail among farmers and will not be fully eliminated as long as human waste is used for agriculture, without adequate disinfection. In the tropical parts of China and along the Golden Triangle border malaria has reappeared, reintroducing old public health concerns.

The immunization program, which played an important role in the decline of infant and child mortality, suffered a degree of relapse during the early stages of the transition to a 'socialist market economy' and the large-scale privatization of primary rural health services. According to some reports, close to universal coverage has now been restored. Nevertheless, the poliomyelitis outbreak in the early 1990s led the Ministry of Public Health to implement a National Immunization Days approach, using the mobilization methods developed in the 1950s.

HIV/AIDS infection is an emerging public health concern. While the primary mode of transmission is through injection of drugs, HIV infection in China is on the increase among the entertainment sector too. The scarcity of adequate sterilization in village clinics may become another factor in the transmission of HIV/AIDS in the future. At the same time, some of the unique features of the PRC and the relaxation of the foreign policy of isolation have enabled China to become the first to enjoy the benefits of new HIV vaccine developments. In 2001–2002, clinical trials will be conducted in three provinces in a joint program of Chinese and Western HIV/AIDS scientists, funded by international agencies.

A program of rapid rural industrialization has been under way since 1981, despite the shortage in professional managers, safety engineers, and experts in occupational health. Because of the accelerated pace of industrialization, health and safety risks associated with a particular industries or plants have only rarely been considered and sometimes deliberately ignored in favor of short-term production considerations. The prevention of occupational hazards and environmental protection are among the challenges currently facing the public health authorities. Until recently, a curative approach to occupational health was prevalent, following the example of the former USSR. Exposure prevention and on-site safety measures are still in their infancy.

The main sources of air-pollution in rural China are rural industry, which uses leaded fuel, and the domestic use of smoke-producing coal, wood, and straw for cooking and heating. Rural industry is also the primary source of untreated waste water, followed by the intensive use of chemical fertilizers and pesticides. Both air and water pollution are increasingly evident in the mortality patterns of rural China. In recent years, China has implemented several environmental protection policies. The investments in these programs and environmental control are described in this chapter.

Road safety is another emerging public health problem related to developing rural industry. These new challenges call for reintroduction of the 'putting prevention first' principles, including health education and mass mobilization.

Chapter 4

Patterns of Health Care Provision

This chapter, and the one that follows, directly address the second objective of our analysis, namely, behavioral patterns typical of the partners in the health dyad. The provision of health care is the focus of this chapter; the behavior of the consumers is presented in Chapter 5.

The primary health services provided in a village depend both on the available facilities and the personnel operating them. As already described in Chapters 1 and 2, the transition to the 'system of household responsibility' ended the ability of most villages to maintain collective clinics and to finance the training and salaries of village doctors. Close to half of the village doctors became self-employed, sometimes renting the village clinic for their private or group practice. The degree to which the type of ownership is related to the technology available in a clinic and to the patterns of care provision is discussed in this chapter.

Another important line of professional differentiation is related to the vocational training and licensing of rural primary care providers presented in Chapters 1 and 2. In this chapter we describe the variations in professional education of the village doctors in HeBei Province and explore whether they can be associated with medical practice and behavior.

Some of the analyses to be presented in this chapter focus on considerations that are unique to rural China, though they have relevance to other developing countries as well. The health facilities and technology available in primary care clinics or the diversity of vocational training of care providers fall within this category. Yet the greater part of the chapter deals with universal issues of health care and patterns of professional behavior that are constantly debated in both post-industrial and industrially developing societies. These include the interrelationships between privatization, professional status and patterns of medical practice, such as prescription policy, fee for services, preventive health care delivery, continuing education, and involvement in community health-related decision-making processes.

The Village Clinic

The preferred location of a village clinic is close to the center of the village, near the village administration buildings. The 387 village clinics we studied in rural HeBei were situated, for the most part, within a radius of 150 meters from the village center. The typical village clinic, 43.7 percent of the clinics in our survey, is privately owned and located in its owner's home. Usually, such clinics consist of two rooms, one used as a reception room, the other containing one or two beds for a short stay. In most clinics the floor was of concrete; in four out of five such clinics water has to be fetched from a tap located in the yard outside the clinic. Indoors, village doctors use an enamel water bowl, decorated on the inside at the bottom. The water in the bowl is changed when the decoration becomes murky. Outhouses for patient use were available in three out of five privately owned, home-based clinics.

Usually, home-based clinics are staffed by one practitioner, the owner of the clinic. The reception room is furnished simply and efficiently, with the doctor's desk in the middle and chairs, benches, or a sofa for the patients waiting for the doctor's attention. The wall across from the doctor's desk is often decorated with paintings offered by satisfied patients and the one behind the doctor is covered by shelves and cabinets, where medicines are stored. None of the village clinics had a locked cabinet for storing drugs, as narcotics are not held in these clinics.

On the average, some 180 types of Western medicines are held in home-based clinics and only a few, an average of 23 different kinds, pre-prepared Chinese medicines and traditional herbs. The explanation for the choice of medicines preferred by the village doctors during our interviews in their clinics was the shortage of space and of time for preparation. Traditional Chinese herbs consume a lot of storage space and proper treatment requires a mixture of several types of traditional materia medica. A single prescription may include more than 20 herbs or other materials, which have to be weighted, sundered, and mixed. However, the fact that the village doctors generate more profit from selling Western medicines should not be overlooked.

Standard equipment in such clinics includes a stethoscope, a mercury sphygmomanometer for measuring blood-pressure, and infusion equipment. As we will see later, injections and infusions are used for many medical complaints, including minor conditions such as the common cold. Despite the frequent use of this equipment and the lack of disposable syringes, however, only half of the clinics are equipped with electric sterilizers. Laboratory equipment is extremely rare. For example, only 5 percent of the home-based clinic in rural HeBei is equipped to perform a urine test.

Another quite common arrangement, almost one in four in our sample, was a group practice operating in a building used only as a clinic. Often, these physical facilities were built to accommodate the old collective clinics and rented by the doctors from the village administration. These facilities, which are much more spacious, typically consist of four or five rooms and are staffed by one to three doctors.

The investment in the physical conditions of the collective clinics prior to the period of the economic reforms is apparent. More than one quarter of these clinics now have tiled floors, 85 percent have running water indoors, and two-thirds are equipped with toilets for patients use, though outdoors. The extra space, however, is rarely used for inpatient services: one clinic in five has no patient bed at all, while the typical clinic of this type has only two or three beds for a short stay.

These clinics, however, are somewhat better equipped than home-based clinics. Beyond the standard equipment of a stethoscope, a mercury sphygmomanometer, and infusion equipment, about one-third of these clinics are able to perform blood or urine tests. Group practices in a specialized physical facility also store a larger variety of medicines. The typical clinic has 215 different types of Western medication, 45 kinds of pre-prepared Chinese medicines, and 55 types of traditional Chinese herbs, double the number kept in a home-based practice. Nevertheless, as with home-based clinics, just half are equipped with an electric sterilizer. Given the common use of injections and infusions and the reuse of needles and syringes, inadequate sterilization may pose a public health risk, as discussed in Chapter 3.

Two other types of clinic are worth mentioning, though they are far less common: branches of hospitals owned by the government and private or group practices that are combined with other businesses. These are relatively rare, close to 5 percent of the clinics in our study, but have drawn some attention in previous discussions of the rural primary care system after the dismantling of the collective village economy.

Branches of hospitals owned by the central or local government comprised 4.9 percent of the clinics in our sample, similar to the national average of 4.5 percent. Many of these branches were established after the economic reforms of 1979 had reached the health sector, stimulated by three main motives: improvement of the quality of health care in the countryside, meeting special or unmet needs of a specific region or population, and devising means for increasing revenues to alleviate financial pressure on the hospitals (Chen et al, 1997).

Newly developed and serving usually more than one village, these clinics are typically located in villages that also serve as the seat of the township administration, at an average distance of 350 meters from the village center. These facilities are larger than those previously described. The average clinic consists of 20–25 rooms and has an average of 18.5 inpatient beds, a pharmacy, and a small operating room that also serves as a delivery room.

Such clinics employ, on the average, 15 salaried doctors and often other medical professionals, such as a pharmacist, administrators, laboratory and other technicians. It is quite rare, however, to find nurses in these clinics. In the great majority of the facilities, the floor is of concrete, running water is available indoors, and in four out of five, outhouses have been constructed for patient use.

The space, however, is not used to increase the privacy of the patients. The doctor's office is similar to that found in the clinics run by group practice and, except for the medication cabinet, similar to home-based clinics. Waiting rooms are not set aside from the doctors' offices and the waiting patients usually sit in the doctor's office. Often, two or more doctors share an office and consultations are conducted in the presence of other patients. Yet, almost each of these clinics has a doctors' conference room, whose walls are decorated with paintings and photographs donated by grateful patients.

Having the space, the technical aid, and a fixed income, doctors in hospital branches are able to practice traditional Chinese medicine more often than their colleagues in private and group practices. On the average, the quantities of Western medicines and pre-prepared traditional Chinese medicines in such clinics are not much greater than those found in group practices, 224.3 and 50.8 different types, respectively. However, the average number of traditional herbs in the hospital branch clinics we investigated is 136.9, more than twice the number held in a typical group practice.

Hospital branch clinics are better equipped than the other types of village clinics. The great majority of such clinics have a laboratory for conducting diagnostic tests, about half own imaging technology. Of the latter, X-ray equipment is most common, followed by ultrasound technology, used mainly in prenatal care. One of the clinics surveyed has EEG technology.

Finally, there are both private and group-practices, whose clinics are attached to shops. Although this type of clinic comprised just 4.1 percent of the village clinics randomly sampled in our survey in rural HeBei, it is of special interest. The decollectivization and privatization of the rural primary health care system raised some concerns regarding the means available to village doctors to maintain a standard of living similar to that of the farmers (Chapter 1). Attaching clinics to shops enables village doctors to combine medical practice with a business, without compromising either. The clinic itself has, on the average, two or three rooms, one of which is equipped with one or two beds for a short stay. One half of these clinics are run by one village doctor, the other by a staff of two or three doctors.

The physical conditions of the clinics attached to shops are similar to those observed in the former collective clinics. One in five has a tiled floor. In half, outdoor toilets are available for the patients. All except one have running water within the clinic. However, they are not as well equipped. Sterilizers are available in just 40 percent of the clinics, laboratory equipment in less than a fifth. The medicines normally found in such shop-attached clinics resemble those found in home-based clinics: on the average, 180 types of Western medicines, about 34 types of pre-prepared traditional Chinese medicines, and 14 different traditional materia medica. Thus, the most business- oriented village doctors are least likely to prescribe traditional Chinese medications, the least profitable form of medication, although their clinics are more spacious than those of the home-based practitioners.

The Village Doctor

The typical village doctor is male (76.2 percent), 42.6 year old, married (92.1 percent) with two children, and head of a relatively large household comprising 4.4 persons, compared with an average of 4.2 for other rural households in HeBei Province. On the average, the village doctors who participated in our study had practiced medicine for more than 20 years, most often in the village where they were working at the time of the survey.

The oldest doctor in our sample was a 72 year old married man, a college graduate who had practiced medicine for 47 years, 40 of them in the village he lived in at the time of our survey. The youngest doctor was a 19 year old unmarried woman, who had started her career with a single year of training in a city hospital after finishing her compulsory nine years of general education, and had been practicing in the village for four years when we interviewed her.

The Professional Training of the Village Doctor

There is great variation in the professional training of the village doctors. As already discussed in Chapter 2, the shortage of care providers at the time the PRC was established led health authorities to initiate massive training programs to staff the planned three-tier health care system. These programs ranged from university training of physicians like that familiar to Western readers to a very basic three month training course in township health centers. University graduates who staffed the third-tier urban hospitals prepared the barefoot doctors for the primary-tier village clinic. Continuing periodic education programs and refresher courses were planned for grass roots health personnel with minimal training to increase the scope and the quality of their vocational competence.

The impact of the economic reforms of 1979 and the decollectivization of the communes and the work brigades on the rural health care system has been discussed in chapters 1 and 2. The same processes that brought about the collapse of the cooperative medical system affected the village doctors, their initial training and continuing education in several ways. With the collapse of the financial base of the village, village doctors had to bear the expense of their training that had formerly been paid for by the collective: tuition, travel expenses, room and board in the county, city or township if remote from their villages, with consequent loss of work days. With the dismantling of the collectives and the relaxation of restrictions on internal migration, the old mechanisms of social control that ensured competence and the updating of practitioners also disappeared.

Aware of the need to ensure quality health care and equally aware of increasing consumer demand for better quality care, the Public Health Department of the central government adopted two measures (Kan, 1990; Hillier and Shen, 1996). The first was the 1985 licensing policy, which required each village doctor to pass a qualification examination to prove that he had the knowledge and competence of a secondary medical school graduate in order to get a permit to practice medicine. No formal prerequisites, however, were set. The examinations could be taken by anybody, whether he had studied medicine solely from books, or as an apprentice in another village doctor's clinic, or had graduated from a medical high school, college, university, or some combination of these possible paths. As a result, there is great variation in the professional training of the village doctors currently practicing, in terms of the source of their professional knowledge, the number of training programs they have participated in, and the total length of their professional training (De Geyndt et al, 1992).

The diversity in professional training of the village doctors in rural HeBei is presented in Table 4.1. Two of the most interesting figures in the table are the number of different training settings and the total time spent in training by the village doctors interviewed during our study in rural HeBei. First, on the average, each village doctor has been trained in at least two programs run by different medical education institutions or health care facilities. Second, village doctors trained in medical schools, colleges, or universities did not necessarily complete the three year curriculum required for qualification as a doctor (Gong et al, 1997).

The second measure taken by the departments of public health of some provinces to improve the quality of health care was to instruct local health authorities to organize monthly refresher meetings on the township level for rural primary care providers. Yet, local authorities had little means of enforcing participation in these meetings, which was largely left to the motivation of the individual village doctors and, in the case of self-employed practitioners, also to their own willingness to bear the costs. It was hoped that market forces, awareness of the doctors of the increasing demands for higher quality health care, and their professional commitment would motivate them to expand their knowledge and skills.

In the following section we explore the professional training of the village doctors and the patterns of their continuing education, based on interviews held with 416 village doctors in HeBei Province between 1996 and 1999. We will concentrate on three attributes of the doctors that, as described above, seem most relevant for such an analysis. First, we will consider the professional training and continuing education of village doctors who first received permits to practice medicine before the economic reforms, between the economic reforms and the 1985 licensing policy, and after 1985. Then we turn to explore the association between the type of employment, that is, private practitioner, member of a group practice, or salaried employee, and the professional training and continuing education of the village doctor.

Table 4.1 The professional training of village doctors, HeBei, 1996–1999 (percent[a], means, and standard deviations)

Type of training	Percent of doctors	Total mean (and S.D.) number of periods	Total mean (and S.D.) number of months
Studied alone	21.6	–	24.4 (23.9)
Trained by a kin village doctor	13.5	–	31.0 (51.7)
Trained by another village doctor	7.7	–	19.0 (21.2)
Trained in the army	9.6	1.9 (2.2)	23.7 (22.6)
Trained in township health center	38.7	1.7 (1.5)	12.9 (11.3)
Trained in another level health center	13.7	1.3 (0.9)	11.6 (10.2)
Trained in a county hospital	41.6	1.4 (0.9)	12.9 (9.5)
Trained in a city hospital	12.7	1.4 (1.0)	13.7 (15.1)
Trained in a county medical school	29.3	1.2 (0.7)	14.8 (10.1)
Trained in a medical college	15.1	–	29.6 (12.6)
Trained in university	2.9	–	32.0 (11.8)
Total	206.4	–	34.0 (33.8)

[a] As many village doctors had more than one type of professional training, the sum exceeds 100%.

Becoming a Village Doctor

Of the doctors interviewed in our study, 144 (34.6 percent) received their first permit to practice medicine before the economic reforms, 80 (19.2 percent) between the decollectivization and the 1985 licensing policy, and 192 (46.2 percent) after 1985. The demographic and social characteristics of the village doctors in these three groups are presented in Table 4.2.

The most striking observation is that there are almost no differences in the general education acquired by the different village doctors, regardless of the period in which they got their first license to practice medicine. The average village doctor had completed just nine years of formal schooling, that is, a middle school education, before beginning his vocational training. Another important observation is the increase in the proportion of women village doctors, from about one in eight before 1979 to almost one-third after the implementation of the new licensing policy of 1985. It appears that the same processes that enabled women to increase their presence in the profession of medicine in industrial societies are at work in rural China too.

In industrial societies, the opportunities for women to enter male-dominated occupations such as medicine were closely related to the emergence of new, alternative opportunities for men. The feminisations of education in Western societies started with technological developments that offered new, more rewarding opportunities to men. The share of women in medicine started to increase when the criteria for candidate selection became more achievement-oriented and the material and symbolic rewards of business administration became more attractive to men. Very similar processes took place in rural China with the economic reforms and the development of the township-village industrial enterprises (TVE)

The economic reforms of 1979 opened new opportunities for individual enterprise initiatives as well as the rapid development of rural industry. Both became highly gender-oriented (see Chapter 7). Most of the privately owned family businesses were established and managed by men and many more men than women left farming for services and industry (Anson and Sun, 2002; Entwisle et al, 1995).

Under the socialist market economy, medical practice ceased to be an economically rewarding occupation. As described in Chapter 1, during the period of collective economy barefoot doctors often enjoyed higher income and more comfortable work conditions. Furthermore, they were nominated by their fellow farmers on the basis of their personal attributes and characteristics, a system prone to be influenced by prejudgment and stereotype. According to data we collected from rural HeBei, the average annual per-capita income of a village doctor fell by 1,268 Yuan below the mean annual per-capita income in his own village.

Table 4.2 The demographic and social characteristics of the village doctors by period of license, HeBei, 1996–1999 (percent, means, and standard deviations)

First Permit Received		Before 1980	1980–1985	After 1985	Total
Sex	(% women)	13.2	22.5	32.3	23.8
Age	mean	49.2	46.1	36.3	42.6
	(S.D.)	(7.5)	(8.0)	(11.0)	(11.1)
Years in practice	mean	28.4	25.4	14.6	21.4
	(S.D.)	(6.9)	(7.4)	(11.0)	(11.1)
Years of formal	mean	9.2	8.2	9.1	9.0
general education	(S.D.)	(7.2)	(1.9)	(5.1)	(5.5)

More than half (n=277) of the 416 village doctors in our study started practicing before the economic reforms, 133 of them without an official permit or license. Such formal recognition was not necessary in those days and their status as barefoot doctors was not challenged by the village committee or their fellow members of the work brigades who nominated them and financed their training. Some (n=55) of these village doctors decided to get an official license to practice medicine upon the collapse of the collective health care delivery system, before the compulsory qualification examinations were required. Most (58.6 percent), however, earned their first permit to practice medicine after it became compulsory under the new policy of 1985.

The different paths one could take to become a village doctor are shown above in Table 4.1 and a simplified model of this complex pattern is presented in Figure 4.1. The figure presents the way in which typical vocational training of village doctors has changed since the two milestone changes in the rural health services: the collapse of the collective health system and the introduction of licensing. The most significant trend has been the decline in the proportion of village doctors trained in local, township level health facilities and the increase of the proportion of village doctors who have acquired some degree of formal medical education. After 1985, most of the practicing village doctors were in whole or in part educated in a medical college, a hospital affiliated with a medical college, or a university.

During the massive extension of the health services into rural China, the typical health vocational education consisted of apprentice-like training in a local health center. Over two-thirds (67.9 percent) of the village doctors currently practicing in rural HeBei started their professional career with such training. On the average, each of these village doctors had completed two training periods and accumulated 12 to 13 months of in-service vocational training before the economic reforms of 1979 ended the collective health care system.

However, the majority of the village doctors who had started their careers as trainees in township or other local health centers sought additional knowledge and skills later on. Most popular were the county or higher level hospitals, where about half of the locally trained village doctors opted for in-service continuing education. Fewer (12.0 percent) attended refresher and upgrading courses at county level medical colleges. By the time they were interviewed, the former barefoot doctors had accumulated, on the average, 2.1 years of professional training, compared with an average total of 2.8 years of medical education acquired by village doctors in a college or university alone, before 1979.

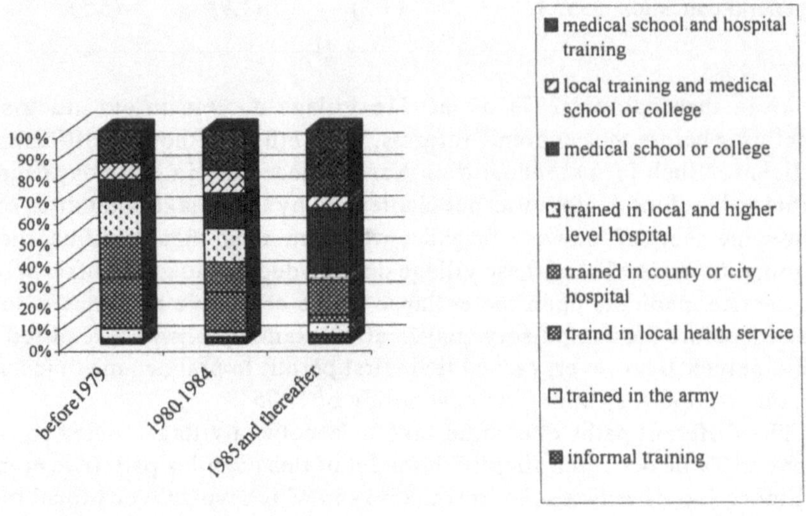

Figure 4.1 The professional training of village doctors by period, HeBei 1996–1999 (percent)

By contrast, just 13.5 percent of the village doctors who commenced their medical practices after the licensing policy of 1985 had been implemented started their careers as trainees in local or township health centers. Another

16.2 percent began in county or city hospitals. After 1985, village doctors typically did their professional training in a county level medical college or university. In HeBei, 60.4 percent of the village doctors who entered the field of medicine during the second half of the 1980s started their medical careers by acquiring such medical education and training.

Like their veteran counterparts, the village doctors who entered medicine in rural HeBei after 1985 with in-service training in local health centers or in county hospitals had completed an average of 2.6 years of training by the time they were interviewed. Graduates of college and universities, on the other hand, had an average of 5.2 years of training. By whatever means, the licensing policy of 1985 increased the access of the rural population to better trained doctors.

Furthermore, the different paths to medical practice offered doctors a variety of opportunities to specialize in one of the fields of medicine. University programs and medical colleges were first in providing specialized training: close to three-quarters of the village doctors with university training and half of those trained in a medical college specialized in at least one of the fields of medicine. By comparison, between 40.0 percent and 43.0 percent of the village doctors trained in health centers or hospitals acquired training in some field of specialization. 30.0 percent of these trained in the army.

Specialization, however, takes a different form in rural China from that of Western societies. Specialization programs of 4–5 years are offered only by hospital-affiliated universities and their graduates are appointed to positions in the third tier, that is, city or county hospitals. The specialized training of a village doctor usually consists of a course, or in-service training in a specialized hospital ward. Under these conditions, it is not surprising that 36.3 percent of the village doctors interviewed in rural HeBei perceived themselves as specialists in two or three fields. Internal medicine was the most popular specialization: 73.6 percent of the village doctors interviewed considered themselves specialists in this field. One-third of the village doctors specialized in traditional Chinese medicine and 20.0 percent to 25.0 percent in surgery, gynecology and pediatrics.

The transition to a market economy and the dissolution of the work brigades and the village as an economic entity which followed are clearly seen in public investment in the training of village doctors. Before the economic reforms, the village bore the training expenses of 59.4 percent of the village doctors and upper level administration paid the tuition fees of an additional 15.5 percent. The figures for village doctors who started practicing in 1980–1984 were 35.2 percent and 11.8 percent, respectively. After 1985, the village fully supported the training of just 2.0 percent of the doctors, upper level administration supported, in whole or in part, the training of 13.7 percent of the village doctors.

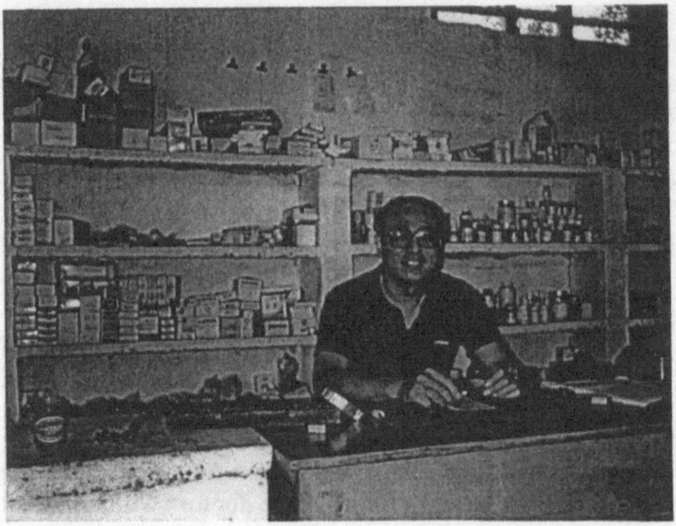

Typical village clinics, HeBei Province, 1995.

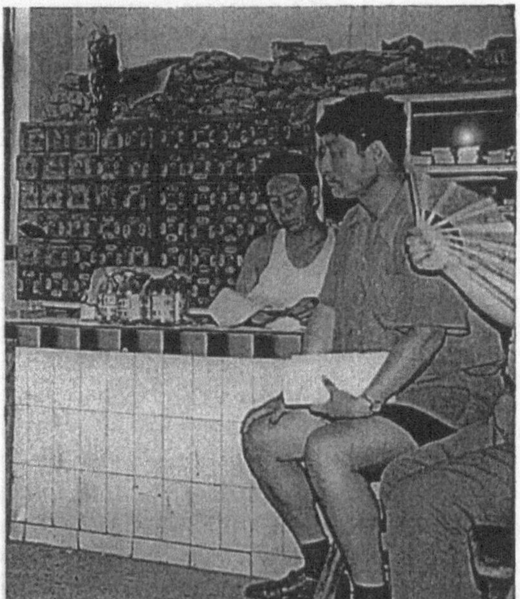

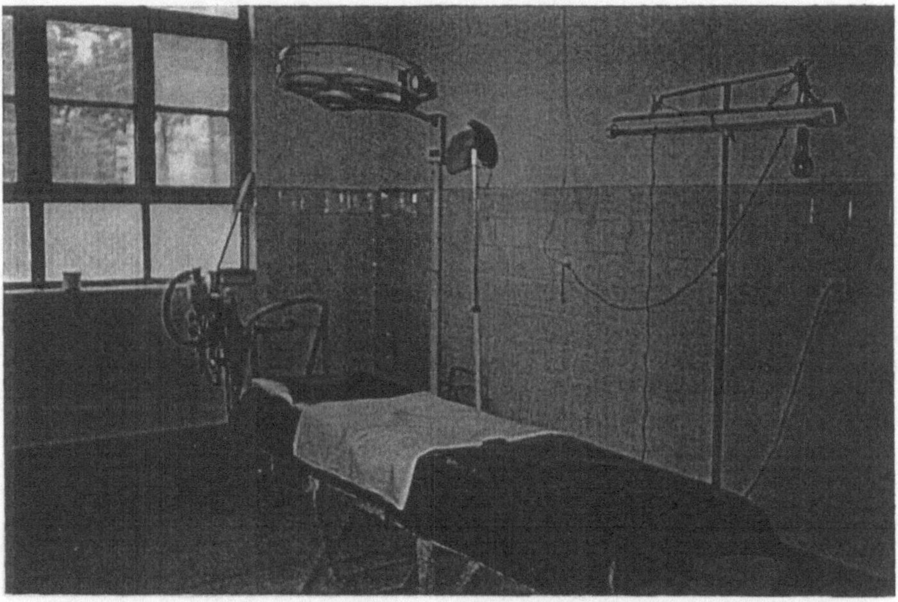

Two typical operating and delivery rooms in township health centres, reflecting the economic level of the townships; Hebei Province, 1995.

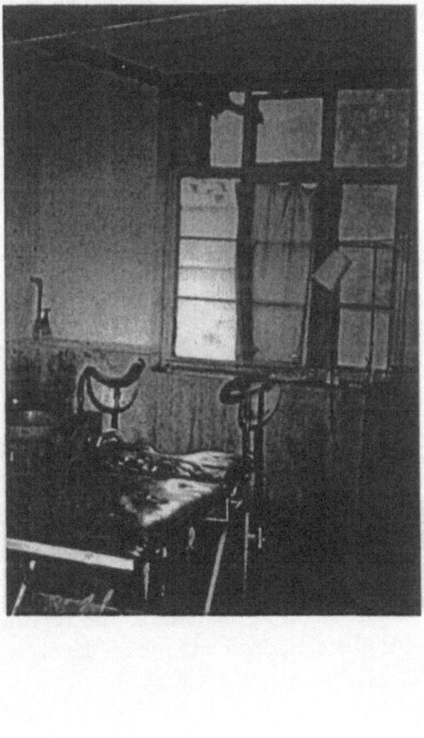

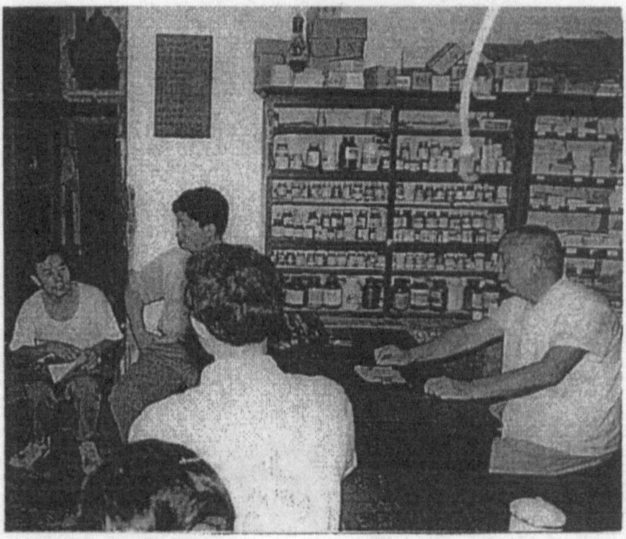

The oldest doctor in our study in his clinic, run by himself and his son. His grandson, aged 18, is being trained in the clinic and intends to take the qualification examinations within a few months; Hebei Province, 1995.

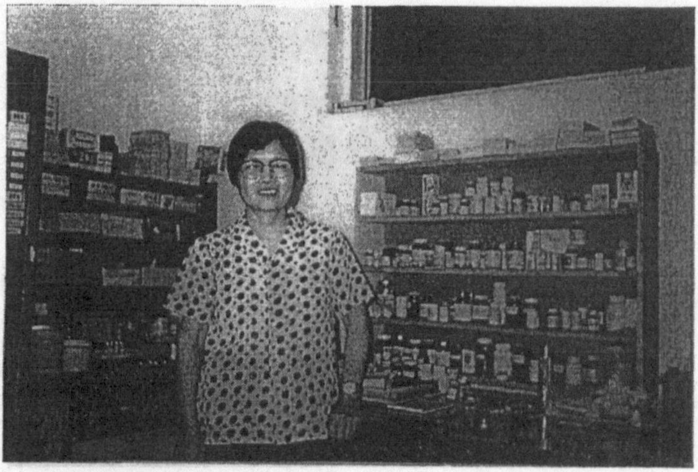

The only MD in our study; she returned to the village after retiring from a city hospital and opened a clinic on the second floor of her sister's house.

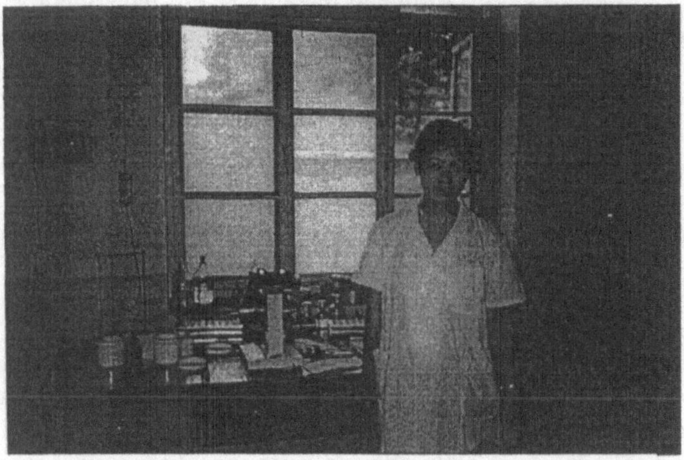

Laboratory and patients' toilets in a township health centre; Hebei Province, 1995.

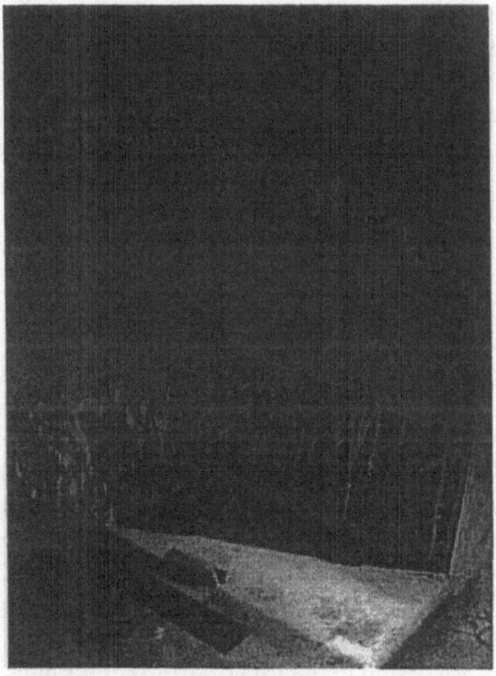

Reproduction: Haggai Anson, Department of Communication, Sapir College

One result of decollectivization and the collapse of the collective medical system was the investment of the village doctors in their own training, which increased steadily. While before decollectivization, 16.4 percent of the village doctors financed their own vocational training, in whole or in part, during the period 1980–1984 fully half of the doctors who started their careers bore these expenses by themselves, and by 1985 most village doctors (84.3 percent) bore the full cost of their own training. Furthermore, the proportion of village doctors who received some financial aid from the village or higher-level administration during their vocational education also declined, from 8.7 percent of those trained before 1979 to 2.9 percent in the transition period and to 1.0 percent after 1985.

The village doctors in rural HeBei do not appear to have sought compensation for this investment in the private sector. They entered private enterprise, group practice, or a government employee status regardless of the source of financing for their medical education. Only one characteristic of the village doctors was associated with the type of practice chosen: those who trained in universities were twice as likely to be salaried employees and to practice in clinics owned by government hospitals. The inclination of university trained village doctors to enter salaried positions seemed to meet both the interests of the hospital branches and the professional needs of qualified doctors.

In line with the government's health policy, hospital branches sought better trained or qualified doctors to deliver high quality health services in the rural areas in general and in places with more pressing health needs in particular. Furthermore, the recruiting of university and college graduates came in response to the population's demand for more competent health care and improved physical conditions. Attracting university and college graduates was also a response to the increasing need of the hospitals to generate income (Chen, et al, 1997).

For their part, university trained doctors found in the hospital branch clinics an opportunity to practice medicine in settings generally better equipped than the typical village clinic. Moreover, the income of salaried village doctors did not fall significantly below that of private practitioners or their counterparts in group practice. Salaried village doctors, then, could save the costs and the risks involved in private or group enterprise, without compromising their standard of living or satisfactory standards of health care provision, in a very similar manner to their Western counterparts (Derber et al, 1990).

Yet, one should be aware of the risks inherent in such a division of professional labor. Intra-professional divisions are often associated with differential prestige attributed to doctors of different training, titles, or working place. One result of such differential prestige could be the help-seeking behavior of the consumers. In some countries, intra-professional variation has lead to greater demand for secondary and tertiary health services (Shuval and Anson, 2000). The demand for higher level care resulted in increased costs both for the health care system and the patients' out-of-pocket health expenditures. Intra-professional division also affected the quality of health personnel drawn to primary care. In Israel, for example, primary care is often provided by health personnel regarded by their colleagues and patients as less competent. Observers of the Chinese health care system have already noted that many farmers prefer to seek help at a level above that of the standard village facility (Liu et al, 1996).

Continuing Education

Continuing education of health personnel presents a serious problem in all societies (see the discussion in the British Medical Journal 1998, but also Gershen 2001a,b; Cahan, 2001; Matos Ferreira, 2001). In most societies, a lifetime license to practice medicine and any of the allied health professions is issued by a legitimate social authority. Some societies, the USA for example, require a periodical renewal of the license, yet the procedure rarely requires proof of competence or additional post-graduate training. Despite recognition of the rapid development of medical science, constantly updated knowledge and new technology, a mechanism which forces health personnel to master and competently implement the latest developments has not yet been devised in any society. Health professionals are expected to internalize the value of life-long learning during their vocational socialization and to continue to develop and update their professional knowledge by reading pertinent scientific literature, attending refresher courses, etc. Many industrial countries have initiated ongoing post-graduate education programs for physicians. Some have introduced incentives for those who take part in these programs. None, however, has a mechanism that empowers an authority to cancel a license to provide medical care of failure on the part of the care giver to update his/her knowledge or to employ the most recent therapeutic technologies.

China, of course, is no exception (Chen et al, 1995). Before the economic reforms, village doctors could participate in training periods in health centers and hospitals free of charge. The village and/or upper level administration bore all expenses, from traveling to the specific location, through room and board during the training period to compensation for the loss of work days. Thus, only 12.4 percent of the village doctors who practiced in HeBei before 1979 remembered paying for refresher courses or advanced training periods by themselves before the economic reforms, and an additional 65.2 percent could not recall that any costs were involved. Similarly, 78.1 percent of them remembered that they were fully compensated with work points while they were updating their knowledge and increasing their professional skills.

Such arrangements, however, were no longer possible after the implementation of the 'system of household responsibility' and decollectivization. Indeed, during the past decade, the village has borne the cost of continuing education for fewer than 10 percent of the village doctors, while higher level administration contributed to the advanced training of another 9.4 percent. Most village doctors (68.6 percent) who have attended upgrading programs during the past 10 years have borne the costs involved alone, including the loss of work days. 8.2 percent chose programs that required no tuition.

The village doctors in rural HeBei, then, like health professionals in many other developed and developing societies, face the universal dilemma of continuing education: the desire for life-long learning and continuous professional updating, as opposed to the need to earn a living and support their families, which limits participation in such programs. How was this dilemma reflected in patterns of participation in continuing education programs?

Over half (53.0 percent) of the village doctors in rural HeBei we interviewed participated in at least one training program after the dismantling of the collectives in the early 1980s. One in three village doctors had participated in a continuing education program during the five year period just prior to the interview. On the average, however, the last training period of the village doctors in our sample had taken place 15.3 years before, and lasted between one month and one year; the average length reported was six months.

The most experienced village doctors, those who started practicing and those who got their first license to practice medicine before the transition to a market economy, were also less likely to have participated in training programs after decollectivization. On the average, they had last participated in a continuing training program 20.3 years before the interview. Their knowledge, experience, and self- teaching skills were sufficient to allow them to pass the provincial Health Department examinations and obtain the newly required license. It was the less experienced village doctors, those who started practicing after 1985, who felt the need to advance their knowledge and skills. On the average, the village doctors in this group had completed their last continuing training program 4.6 years before the survey.

Formal professional socialization in China succeeded in conveying the value of life-long learning more than the older, apprenticeship system. Our data indicate that village doctors with formal college, secondary medical high-school, or university medical education were most likely to participate in continuing education programs, while their locally and army-trained colleagues were least likely to do so. This tendency was not the result of the effect of professional experience (Table 4.3). Practical experience did explain some of the diversity, but the differences between village doctors with formal professional education and village doctors with only on-the-job training continued to be statistically significant, even after professional experience is taken into account.

The dilemma of the village doctors becomes clearer when the relationship between continuing education and employment status is examined (Table 4.3). As may have been expected, self-employed practitioners found it most difficult to leave their practice for additional training; salaried employees were more easily able to do so. As far as can be judged from interviews with village doctors in HeBei Province, it was not the direct or the indirect costs that kept private practitioners away from refresher training programs. Rather, it appeared that the commitment to another professional code, the code that demands they be available to their patients, was the explanation for the difference between self-employed village doctors and salaried employees.

Table 4.3 The timing of the last continuing education training period (mean number of years before 1997)

	Number of years (unadjusted)	Number of Years (adjusted)
Started practicing		
Before 1979	20.3	19.7[a]
1980–1984	11.4	11.8
1985 and thereafter	4.6	5.7
Professional training		
Informal	21.5	20.8[b]
Army	22.3	19.1
Local health center	20.8	17.2
Upper level hospital	16.7	15.3
College University	12.2	14.5
	8.9	12.6
Employment status		
Self employed	16.4	15.9[c]
Group practice	13.7	14.5
Employee	12.4	16.0

[a] Adjusted for level of education.
[b] Adjusted for years of experience.
[c] Adjusted for number of doctors in the village, professional training, and professional experience.

Three characteristics of the village doctors help to explain the differences in the timing of the last training period between private practitioners, doctors in group practice, and employees in hospital branch clinics: experience, professional education, and the number of colleagues practicing in their village. The less experienced doctors, those who were trained in city hospitals, colleges, or universities, and doctors who could leave the village knowing that their patients' needs could be met by other care provider(s) have participated in more recent upgrading programs. Moreover, the number of doctors in the practitioner's own clinic was unrelated to continuing education. In other words, the village doctors in our study appeared to be less worried about the possibility of losing business to competing clinics and more concerned that urgent health needs might not be met. Continuing education by means of relatively long training periods in health centers or hospitals, away from daily practice, was breaking down. This process was not unnoticed by the Chinese health authorities, who were concerned about the quality of care in the rural areas (see Chapter 2). An alternative continuing education has been designed in HeBei Province, one that does not require that village doctors be absent from their clinics for long periods at a time. Township health centers or county hospitals have been instructed to organize monthly academic meetings for rural primary care providers. Each of these meetings is devoted to a specific topic, and new developments in medical knowledge and therapeutic technology are presented.

As with other means of continuing education around the world, there is no way to force village doctors to take part in the academic meetings. Two out of five village doctors in our sample did not attend any such meeting during the year prior to the interview and most of those who did attend, did not do so regularly. On the average, village doctors who went to the academic meetings at all went once in three months. At the same time, some of the doctors were highly committed to advancing their knowledge and attended these professional meetings religiously. About 10 percent of the doctors in our sample participated in more than 10 such meetings during the year before the interview. Twelve of them sometimes took the opportunity to participate in meetings held in more than one health center.

Surprisingly, we were not able to discover any consistent pattern of participation in the academic meetings. Professional experience, training, and the number of doctors in the village, which affected participation in the continuing education programs, had, in contrast, no effect on attendance at these academic meetings. Nor did the distance of the doctor's village from the township health center or the county hospital account for the degree of participation in the meetings. Absence from or attendance at the academic activity seems to cut across all village doctor categories, regardless of social, professional, and residential criteria.

Sources of Income

The economic, political, and social processes which led to privatization of most rural health services have been described in Chapter 1. Our purpose in this section is to evaluate some of the hopes and concerns raised by students of the rural Chinese health care system.

One of the most important concerns was the implication of privatization for access to health care. The wish to keep the comparatively high standard of living of the collective period and/or the need to return the capital invested in training and maintaining a clinic, it has been argued, would lead village doctors in private practice to focus on making a profit. Thus, they might neglect their medical practice for agriculture during the labor intensive seasons, or perform expensive procedures, which patients may not be able to afford, more often than practitioners working under other arrangements.

We chose to evaluate the degree to which the income and the sources of income of private practitioners in rural HeBei differed from those of village doctors in group practice and salaried employees in clinics run by government hospitals. First, we observed that the village doctors in our study indeed had some difficulties in maintaining a standard of living similar to that of their neighbors, the farmers, and that their annual per-capita income was generally lower than the village averages. In particular, the annual net income of village doctors in group practice fell behind the average income in their village, probably because of the costs of their larger, often rented, clinics (Table 4.4).

While the mean annual net income of village doctors of varying employment status was quite uniform, the sources of the income varied significantly. Medical practice was the main source of income for only half of the private practitioners and the doctors in group practice, while in contrast, almost all salaried doctors were dependent on medical practice for their living. The majority of self-employed village doctors had further income from agriculture or business, a source of income which was less common among doctors in group practice and least so among salaried employees. On the other hand, patients' fees comprised practically all of the income generated by medical practice of self-employed village doctors and most of the income from medical practice of doctors in group practice.

By contrast, patients' fees accounted for just 30 percent of the income of village doctors employed in government owned clinics. It should be noted that this income was not divorced from the medical practice of salaried village doctors. Hospitals and township health centers reacted to the pressure to generate an increasing share of their running budget by encouraging their staff to increase productivity and generate income for the hospital. A system of incentives has been implemented, by which the medical staff is entitled to an annual bonus according to their individual contribution to the hospital's revenues (Gong et al, 1997; Wong and Chiu, 1998). As already mentioned, hospitals and health centers, like private and group practices, generate most of their income from patients' fees for drugs, medical procedures, and the use of diagnostic technology. In rural HeBei these bonuses amounted, on the average, to almost one-third of the government employed doctors' annual income.

Table 4.4 Sources of income by employment status, HeBei, 1996–1999 (percent, means, and standard deviations)

	Self employed	Group practice	Salaried employee
Doctor's per-capita income compared to village's average – mean (Yuan)	-1,160.1	-1,470.0	-950.5
S.D.	(1,455.6)	(1,170.3)	(1,255.9)
Doctor's net income in previous year – mean (Yuan)	4,723.3	4,415.9	4,845.0
S.D.	(3,402.7)	(3,436.3)	(1,975.8)
Percent of income generated from medical practice – mean	49.9	51.3	76.0
S.D.	(28.0)	(29.7)	(29.3)
Involved in agriculture or business (%)	76.0	65.4	38.1
Patient' fees are most important source of income from medical practice (%)	95.9	79.5	30.0
Weekly hours devoted to medical practice in the *less intensive* agriculture season mean	104.1	104.2	94.5
S.D.	(47.6)	(46.9)	(53.6)
Weekly hours devoted to medical practice in the *intensive* agriculture season mean	80.8	84.2	84.6
S.D.	(57.0)	(52.2)	(60.3)
Percent of procedures usually charged for mean	67.8	61.9	84.8
S.D.	(24.9)	(22.9)	(18.6)

Yet, the suggestion that village doctors in private practice prefer business or agriculture to medical practice and that health care would be less accessible during the intensive agriculture season seemed to be far-fetched, at least in HeBei Province. The agricultural cycle did affect the work pattern of the village doctors, but the effect on all of the doctors was the same, regardless of their employment status. Village doctors in all three main practice settings doubled the time they devoted to agriculture during the intensive seasons, from 2.0 to 4.1 hours a day in the fields. They also devote fewer hours to medical practice during the intensive agriculture season, again, regardless of the type of employment status (Table 4.3).

The social context of rural China has to be considered in order to understand these figures. The doctor who lives in a village, whose residence is often attached to the clinic, is always on call and always available, except when she temporarily leaves the village. Indeed, almost all of the village doctors we interviewed (91.2 percent) worked seven days a week, even during the less intensive agriculture season; one-third reported practicing medicine twenty-four hours a day.

During the two intensive agriculture seasons, all available hands are recruited to do the work that needs to be done in the farm. The village doctor who received his share of the collective land with the transition to the 'system of household responsibility' is no exception. Yet, she remains on call and available. He can easily be found and driven to the patient's home or to the clinic. Of the village doctors who participated in our study in rural HeBei, 72.3 percent said they continue to practice medicine seven days a week during the intensive agriculture season and 25.0 percent reporting doing so 24 hours a day. It would appear that it was the demand for health services, rather than the supply, that declined during the intensive agriculture season.

In the same manner, the variability in the fee structure of the village doctors reflects the social context of the village and the changing nature of medical practice more than the motivation to generate income. Self employed doctors and doctors in group practices, whose income from practicing medicine was mainly dependent on patient fees, tended to wave the charges for one out of three medical procedures they performed. On the other hand, salaried employees, who worked for hospital branches, charged for almost all procedures they perform.

Private and group practitioners often refrain from charging for procedures not perceived as curative in nature. Measuring blood-pressure or other diagnostic tests, home visits, and the use of an inpatient bed were the three procedures for which these doctors tended not to charge their patients. On the other hand, regardless of their employment status, doctors tended to charge for bandaging wounds, giving injections or infusions, and dispensing medicines. As one self- employed village doctor told us, "We live in the same village, how can I ask money from someone who just came to talk to me?". Another doctor treated a boy who cut his foot while playing in the street in front of the clinic and sent him home with best wishes to the parents. "He is just a child," he said, when we asked about the fee. Good relationships with neighbors seemed more important than the extra pay.

The hospital-branch clinic is different from private and group practices in two important ways. First, the medical and administrative functions are managed separately. The administrative staff, rather than the doctor, collects the fees. This separation of treatment and administration enables the village doctors in a practice of this kind to list all procedures performed for each patient, who is then charged by another staff member as he leaves the clinic. Second, such settings allow for greater social control over the doctors, exercised both by their colleagues and the administration. Indeed, almost all village doctors in hospital branches keep detailed records on all of their patients, compared with two-thirds of the doctors in group practice and about half of the private practitioners.

How were these differences in sources of income and charging reflected in the medical practice of the village doctors? Some observers of the Chinese rural health care have argued that the dependency of private practitioners on patient fees has led to over-prescription of medicines and to the neglect of preventive care. It has been suggested that medicines composed some half of China's national expenditure on health, mainly because this was the main source of earnings for private rural practitioners as well as for upper level health care facilities (Gu et al, 1993; McGreevey, 1995a, 1995b; Umland et al, 1992). As we have seen, all village doctors in HeBei Province charged patients for medicines and were more likely to charge for direct curative care, while self-employed doctors and those in group practice were quite often not paid for procedures that were diagnostic in nature. As China goes through the epidemiological transition, preventive cardiovascular health is gaining in importance. It may, nonetheless, be neglected by village doctors, who are dependent solely on patient fees, if generating income is indeed their primary motive. These issues are addressed in the next section.

Medical Practice

Evaluating adequate medical practice is extremely difficult. Different health conditions may cause similar symptoms and a given health problem may be manifested in a variety of ways by different individuals. Moreover, there is a plethora of ways in which similar symptoms, such as discomfort, pain, or general malaise, can be described by patients. In fact, this idiosyncrasy is one of the sources of power of the profession of medicine.

In our study, we have tried to compensate for these problems by examining the diagnosis and treatment provided by village doctors for two prevalent conditions: the common cold, which is an acute health problem, and hypertension, a chronic condition considered to be asymptomatic and easy to diagnose and treat. We investigated the variation in patterns of medical practice and preventive care among village doctors in the context of the two most important changes in rural health care in the past two decades: the rise of private practice and the transition in medical training.

Of the 1,262 patients whose records were collected from village doctors during our research in HeBei Province, 476 were diagnosed with common cold. The condition of most of them (326), as may have been expected, were evaluated by the village doctor as 'not serious at all'. What treatment was offered these patients? All were interviewed by the doctor and most (89.6 percent) had their lungs checked. More than half of the patients (58.8 percent) underwent a physical examination and pulse, an important diagnostic technique in traditional Chinese medicine, was measured in 39.2 percent of the cases. Some had their blood-pressure measured (28.2 percent), fewer had a blood test (10.7 percent). Ears were rarely checked (1.2 percent). On the average, a patient whose problem was diagnosed as uncomplicated common cold went through 3.4 diagnostic procedures.

Only one in ten common cold patients was sent home without any treatment, all by private practitioners or group practice doctors. All other patients received at least one Western medication and the majority (81.6 percent) got an injection before being sent home. Some patients got an infusion (19.7 percent), a few (6.3 percent) were treated by acupuncture or some other traditional manipulation. Patients were treated with an average of 2.2 different technologies and 3.3 different Western medicines. Most patients were supplied with medicine for three days, after which they were asked to return to the clinic for re-evaluation.

Fewer patient records were available for hypertension patients (192). Again, most patients (181) were evaluated as 'not serious' cases of hypertension by the village doctor. In the clinic, most patients were interviewed and all had their blood-pressure measured. Doctors listened to the heart beat and took the pulse of two out of three patients, but only one-third had their eyes checked on the visit recorded.

Western medicines were administered to almost all hypertension patients (95.4 percent). On the average, four types of Western medication were prescribed for two to three weeks and 86.1 percent the patients were instructed to maintain a salt-free diet. However, many patients (63.0 percent) also received infusions and 31.2 percent were given an injection while in the clinic.

While the treatment provided by the village doctors we interviewed in rural HeBei was very similar to that provided in other parts of China (Dong at al, 1999a), it was considerably different from the treatment usually provided for these two conditions in the West. In Western medicine, uncomplicated common cold is treated as a self-limiting condition and one or two medicines, at most, are prescribed to ease the discomfort caused by this condition. More than one anti-hypertension medication is provided in only the more complicated cases, when one drug fails to stabilize blood pressure at 140/90 mm Hg (Paran et al, 1998). Injections and infusions are not administered in non-severe cases of either of these two conditions.

There was, however, quite a wide variation in treatment by village doctors in different types of practice (Table 4.5). Moreover, the differences, were not what might have been expected on the basis of assumptions derived from the dynamics of the market economy (Hillier and Shen, 1996). Judged by the data we collected in rural HeBei, it is not the private practitioners who are responsible for the intensive use of medicines, nor are they over-utilizing other profit-generating procedures. Rather, it was the salaried doctors in clinics set up by government hospitals who were using significantly more diagnostic and treatment technologies, followed by the village doctors in group practice. These patterns of medical practice may indicate a greater inclination of salaried employees to comply with the base-hospital policy, designed to meet its need to increase income (Chen, et al, 1997). To meet this need, hospitals have updated their medical technologies in order to attract more patients and invested in technologies for which patient fees are not controlled by the government. They then encourage their staff to recommend the use of these new technologies to their patients. As described above, clinics in government hospitals are indeed better equipped than private enterprises and group practices. At the same time, while the utilization of more technologies by salaried employees reflects administrative pressure to use the technologies available, it may similarly reflect patient demand.

Assumptions about the market economy have also led observers of the rural health services in the PRC to suggest that privatization will have a negative effect on preventive health. It has been suggested that fee-for-service may lead to concentration on income-generating curative care, neglecting the less profitable preventive medicine and health education (Chapter 1). No indications for differential investment in preventive health were found in our data. For example, the blood pressure of half of the patients above the age of 45 was taken, regardless of the purpose of their visit, in all types of clinics, and a similar proportion of patients were advised on diet, hygiene, and physical activity, regardless of the type of clinic they visited.

Surprisingly, the patterns of medical practice of the village doctors in rural HeBei were not related to their professional training. Does this mean that the transition in professional training from relatively short periods of an apprenticeship-type training to longer periods of medical education has no effect on the provision of health care? There is no clear cut answer to this question, because the similarities in vocational behavior of village doctors with different professional training can be the result of several factors.

Table 4.5 Treatment of common-cold and hypertension in different practices, rural HeBei, 1996–1999 (percent, means, and standard deviation)

	Self employed	Group practice	Salaried employee	Statistics
a) Common Cold				
Diagnostic procedures				
mean number	3.2	3.6	4.3	F=5.5
S.D.	(1.3)	(1.5)	(1.3)	(p<.01)
Number of treatment technologies used				
mean number	2.0	2.3	2.6	F=5.3
S.D.	(0.7)	(1.0)	(0.8)	(p<.01)
Number of Western medications prescribed				
mean number	3.2	3.5	4.5	F=5.9
S.D.	(1.6)	(1.9)	(1.5)	(p<.01)
b) Hypertension [a]				
Number of diagnostic procedures				
mean	4.3	4.4	4.7	F=0.5
S.D.	(0.2)	(0.2)	(0.6)	(NS)
Number of treatment technologies used				
mean number	2.3	2.5	3.0	F=1.3
S.D.	(0.1)	(0.1)	(0.4)	(NS)
Number of Western medications prescribed				
mean	3.6	4.3	6.6	F=8.2
S.D.	(0.2)	(0.3)	(0.8)	(p<.001)

[a] Adjusted for level of severity (light or moderate).

First, it has been long recognized that graduates of hospital-affiliated medical schools are over-trained for the treatment of most common medical conditions and for the provision of preventive care. Many of the prevalent health problems can be properly cared for by providers trained to apply standardized diagnostic and treatment protocols. Para-professionals and auxiliary personnel can efficiently implement public health policy, screen for early detection of cancer and cardiovascular health risks, and provide health education. The improvement in the health status in the PRC in general and in rural China in particular as well as the experience of the early years of the Soviet Union strongly support this argument. Recent developments in the provision of health services in United States and the United Kingdom reflect the same reasoning, while sociological analysis of these processes and recent developments in the sociology of professions offer a theoretical explanation.

The introduction of two new health professions in the USA, the nurse practitioner (usually a female) and the assistant physician (mainly men), the employment of nurses as case reviewers by insurance companies, and the transfer of some therapeutic decisions and tasks from physicians to nurses in the UK are particularly pertinent to this argument. These three developments would not have been possible without the recognition that an MD degree is often not necessary for the provision of high quality care. In all of these examples, medical doctors have maintained formal professional authority and supervision, either by legal responsibility or as final decision makers in cases of uncertainty or appeal. The source of this authority, however, is embedded in the power of the profession of medicine, its success in achieving social monopoly over the right to penetrate the patient's body, and autonomous decision making, rather than in the mastering of an esoteric competence (Annandaile, 1996; Freidson, 1986, 1994).

Second, research in medical education has also consistently indicated that medical practice is shaped primarily by the work setting in which it takes place and that practices and attitudes acquired during the process of professional socialization have been modified by the behavior and the attitudes of colleagues and the administrative demands of the work environment (Annandale, 1998). Concurrently with this research, the medical practice of the village doctors in rural HeBei is being shaped by the various work settings – private clinic, group practice, and hospital branch – rather than by their medical training.

Finally, excess use of medication and other forms of treatment could be the result of patient demand, as has been observed in other societies (Zhan et al, 1998; Dong et al, 1999c). These demands are often rooted in health-related beliefs, which attribute supreme efficiency to medicines, particularly those administered directly into the body (injection) or the blood stream (infusion) (Hardon, 1992). Coping with patient demands, particularly those inherent in cultural attitudes and beliefs, is not a simple task (Shuval and Anson, 2000). From the point of view of medical ethics, the best interest of the patient requires that his/her perceptions and expectations be considered. Ignoring the patient's perceived needs may result in noncompliance, negligence of ill-health, and possibly a deterioration in the patient's condition. Nonetheless, regardless of the work setting, losing a patient to another care provider is contrary to the provider's economic interests in all three types of clinic.

Summary

This chapter addresses the second of the three specific goals presented in the introduction. It deals with the behavior patterns of village doctors, as shaped by their work setting and professional training.

We start the chapter by describing the typical village clinic. In rural HeBei the typical clinic is home-based, occupies one or two rooms, and is run by its owner. Less common are group practices located in specialized units or in a clinic that formerly served the collective village. Least common are branches of government hospitals and clinics attached to shops or other forms of business.

The physical conditions and the equipment available in each type of clinic are described. There is considerable diversity in the availability of running water, toilets, sterilizing equipment and the medicines kept in the different types of clinics. Medicines differ in their requirements for storage space and preparation time, and in the profit generated by their sale. Western medication can be considered the "best deal": easy to store, ready made, and generates relatively high profit. Traditional Chinese herbs, on the other hand, are the poorest deal. They require extensive storage space, time-consuming preparation, and are just moderately profitable. While the number of different medicines of all kinds kept in a typical clinic increases with its physical size, the tendency of private doctors to acquire and store more Western-type medicines suggests that profit generating was not an uncommon consideration in the choice of the medicines sold in the clinic.

The economic reforms and new licensing policy gradually increased the access of the rural population to better trained village doctors. In HeBei Province, a clear transition was observed from doctors trained as apprentices in health centers and/or hospitals to village doctors trained in county colleges or university-affiliated hospitals. Moreover, the latter were more likely to have specialized in one or more fields of medicine, bringing these specialized services to the village, along with adequate quality primary care.

Graduates of universities and medical colleges prefer to practice as employees in clinics established by government hospitals. This arrangement seems to meet the interests of both parties: the clinics are able to improve the quality of rural health care and meet the needs of under-served villages; the village doctors receive a stable income and work in well-equipped clinics, without having to make heavy investments in the equipment necessary to practice medicine in accordance with their training.

In almost all countries, very few health professionals participate regularly in continuing professional education and village doctors in rural HeBei are no exception. We discuss factors affecting the degree of their participation and show that this is not related either to costs or to employment status (as employees or self-employed). The practitioners we interviewed in HeBei expressed a high degree of commitment to a professional code of ethics, to their patients and to the value of ongoing learning, but in practice those who were sole practitioners in their village were less likely to participate.

The sources of income of village doctors vary considerably, according to the employment status of the practitioner. This variation, however, does not seem to affect the time devoted to medical practice, as suggested in earlier studies of the Chinese health care system after the economic reforms. Moreover, village doctors in private practice, whose income from practicing medicine is completely dependent on patient fees, charge for fewer procedures than salaried employees, whose income is least dependent on fee-for-service. The differences between the types of practice and fees were most obvious for procedures not perceived as directly curative. These behavior patterns are discussed in terms of the social context of both the village and the clinic.

Private practitioners, doctors in group practice, and salaried employees present quite different patterns of medical practice. Nonetheless, contrary to what may have been expected, the professional behavior of the typical village doctor can not be interpreted strictly in terms of profit generation. Doctors employed in clinics established by hospitals use diagnostic and treatment technology with far greater frequency and charge for each of these. Preventive health care, the least profitable service, was similarly provided in all types of clinics, regardless of the employment status of the practitioner.

Professional training was not related to diversity in forms of medical practice. These findings are presented in the context of recent empirical evidence and theoretical developments in the field of medical sociology and the sociology of the professions.

Chapter 5

Patterns of Lay Behavior

In this chapter, patterns of health-related behavior and patterns of utilization of health services are presented. Seeking medical help and health-related behavior are both socially shaped, learned through the process of socialization and subject to social norms, pressure, and control, like any other form of human behavior. The consumption of tobacco and alcohol, like careful driving and other types of risk avoiding have social and cultural meaning. The social meaning attributed to any particular behavior largely determines which social groups are encouraged to adopt it and which are discouraged or forbidden from adopting that particular form of behavior.

In all societies, the access to, and the consumption of, goods and services is unequally distributed. Patterns of nutrition and utilization of health care are socially constructed, reflecting both position in the social structure and cultural perceptions. Social status often determines who will have access to the available social resources, such as health-related knowledge, food, and health care. Accepted cultural attitudes and perceptions define dietary preferences and the health conditions for which medical intervention is legitimately sought.

In this chapter, we look at the social distribution of four forms of health behavior in rural China: cigarette smoking, alcohol consumption, nutrition, and the utilization of health services. The patterning of each behavior by age, gender, and social class is examined to the extent enable us by the available data.

The Consumption of Alcohol

Alcohol use in China was first mentioned during the Shang Dynasty, 1600–1100 BC (Hao, 1995; Hao et al, 1999; Li, 1996). Alcohol has an important place in festivities and special occasions. Drinking alcoholic beverages is an integral part of social life, of socializing and getting together. Alcohol is also perceived as an effective medicine and used extensively in traditional medicine, mixed with other materia medica. Symbolically, drinking alcohol is associated with masculinity, maturity, and courage. In social gatherings participants, typically men, challenge each other to drink the full content of the glass in one go (gan-bei – "bottoms-up"), before refilling it to the top.

Alcohol consumption, as a public health risk, have entered the research agenda in China during the past decade. It became clear that alcohol consumption has increased dramatically since the economic reforms of 1979, and was directly relation to the economic prosperity that followed the transition to market economy.

According to some sources (Hao et al, 1999), between the cultural revolution and 1995 the consumption of alcoholic beverages increased by a factor of ten. Annual average national production of alcohol increased by 7.2 percent between 1952 and 1978, while the annual population growth actually declined from 21.9 percent to 12.5 percent in the same period. Following the transition to a socialist market economy, however, the production of alcohol increased in proportion to population growth. Between 1982 and 1995, the production of alcohol increased by an average of 13.3 percent annually, similar to the mean annual growth of the population. In 1993 the per-capita annual consumption of alcohol was 3.95 liters, compared with 1.91 liters in the European Union and 2.91 in Central and Eastern Europe (World Health Organization, 1997).

With the increase in disposable income of rural households alcohol became a common commodity in the countryside. Within 15 years, the annual per-capita consumption increased almost six-fold, from 1.2 liters in 1981 to 7.1 liters in 1996 (see Table 5.1, p.5–11). In 1999 annual per-capita alcohol consumption in the rural PRC was 7.0 liters (China Yearbook, 2000), indicating, perhaps, that the increase in alcohol consumption has reached a plateau.

Observers of patterns of alcohol consumption in developing countries have noticed a curvilinear pattern of consumption over time: a steady increase in the quantities of alcohol drunk that peaked during the early 1980s and generally declined thereafter (Edwards et al, 1994). It is too early to say whether alcohol consumption in China has reached this stage or not. However, if it has, it has stabilized at a level higher than that of the post-industrial societies but lower than of many developing societies.

With the increase in alcohol consumption, alcohol-related problems seem to have increased as well (Hao, 1993). A national survey conducted in 1993 discovered that, based on DSM-III-R definition, the prevalence of alcohol dependency or alcohol abuse was 8.1 percent among men and 0.2 percent among women. In the same year, 2.2 percent of patients discharged from hospitals were diagnosed with alcohol-related conditions, an increase of 0.5 percent from 1991. These figures, however, do not necessarily indicate an increase in alcohol dependency, abuse, or related problems. No comparative data regarding alcohol abuse or addiction are available before 1990, and the increase in alcohol related hospitalizations could be the result of a greater awareness of such problems and/or changes in attitude toward mental disease and problematic behavior.

As stated above, drinking alcohol is socially patterned. Its cultural meaning encourages some social groups to consume alcohol, while constraining the drinking of alcohol in other groups. In a culture where alcohol consumption symbolizes masculinity, courage and maturity, men are more likely to drink than women. Indeed, in our sample of men over the age of 15 in rural HeBei, 39.8 percent had consumed some alcohol during the two weeks before they were interviewed, while only 1.2 percent of the women had done so.

Alcohol consumption is also associated with age (Figure 5.1). In fact, in our data the age of the respondent explained 19.4 percent of the variance in alcohol consumption. Men start drinking as they reach adolescence and prevalence increases with age. In rural HeBei, more than one-third of the men aged 25–29 had consumed alcohol in the two weeks prior to the interview, more than half of the men aged 35–54 had drunk some alcohol during the same period. After the age of 55, the prevalence of alcohol consumption starts to decline and it becomes relatively rare among the aged. The quantity consumed follows a similar pattern: in rural HeBei, of those who drank any alcohol at all the young had consumed 10.7 gr. of alcohol in the two weeks prior to the interview, persons aged 50–54 had consumed 26.1 gr., and the elderly had consumed 20.2 gr.

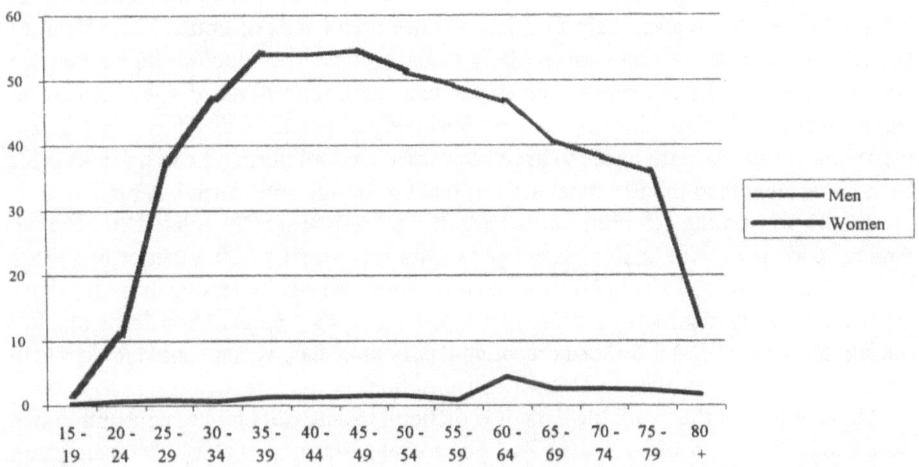

Figure 5.1 Alcohol consumption by age and sex, HeBei, 1996–1999 (percent consumed in the past two weeks)

Among women, the association between age and alcohol consumption takes on a different pattern. In rural HeBei, the prevalence of alcohol consumption among women reached a peak of 4.4 percent at the age of 60 and, although it declined thereafter, remained high relative to the prevalence among younger women, until they reached the age of 80. It seems that at older age, both men and women are less affected by the social aspect of drinking. Men no longer have to prove their masculinity, women become relatively free of social constraints and can afford to take part in socialized drinking.

In Chinese culture, alcohol is consumed in company, usually during meals, while solitary drinking is strongly discouraged (Hao et al, 1999). Accordingly, though unlike reports from Western societies (Curran et al, 1998), alcohol consumption is more prevalent among married men, 48.9 percent of whom had consumed alcohol during the two preceding weeks, less prevalent among the formerly married (29.6 percent), and least prevalent among the never-married (8.2 percent). Adjusting for age, the odds of married men consuming alcohol were 3.5 times higher than those of adult never-married men and 1.4 higher than these of formerly-married men.

There were two additional indications in our data from rural HeBei that alcohol consumption is a symbol of maturity and masculinity among men. First, at all ages, dependent men, that is, men who lived with their parents-in-law, adult children, or other relatives, were less likely to drink alcohol than heads of households. Head of households were three times more likely to have consumed alcohol during the two weeks preceding the interview than dependent men, regardless of age and marital status. Second, alcohol consumption was positively associated with education. Literate men were 1.5 times more likely to have consumed alcohol during the two weeks prior to the interview than the illiterate, after adjusting for age and marital status.

At the same time, alcohol consumption was only partially related to income. Among poor men with an annual net per-capita income of 1,000 Yuan or less, 35.2 percent had consumed alcohol during the preceding two weeks; among the rich, whose annual per-capita income was more than 2,700 Yuan, 43.7 percent had drunk alcohol during the same period. Furthermore, annual per-capita income accounted for less than 1.0 percent of the variance in alcohol consumption.

On the basis of the available data, it is difficult to assess if alcohol consumption is becoming a social problem in the PRC. The social patterning of alcohol consumption observed in HeBei Province resembles that prevailing in industrial societies, though national average consumption seems to have stabilized on a somewhat higher level. Currently, China has no anti-alcohol policy, partly because of other health problems, which are regarded as more urgent and thus receive priority consideration, and partly because alcohol production is a nationwide industry that supports a large number of families and generates handsome revenues for the government (Hao, 1995). This situation is not unique to the CCP, but common in many other industrially developed and developing societies (Shuval and Anson, 2000).

Smoking

As with alcohol, cigarettes consumption also increased faster than the population growth, following the 1979 transition to market economy. In 1984, 61 percent of all men reported being regular smokers; among men aged 45–64 the prevalence increased to 75 percent within one decade (Yu et al, 1995). As we have shown, this is also the age group with the highest prevalence of alcohol consumption.

In 1995, 30 percent of the world's cigarettes were consumed in the PRC, where 20 percent of the world's population lived (Niu et al, 2000). During the late 1980s, the prevalence of cigarette smoking in the PRC was one of the highest in the world, second only to that observed among men in Mauritius (Berrios et al, 1997). As a result, smoking-related morbidity and mortality are on the increase and seem to explain the increased mortality rates among men of working age (Banister, 2000). It has been estimated that the consumption of cigarettes accounted for 30,000 deaths in 1975, a number expected to reach 900,000 by the year 2025.

Cigarette smoking is a social, learned behavior and is thus socially patterned. In all developing societies smoking is more prevalent among men, as it was at the turn of the 20th century in the United States and Western Europe. Gender differences were observed in the PRC as well: the prevalence of smoking in our sample of rural HeBei was 53.3 percent among men over 15 years of age and 4.8 percent among women of that age.

The association between age and the prevalence of smoking in rural HeBei is very similar to that of alcohol consumption (Figure 5.2). Very few men start smoking before they reach the age of 20 (2.3 percent), but the prevalence steeply increases after this age. The prevalence of smoking peaks in the 40–49 age group and declines among older men. Almost one in four men aged 20–24 smokes; among 40–49 year old men, 70.8 percent smoke regularly.

Among women, the increase of the prevalence of smoking with age is much more moderate than that of men. As with alcohol consumption, very few women (1.7 percent to 2.7 percent) smoke before the age of 40. After that age the prevalence of cigarette smoking increases, reaching a peak of 17.1 percent among women aged 60–64 and declining gradually among older women.

In general, women smokers consume fewer cigarettes a day than men: an average of 11.6 compared with 15.5, respectively. Among women, the number of cigarettes consumed daily does not vary by age. However, for men the distribution of the daily number of cigarettes consumed by smokers follows the pattern of the prevalence of smoking. Male smokers younger than 20 consume an average of 10.3 cigarettes a day; as age proceeds, the number of cigarettes consumed increases, and men smokers aged 45–49 smoke an average of 17.1 cigarettes a day. The number of cigarettes consumed by older men declines steadily with age to 10.1 cigarettes a day among smokers over 80 years of age.

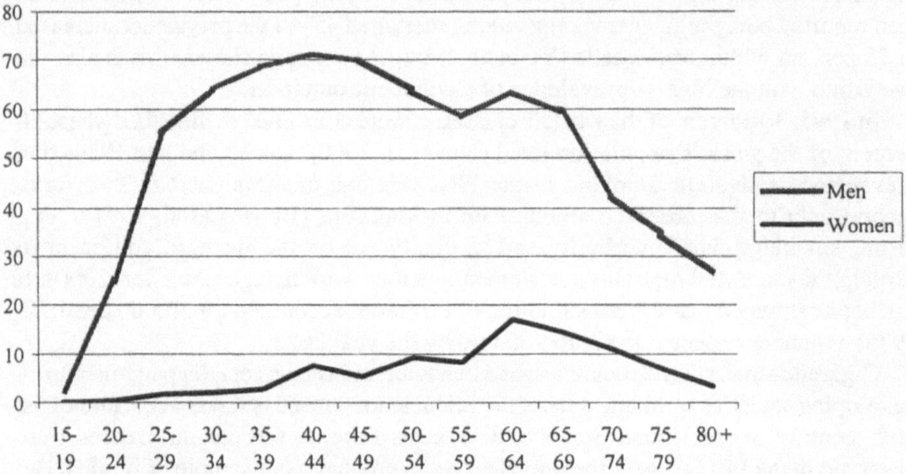

Figure 5.2 Prevalence of smoking by age and sex, HeBei, 1996–1999 (percent who smoke regularly)

This pattern is quite different from those observed in industrial societies (World Health Organization, 1997; Shuval and Anson, 2000; Bietlot et al, 2000). First, the prevalence of smoking among rural Chinese men was similar to that observed in Eastern Europe, which in turn is higher than that reported for Western European and the USA. Second, the smoking habits of Western men and women started to converge since the 1980s, so that the prevalence of cigarette consumption among rural Chinese women is much lower than that reported for industrially developed societies. According to the World Health Organization (1997), the largest gender difference in smoking during the mid 1990s was observed in Albania, where 49.8 percent of the men, but just 7.9 percent of the women, were regular smokers; the smallest gap was observed in Denmark, where the prevalence among men was 41.0 percent and among women 37.0 percent. Third, in Western Europe about half of the regular smokers consume 20 or more cigarettes a day, regardless of their gender. In the PRC this is true for rural men who are regular smokers, but not for women, 62.2 percent of whom consume fewer than 20 cigarettes a day.

Finally, the pattern of association between the prevalence of smoking, age and sex that we observed in rural HeBei was not reported in Western countries. In industrial societies the prevalence of smoking is fairly similar for men between 15 and 54 and declines gradually thereafter. For women, the prevalence increases up to the age group of 35–44 and then starts to decline (Bietlot et al, 2000).

How can the unique association between the prevalence of cigarettes smoking, age, and gender in rural China be explained? It seems that smoking, like drinking alcohol, is a symbol of masculinity and maturity. At a younger age, before men are considered adults, few adopt this behavior. As men accept adult social roles, more of them start smoking. For women, social control and the cultural definition of acceptable behavior for women constrain smoking until later in life.

This interpretation was supported by further analyses of the social patterning of smoking in rural HeBei. For example, as with drinking, never-married men and men who were dependent on their families were less likely to smoke, regardless of their age. On the other hand, women heads of household were significantly more likely to consume cigarettes than any other group of women, after the effect of confounding variables such as age and marital status is accounted for.

Smoking is not related to income in rural HeBei, but the prevalence of smoking declines as the level of education rises. In all ages, each added year of schooling increased the odds against smoking, by 3.6 percent for men and10.0 percent for women. Thus, if the average level of education continues to rise gradually, the prevalence of smoking is likely to decline in accordance.

Currently, however, cigarette smoking is emerging as a serious public health problem in rural China. The health authorities are not unaware of the risks involved, but 450,000 people were employed in the tobacco industry in 1994 and the tax on cigarettes comprised 7.0 percent of the government's total tax revenues in that year. Nonetheless, a Chinese Association on Smoking and Health was established in 1990 and a law aimed at regulating cigarette consumption came into effect in January 1992. It is due to this law that warning labels, similar to those introduced in the USA and Western Europe, now appear on Chinese made cigarette packs. The law restricts tobacco promotion, advertising, and use in some public places, such as schools and public transportation. It has also regulated the level of tar and other damaging substances in tobacco products.

Yet the enforcement of such a law in rural areas calls for extensive resources and without a major investment in health education and rehabilitation programs, and unless health workers are provided with adequate methods and skills to help the smokers in their community, smoking will remain a major risk for rural men. With modernization and a decline in the power of traditional mechanisms of social control this behavior may spread to social groups that so far seem relatively protected, women and youth in particular.

Nutrition

Before the establishment of the People's Republic of China, the majority of the population lived perpetually on the verge of hunger, if not starvation. Landlords, administrators, and warlords were the only exceptions. The communist revolution and the establishment of the communes put an end to centuries of extreme poverty and shortage of food. During the early years of Mao Ze Dong's regime, collective agriculture production increased dramatically, and for the first time Chinese farmers produced more food than they could consume (Smith, 1993).

The prosperity of the 1950s ended in a devastating famine following the period of the 'great leap forward' (Chapter 1). From the mid-1960s onward, agricultural production increased steadily, but the availability of food was not restored to the level of the first post-revolution years until the completion of the redistribution of communal land under 'the system of household responsibility' in the early 1980s.

The increase in average income in rural China has been described in Chapter 1. One result of the increase in disposable income was improvement in the standard of living and an increase in the consumption of food products (Table 5.1). During the first decade of the economic reforms, the consumption of all main nutrients increased steadily, except for grains and vegetables. The consumption of other products – meat, fish and seafood, oil, eggs, sugar, and alcohol – doubled or more than doubled. In keeping with the old saying "a poor man eats three bowls of rice and one bowl of meat, a rich man eats three bowls of meat or fish and one bowl of rice," the consumption of oil, meat and fish or seafood products continued to increase steadily in the 1990s, while the consumption of grains declined by 4.8 percent and that of vegetables by 16.2 percent.

Examination of the changes in food consumption in rural China in light of currently accepted dietary recommendations suggests that the trends observed in the past decade may have mixed health consequences. Most alarming is the decline in per-capita consumption of vegetables, the increase in the consumption of eggs and egg products, and the increase in the consumption of alcohol as discussed above. On the other hand, the increase in the consumption of poultry, fish, and seafood products and the decrease in sugar consumption is consistent with current scientific beliefs. It should be noted, however, that poultry comprises just 14.8 percent of the meat consumed, and the consumption of beef and pork products is still on the increase.

The increase in the consumption of sugar with the prosperity that followed the economic reforms of 1979 in China's countryside seemed to have leveled at a much lower rate than that of other Asian societies (Ismail et al, 1997). Moreover, the per-capita consumption of sugar in China remained far below the "dentally safe" level of 10.0 Kg per year.

While the standard of living and the access to food increased throughout rural China, there was and still is considerable regional variability in the availability and consumption of food. Thus, for example, while in 1999 the national average per-capita consumption of vegetables in rural China was 109.0 Kg, country dwellers in Tibet and

Gansu consumed less than 35.0 Kg, and the per-capita consumption of the rural population in Liaoning Province was above 200 Kg. The consumption of meat varied by 41.5 percent of the national per-capita average of 15.3 Kg: farmers in the province of Shanxi consumed close to one-third of the national average (5.4 Kg per person), while in the affluent Guangdong Province consumption was 28.4 Kg, more than five times higher.

Table 5.1 Per-capita consumption of food products, rural China, 1981–1999* (mean)

	1981	1987	1996	1999
Grains (Kg)	248.0	259.0	256.2	249.3
Vegetables (Kg)	142.0	130.0	106.3	109.0
Addible oil (Kg)	2.0	4.7	6.1	6.1
Meat (Kg)	5.8	11.7	12.9	13.2
Poultry (Kg)	0.3	1.2	1.9	2.3
Eggs and related products	0.8	2.3	3.4	4.1
Aquatic products (Kg)	0.8	2.0	3.7	3.7
Sugar (Kg)	0.7	1.7	1.4	1.4
Liquor (Lit.)	1.2	5.5	7.1	7.0

**Sources*: Smith, 1993; China Yearbook 1997, 2000.

Inequitable access to food presents the government and health authorities of the PRC with a full range of nutritional health problems. On the one hand malnutrition, characteristic of developing societies, is not yet fully under control. On the other hand health problems related to excessive weight, obesity, and eating disorders, which prevail in post-industrial societies, start emerging, particularly among urbanites and the better off.

Malnutrition among children of all ages declined during the 1990s but remained a public health concern in the PRC (Shen et al, 1996; Chang et al, 1994). In the early 1990s, 16.5 percent of all Chinese children under five were underweight for their age and 31.4 percent did not achieve expected height (stunting). However, compared with other developing countries, the PRC can claim a remarkable achievement in eradicating childhood malnutrition. The prevalence of weight per age deficiency among Chinese children was less than half that reported by some other Asian societies, such as Viet Nam (40.0 percent) and Sri Lanka (37.7 percent), though it is still higher than that reported for Mongolian children (12.3 percent). The prevalence of stunting in China was lower than in India (53.1 percent) and Viet Nam (36.0 percent), but higher than in Sri Lanka (23.8 percent) and Mongolia (26.4 percent) (World Development Indicators, 2000).

Naturally, the prevalence of malnutrition among preschool children is related both to the economic development of the region in which they live and to the social characteristics of their parents (Chang, 1994). Thus, malnutrition is more common in rural than urban areas and in poor regions it greatly exceeds the national average. Close to one-quarter of the variation in child malnutrition is explained by per-capita household income. Yet, income was not the only characteristic related to growth and development in preschool children. Literacy decreases the odds of stunting by about half and the odds of children being underweight by one-third. The prevalence of malnutrition was similar for boys and girls and both sexes alike benefitted from parental economic status and educational achievements.

Whether the economic reforms brought about a sharper decline in malnutrition among children under the age of five or continued the trend which had started earlier cannot be evaluated, because of the absence of data from the early years of the PRC. However, the lower prevalence among children from wealthier regions, better-off households and literate parents suggests that if the current development of the rural economy and the eradication of illiteracy continue and spread to the remote, poorer, rural regions, childhood malnutrition will continue to decline.

A similar decline in the prevalence of malnutrition has been observed among Chinese adolescents (Wang et al, 1998). During the early 1990s, the prevalence of stunting among rural adolescents decreased from 26.7 percent in 1991 to 21.3 percent in 1993. The prevalence of underweight children, however, remained unchanged during these two years: 12.6 percent and 12.8 percent of the adolescents, respectively. These figures are lower than those observed among preschool children, and among adolescents themselves stunting and underweight were more common among 10–13 year olds than among 14–18 year olds. It appears that under-nutrition in the PRC is associated with age and that it declines as age proceeds.

The source of about 70 percent of the energy consumed by rural adolescents is cereals and other carbohydrates. Lipids comprise 20–23 percent. Between 1991 and 1993, a slight decline appeared in the proportion of grain-based energy, while the proportion of calories derived from fat increased (Wang et al, 1998). In 1991, 15.8 percent of rural adolescents were on a high-fat diet, that is, they obtained more than 30.0 percent of the energy they consumed from lipids. In 1993 this figure increased to 20.8 percent. During these two years, the percentage of adolescents who acquired more than 10.0 percent of the energy they consumed from saturated fat increased from 8.8 percent to 12.1 percent.

As with preschool children, stunting and underweight conditions were less frequent among adolescents from high income families, but adolescents from such families consumed more lipids (Table 5.2). The proportion of high income family adolescents on high-fat diet increased by 33.7 percent between 1991 and 1993. Furthermore, within the same two years, the prevalence of a high level of *saturated* fat diet among adolescents increased by close to 70 percent among the better off and by less than 10 percent among the poor.

Table 5.2 Consumption of fat among rural adolescents by family income, China, 1991–1993* (percent of the study population)

	Total fat				Saturated fat	
	Insufficient (< 10% of total energy)		High (> 30% of total energy)		High (>10% of total energy	
	199 1	199 3	199 1	1993	1991	1993
Family income:						
High	3.6	4.9	29.1	38.9	14.0	23.7
Middle	11.4	10.1	13.8	19.7	8.5	9.5
Low	16.4	18.9	8.4	8.7	5.6	6.1
Total	11.3	12.0	15.8	20.8	8.8	12.1

**Source*: Wang et al, 1998.

As dietary habits acquired during adolescence generally persist through adulthood, these findings should alarm the public health authorities. The reliance on fat and saturated fat increased considerably within a short period of two years, particularly among well-to-do rural families. This trend suggests that animal fat is considered culturally as a symbol of prosperity, and as more farmers grow out of poverty these figures are likely to increase.

Currently, overweight conditions and obesity are quite rare among adolescents in rural China: 3.5 percent in 1991 and 3.8 percent in 1993. Nonetheless, there were some indications that Chinese teenage girls are beginning to show concern about their weight, similar to their sisters in Western societies (Wang, 1998; Lee and Lee, 1999). For the moment, body dissatisfaction is more prevalent in urban China than in the countryside. However, it is very possible that the processes of modernization and globalization will bring eating disorders to rural China as well, presenting the public health authorities with yet another challenge.

Among rural adults malnutrition, defined by underweight, seemed to have leveled at about 8.0 percent during the late 1980s (Popkin et al, 1995). The findings of several studies, however, suggested that the prevalence of overweight have increased moderately but steadily since then (Popking et al, 1995; Qu et al, 1997, 2000; Yu et al, 1999).

As with rural adolescents, between 65.0 percent and 70.0 percent of the energy consumed by adults is derived from plants and carbohydrates. However, Qu et al (1997, 2000) argue on the basis of their own studies and extensive literature review that nutrient intake among rural adults is insufficient. The average energy intake they observed among adult women during the late 1990s was 1826 kcal/day, lower than the 2700 kcal/day recommended by the Chinese nutrition authorities for women of working age in the mid-range exercise level. Further, the intake of protein, calcium, and vitamins A, B1 and B2 of some half of the women in their two rural samples was insufficient by the Chinese RDA criteria. The major source of protein in the countryside, however, was plant-based (60.0 percent), with soy beans in first place. Animal fat, currently considered a risk-factor for cardio- and cerebrovascular diseases, comprised less than 10.0 percent of the total protein intake but was an important source of lipid intake. Excess consumption of lipids was observed among 10.0 percent to 20.0 percent of the rural women.

Although these findings are based on rather small samples, it appears that heath education and health campaigns that focus on adequate nutrition are called for. Such measures were taken under the CCP during the pre-economic reform period and proved very successful in reducing morbidity and mortality from infectious diseases. While the epidemiological transition proceeds in rural China, special attention to the risks which accompany economic development and the increasing availability of food in industrial societies is required.

Utilization of Health Services

In all societies, utilization of health services is greatly influenced by both cultural attitudes and structural factors (Turner, 1995). It is culture that defines the problems considered to be health conditions and the level of discomfort that legitimizes seeking medical help. Cultural perceptions also attribute priorities to different health problems and social groups when help is sought (Carmel et al, 1990). Structural factors, such as the availability of health services, instrumental and psychological barriers to care, and one's position in the social structure determine the accessibility of care. Thus, structural factors mediate between the cultural definition of health needs and actual help seeking for health problems.

Some of these issues are addressed in this section. Using the data collected in rural HeBei, we first explore the health conditions for which farmers tend to seek medical help. Second, we look at structural factors which may present barriers to medical treatment and limit access to care. Finally, we search for the social groups which are either more or less likely to seek help. That is, the degree to which individual parameters, particularly sex and age, are associated with seeking help. The relationship between utilization of health services and social class position are discussed in detail in Chapter 6, which is devoted to health inequalities.

Health Status

The first step on the road to care is the perception of a real need, whether defined by the individual or by his/her social environment. In China, utilization of health services is strongly related to the way people perceive their current health status (Li and Fielding, 1995). On the other hand, the way people evaluate their general health, reflecting a more general and long-term perception of their health status and quality of life, is only a poor basis for predicting their behavior with regard to seeking help.

For the farmers in rural HeBei, acute health conditions are the health problems which require immediate medical attention (Figure 5.3). Over half of the farmers who experienced an acute condition, either as a unique health problem or coming in addition to a long-standing, chronic health condition, sought medical help within a few days of the onset. Chronic health problems, on the other hand, were not perceived as urgent and some one-third of the chronically ill did not visit a health care provider for over a year.

Further examination of the data indicated that HeBei's farmers were more likely to seek medical help when new health problems interfered with their daily activity, particularly when these restricted the normal fulfilment of their social roles (Figure 5.4). Visits to doctors related to long-term health conditions were considerably delayed, even when the delay caused disability and interfered with daily activity. In other words, farmers were unlikely to seek help for health conditions that limited their daily life for a lengthy period of time but did not result in a sudden, noticeable, ability to perform their regular duties. Similarly, newly apparent psychological difficulties were not seen as legitimate cause for consulting the health services.

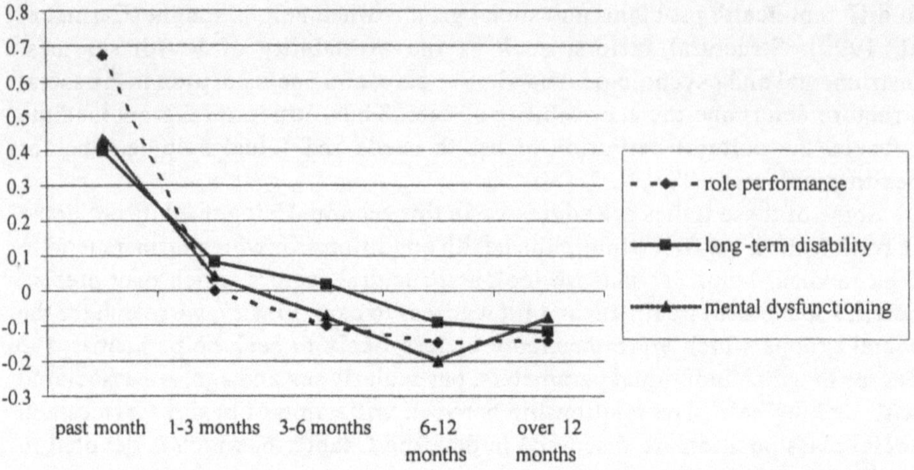

Figure 5.3 Last doctor visit by acute and chronic health conditions, HeBei, 1996–1999 (percent)

The use of medication follows a similar pattern, reflecting the priority attributed to acute conditions and to the need to restore the usual level of function (Li and Fielding, 1995). In rural HeBei, the great majority (80.8 percent) of people who reported a recent acute health problem were taking medication, but less than half (46.0 percent) of the chronically ill were receiving chemotherapy or any other type of treatment when interviewed. On the average, acute conditions were treated by 2.4 kinds of medication, and by 3.89 drugs if the acute episode occurred to a chronically ill person.

Given that most village doctors charge for the medication they prescribe and sell, the medical expenses of the farmers varied according to the nature of their problems. Chronically ill respondents who also suffered an acute condition had the highest expenses: a mean of 11.0 Yuan during the two weeks preceding the interview. Respondents who had only an acute health episode spent, on the average, 5.1 Yuan during the same period, but those with only a chronic health problem spent just 1.9 Yuan.

It appeared that acute health problems, which bring about an unexpected decline in daily function and role performance, are considered the most legitimate reasons for seeking medical help. These conditions legitimize not just consulting the doctor, but also buying medication. Chronic health problems, disability, and poor psychological well-being are largely neglected by rural people and are likely to be treated only upon the onset of an unrelated acute health problem.

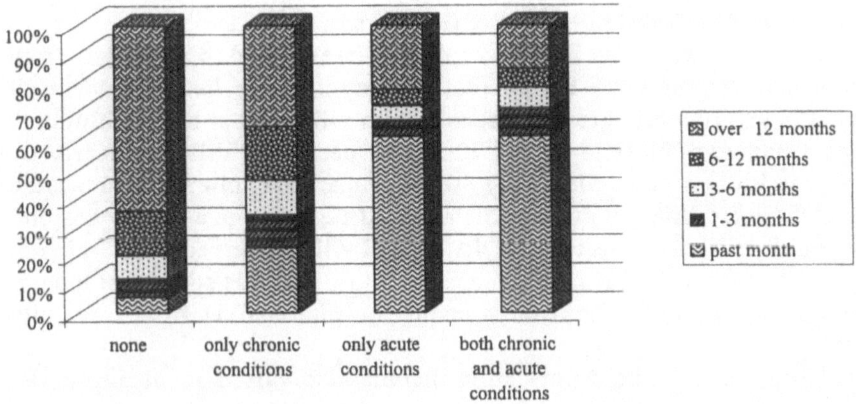

Figure 5.4 Last doctor visit by subjective evaluation of health, HeBei, 1996–1999 (mean, adjusted for age and sex)

* A higher score indicates poorer health.

Structural Factors

One of the basic structural factors which determines seeking help is, of course, the availability of health services and the practical and psychological costs involved in reaching these services. The higher the cost, the higher the barrier to the utilization of medical care. Access to health care is usually defined in terms of the distance to the available services, the expense involved, and the psychological costs of utilization (Shi, 1996).

Currently, the number of doctors practicing in a village is regulated by the village size (see Chapter 6). Thus, for some villages primary health services are provided by the clinic in a neighboring village, a geographical distance which may increase both practical and psychological costs. The type of clinic or clinics available in a village may further influence the costs of unitization. As shown in Chapter 4, fee policy and practice varied with the clinic's type of ownership. The degree to which these variables affect the behavior of farmers in seeking help in rural HeBei is discussed in this section.

Of the 288 villages surveyed in HeBei Province during 1996–1999, 11 were dependent on other villages for the provision of health services. This structural characteristic considerably increased the distance to the closest primary service (Table 5.3). In these villages, farmers had to travel twice as far to meet their health needs, although in HeBei, as in other parts of China, the closest primary service is about half a kilometer away (Henderson et al, 1995).

At the same time, villages without a clinic were located relatively far from the third layer of the three-tier system. County and city hospitals were all located at a significantly greater distance from villages that had no clinic, at average distances of close to 30 and 70 Km, respectively. Villagers served by private practitioners and collectively owned primary care clinics were located closer to these facilities, at average distances of 12 Km from a county hospital and 45 Km from a city hospital. The distance of villages served by a clinic run by a government hospital from the respective hospitals was somewhat longer, on the average, about 20 Km from a county hospital and 51 Km from a city hospital.

Furthermore, household per-capita income also varied according to the size of the village and thus by the types of clinics available within the village itself (Chapter 6). On the aggregate level, the poorest households in rural HeBei were found in villages with no clinics at all, the wealthiest in villages served by government hospital branches. Surprisingly, these structural factors were hardly reflected in the psychological costs of utilization of care, measured here by level of satisfaction with the available primary care services (Table 5.3). Despite the observed variability, statistical analysis revealed only two significant differences. The availability of choice, i.e. the number of different types of clinics in the village, was associated with greater satisfaction with the service and farmers living in villages with both collectively owned clinics and private practitioners were more satisfied with the quality of the health care offered in their village. Second, farmers were significantly less satisfied with the doctor-patient relationship in clinics operated by government hospitals.

Moreover, physical distance did not cause differential health expenditures. Total out-of-pocket expenditures during the two weeks preceding the interview, however, were related to the types of clinic available in the village. In villages where both collective and private clinics were available, the farmers' expenses were significantly higher: 21.4 Yuan, compared with an average of 11.9 Yuan. Thus, competition does not necessarily guarantee the best deal for consumers.

The structure of the health services in the village was not related to the utilization of medical care, yet, the reasons named by the 1,376 respondents who did not seek medical help, although they felt ill, varied according to the type of clinic in their villages. The typical reason offered by 67.3 percent of the respondents for avoiding a consultation with a doctor when needed was that the health condition experienced was not serious enough. Relatively few (17.7

percent) named lack of money as the primary reason for refraining from meeting the need. Severity of the discomfort, however, was mentioned significantly more often in villages where both collective and private clinics operated. As seen above, in these villages out-of-pocket health expenditures tended to be comparatively high. In villages where governmental clinics were available, instrumental difficulties, such as lack of money or time, were mentioned with significantly greater frequency.

Table 5.3 The availability of rural health services, HeBei, 1996–1999 (means and standard errors)

	Geographical distance to closest service (Km)				Household per-capita income	Satisfaction [a]	
Clinic type	Village clinic	Township health center	County hospital	City hospital		Service	Doctor-patient relationship
No clinic	0.47 (0.02)	3.19 (0.13)	28.60 (0.58)	73.10 (1.74)	1348.12 (305.78)	-0.09 (0.07)	-0.05 (0.06)
Private only	0.24 (0.004)	1.99 (0.03)	15.73 (0.14)	58.14 (0.42)	1984.90 (80.89)	0.01 (0.02)	0.02 (0.02)
Collective only [b]	0.23 (0.01)	2.33 (0.05)	15.31 (0.22)	57.44 (0.66)	2372.32 (128.99)	0.09 (0.03)	0.02 (0.03)
Private and collective [b]	0.23 (0.01)	2.29 (0.05)	10.96 (0.25)	44.69 (0.73)	2550.57 (137.73)	-0.10 (0.03)	-0.07 (0.03)
Government branch	0.25 (0.02)	2.68 (0.14)	20.67 (0.63)	51.00 (1.89)	3498.08 (335.18)	-0.17 (0.08)	-0.14 (0.07)
F (clinic type, d.f.=4) P	46.80 0.00	31.45 0.00	230.29 0.00	93.49 0.00	9.52 0.00	6.43 0.00	2.93 0.02

[a] The higher the score, the higher the level of satisfaction.

[b] Collectively owned clinic, or clinic run by group practice.

It has been argued that the transition to a market economy, the dismantling of the collectives, and the privatization of the rural primary health services limited access to care in rural China (Carrin et al, 1996; Wong and Chiu, 1998). Overt expression of the connection between unmet health needs and economic hardships was rare in rural HeBei, though our data indicate that farmers were more likely to refrain from seeking help in villages where treatment was, on the average, more expensive.

Non-compliance with the village doctor's referral to a higher level health facility followed a similar pattern. During the year prior to our health survey in rural HeBei, 234 respondents were referred to a township health center, but did not go there. Again, the modal reason was their own perception that the health problem was not serious enough, though this was mentioned less often – by 44.4 percent of the noncompliant interviewees. Shortage of money was named by 29.5 percent of the respondents, which is quite a high figure when compared to that for non-utilization of primary care.

Reports that the rising cost of hospital care for inpatient as well as for outpatient services limits the access of peasants to tertiary services (Chen, et al, 1997; Liu et al, 1999) were only partially supported by the interviews conducted in rural HeBei. During the year before the interviews were held, 156 respondents were referred to a hospital but did not go. Only a few of them (15.4 percent) did not comply with the village doctor's recommendation because they felt their condition was not serious enough. An additional 14.7 percent could not afford the expected expenses. Forty-six (29.5 percent), however, could not comply because of transportation difficulties. A similar proportion (28.8 percent) expressed distrust and alienation from the hospital staff as the main reason for not complying with the referral.

Structural factors, then, did not increase the practical or psychological costs of seeking help. Mainly, it was the perceived health needs that determined the utilization of primary and, though to a lesser degree, secondary health services. Non-compliance with referral to a hospital, however, emerged as related to a psychological distance rather than to a geographical one.

Understanding Utilization of Health Services in Rural HeBei

In all societies, the position of the individual in the social structure either eases or constrains access to care. Social class is one such characteristic, consistently found to determine one's health and the ability to purchase health care when needed. Yet, access to material resources is by no means the only personal attribute which determines behavior with respect to seeking help. Age, gender, ethnicity, and race are other, equally important, social categories defining one's social position and consequently access to health care and other social resources (Anson et al, 2003; Carmel et al, 1990; Tipping and Segall, 1995; Shuval and Anson, 2000; Anson, 2000).

Earlier in this chapter, we showed that acute health conditions are perceived as requiring medical help. In Chapter 3 we discussed the cultural attitudes which emphasize the importance of medication in restoring health. In this section we have chosen to focus on patterns in seeking help and utilization of medication by persons who experienced an acute health problem or problems during the two weeks preceding the survey. Using a multivariate statistical method, we searched for the role of personal characteristics and for the way these interact with structural and psychological factors in patterning behavior with respect to seeking medical help in rural China. We look first at the inclination to use the primary health services offered by the village doctor and then at the use of medication.

Of the persons interviewed during the health study in rural HeBei, 2,006 reported they had had an acute condition in the past two weeks and 468 of these (23.3 percent) did not seek professional help for that particular condition. The age of the sick person is the most important determinant of behavior with respect to seeking help (Table 5.4). Children were most likely to be taken to the clinic: almost all of the preschoolers (98.5 percent) and the great majority of school aged children (93.8 percent). The inclination to seek a doctor's help declined with age and leveled off at adulthood. Culturally, it appears that the health of children is perceived as most valuable and their health problems should be attended to as they emerge.

Neither the sex nor the educational level of the ill person served as a basis for differentiating between those who sought help for an acute health problem and those who did not. Per-capita household income, however, was positively associated with seeking help. A rise of 1,000 Yuan in annual per-capita income increased the probability of consultation with a doctor by 13.1 percent.

Of the structural variables, only the distance from the nearest primary care clinic proved to be an important factor. The farther the clinic, the less likely were farmers to see a doctor when necessary. The distance from a clinic, however, did not modify the odds against different age, sex, education, and income groups of visiting a doctor. Personal characteristics and structural factors appeared to affect help seeking decisions independently of each other. As with the level of satisfaction with the health services, the types of primary care services available in the village were not considered when the time came to decide whether or not to consult a doctor.

Table 5.4 Predicting the utilization of health services for acute conditions, HeBei, 1996–1999 (odd ratios extracted by logistic regression analysis)

		Personal characteristics	Structural factors (added)	Psychological costs (added)
Age	0 – 5	21.12*	17.44*	17.60*
	6 – 14	5.03*	6.93*	5.96*
	15 – 24	2.96*	4.15*	4.20*
	25 – 44	0.81	0.81	0.82
	45 – 59	0.86	0.87	0.88
	60 and over	1.00	1.00	1.00
Sex	(women)	0.87	1.02	1.02
Education		1.01	1.00	1.00
Per-capita income		1.15*	1.13*	1.13*
Clinic Type				
	Private only		0.72	0.71
	Collective only		0.78	0.78
	Private and collective		0.60	0.60
	Government		0.72	0.72
	No clinic in village		1.00	1.00
Distance from nearest clinic			0.70*	0.70*
Satisfaction with				
	Service			1.05
	Doctor-patient relationship			1.01
Log Likelihood Ratio		1934.86	1634.02	1633.36

*A statistically significant difference.

Most often, medical help was sought from the local village doctor. The behavior of the farmers seeking help in HeBei Province did not support the argument that the increase in the disposable income of rural households since the implementation of the 'system of household responsibility' in the early 1980s generated a greater demand for higher quality health care (Chapters 1 and 2). Some have suggested that wealthier farmers prefer the services provided by county or city hospitals to those provided by the village doctor and the township health center. In rural HeBei, however, this was hardly the rule, according to our respondents. One in five persons indeed sought help in a higher-tier, rather than in a village health facility, without consulting the village doctor first. Nevertheless, about half of these turned to the township health centers, almost all from villages where no primary care services were available.

The services offered at upper level facilities, that is, county or city hospitals, were clearly preferred only by older men with high a income level. A higher income enables men above the age of 50, those who are generally reluctant to seek medical help at all, to look for treatment in a city or a county hospital, regardless of its distance from their home. It is very possible that the decision to seek professional consultation is dependent on the perceived seriousness of the health problem. When defined as serious enough to be treated at all, older men, though not women, prefer to travel to a hospital if they can afford it. Higher income enabled them to cover the costs of traveling, hospital registration and treatment.

The use of medication for an acute condition took on a different pattern (Table 5.5). The need to relieve the discomfort caused by an acute illness and to restore the ability to perform one's regular roles cut across all age groups. In this respect, children were not treated differently from adults, though adults between 45 and 59 years of age were significantly less likely to use medication for such conditions, whether or not they sought medical help.

Higher level of education, which was not affect the tendency to consult a doctor, decreased the inclination to use medication for acute illness. The better educated may be better equipped and sufficiently confident to wait for spontaneous recovery, which is often the case with acute diseases and, as we will see in Chapter 6, to apply self care. Moreover, seeking professional help did not change this tendency, though persons who turned to a doctor were generally more likely to use medication. Thus, the level of the patient's education appeared to be a serious consideration in the doctor's decisions, in two possible ways. First, it seems that primary care providers trust the better educated persons' ability both to apply self-care and to monitor the condition of their own health. These patients can be trusted to seek further medical help if the condition deteriorates. Second, the prescribing behavior of village doctors is sensitive to the patients' wishes and demands, as discussed in Chapter 4.

Table 5.5 Predicting the utilization of medications for acute conditions, HeBei, 1996–1999 (odd ratios extracted by logistic regression analysis)

		Personal characteristics	Doctor visit	Structural factors	Psychological costs
Age	0 – 5	0.89	0.78	0.93	0.95
	6 – 14	1.27	1.16	1.20	1.23
	15 – 24	1.10	1.03	0.98	1.02
	25 – 44	0.75	0.77	0.88	0.85
	45 – 59	0.65*	0.66*	0.72	0.74
	60 and over	1.00	1.00	1.00	1.00
Sex	(women)	0.92	0.93	0.93	0.92
Education		0.96*	0.96*	0.94*	0.94*
Per-capita income		1.08*	1.07*	1.12*	1.12*
Visited the doctor for condition			1.62*	1.67*	1.66*
Clinic Type					
	Private only			1.08	1.06
	Collective only			1.37	1.36
	Private and collective			0.94	0.93
	Government			0.74	0.83
	No clinic in village			1.00	1.00
Distance from nearest clinic				1.83*	1.81*
Satisfaction with					
	Service				1.08
	Doctor-patient relationship				0.96
Log Likelihood		2052.53	2037.61	1624.74	1623.00

*The difference was statistically significant.

Higher income, which facilitates consumption of all kinds, also facilitates the use of medication. The higher the per-capita income, the greater the likelihood that the farmers will take medication to relieve an acute condition. This tendency was not affected by other social characteristics of the patient, whether or not he consulted a doctor, by structural factors, or by the psychological cost of dissatisfaction with available health services.

Of the structural factors, only the distance from the nearest clinic was related to the use of medication. The farther a patient lived from a clinic, the more medication he took to treat an acute health problem. Both patients and doctors seemed to have recognized the cost in time and inconvenience of living at a distance from the clinic. When doubts regarding the necessity of drug therapy arose, for example, medication was prescribed in order to avoid repeated visits to the clinic.

The pattern that emerges is that in treating acute health episodes, village doctors prefer to delay the suspension of medication until further developments can be observed. This preferred practice is modified by the characteristics of the patient treated. The better educated are more likely to appreciate such an approach and to comply with the recommended practice. The less educated, on the other hand, may demand immediate medical intervention, in line with the cultural belief in the power of medication (Chapter 4). The distance of the patient's residence from the clinic is another consideration in the decision making process. The greater the distance, the higher the costs involved for an additional visit to the clinic and the higher the risk taken, should the patient's condition deteriorate.

Summary

This chapter deals with the patterns of four types of health-related lay behavior: the consumption of alcohol, tobacco, nutrition, and the utilization of health services. Health-related behavior is a social behavior and, as such, is socially and culturally constructed and learned during the process of socialization. It is for that reason that we consider how these kinds of behavior are influenced by social categories, in particular age, sex, and social class.

The prosperity that followed the economic reforms of 1979 brought about a substantial increase in the consumption of alcohol in the PRC. The rate of production increased faster than that of population growth and consumption of alcohol in rural households increased almost six-fold within 15 years. Nonetheless, there is some indication that this consumption has reached stability at a level somewhat higher than the European level, but lower than that of other developing societies.

Chinese culture largely limits the consumption of alcohol by women, but strongly encourages social drinking among men. Just a negligible number of women in rural HeBei consumed alcohol, while in some age groups over half of the men did so. It appears that in rural HeBei, drinking is relatively rare among youngsters and the elderly but very common among men of working age.

Alcohol consumption emerged as a status symbol among men. The better educated and heads of households were significantly more likely to consume alcohol than illiterate men and men dependent on their families, regardless of age. Unlike reports from the USA, alcohol consumption was higher among married rural men than among the formerly married, and least prevalent among the never-married.

China's share of the amount of tobacco consumed worldwide is considerably higher than its relative proportion of the world's population. Cigarette smoking observed in rural HeBei is widespread among men but relatively rare among women. The pattern of smoking, broken down by age and sex, differs significantly from that reported by industrial societies. Among young men, the prevalence is relatively low, but almost three in four men in their prime, aged 40–44, smoke regularly. Among women, the highest prevalence was observed at the age of 60–64, similar to the pattern of alcohol consumption. As with alcohol consumption, it appears that smoking is a symbol not only of masculinity, but also of social maturity.

The consumption of cigarettes presents a severe public health risk. Current legislation in effect may not be sufficient to effectively cope with this risk, which seems to be reaching epidemic proportions among rural men. As the power of traditional mechanisms of social control erodes with modernization, smoking may spread to women and younger men in the near future.

The level of nutrition in rural China improved considerably after the economic reforms. Nationwide, food consumption has doubled since the early 1980s, but access to food is unequally distributed. The PRC thus faces a double-edged sword: malnutrition in some poor regions on the one hand and the emerging problems of the affluent, such as excessive weight and eating disorders on the other.

Malnutrition is on the decline and the prevalence of underweight children and stunting is lower than in many other Asian societies. Its prevalence declines with the child's age and the level of education of the parents. Malnutrition is related to the economic condition of the region and the child's family. It seems, therefore, that malnutrition will continue to decline as long as rural economic development and access to education continue.

At the same time, there are some alarming signs. The consumption of vegetables is declining and the consumption of fat is increasing. This transition is more rapid among the better off than among the poor, suggesting a cultural preference that, according to currently accepted knowledge, entails health risks. Obesity and eating disorders are relatively rare in rural China but starting to emerge as public health problems in the cities. These will probably spread to the countryside in the foreseeable future.

In rural HeBei, acute health conditions which abrupt the fulfilment regular social roles constituted the main reason for utilization of health services. This pattern emerged from analyses of visits to a doctor, use of medication, and medical expenditures. Long term health conditions and psychological difficulties were treated less frequently and were more likely to be attended to when accompanied by an acute health problem.

Structural factors such as the services available in the village and the distance from an upper level facility hardly affected access to care or utilization of primary health services. Nor did these structural factors increase the practical or psychological costs of seeking primary medical care. Nevertheless, several social categories are more likely to consume health services than others: children, more affluent adults, and those residing close to a clinic are more likely to visit a village doctor when they feel they should.

Consumption of medication takes on a different pattern. It is related to both structural factors and individual characteristics. The further the patient's residence from the nearest clinic, the greater his chances of using medication. Both the poor and the better educated patients were less likely to use medication in cases of acute health conditions, even if they sought medical help.

Our data suggest that educational level allows both doctor and patient to rely on self-care by the patient and to avoid or delay drug therapy when possible. Moreover, it appears that both doctors and patients take into consideration the costs involved in the distance to the service when making treatment decisions. The preferred practice seems to be to delay or suspend medication until further developments can be observed.

The health behavior of men aged 45–64 is causing some concern. A high proportion of men in this age smoke and consume alcohol, but they consume fewer health services and tend to avoid medication. The combination of risky health behavior and neglect of treatment for medical conditions may result in loss of health as these men reach old age.

Evidence for the preference of upper-level health services, as suggested in previous studies, was very weak in rural HeBei. High income indeed facilitated consumption of services available at upper level facilities, an opportunity which was rarely taken up by persons younger than 50 years of age or by women of any age. This preference prevails among older men, those who are generally quite reluctant to consume primary health services and medication. When people of this age do decide to seek medical help, they prefer a hospital to a village clinic or township health center.

Chapter 6

Patterns of Inequality

In all societies, resources are scarce and unequally distributed. Health and health care are examples of such resources. In any given society, some members are healthier than others, some enjoy easier access to health services and their health care needs are met to a larger extent than those of others in the same society or social group. The sociological question, however, is whether the unequal access to health and health care follows other types of social divisions, and the degree to which health inequalities overlap patterns of differential accessibility to other social resources.

In many post-industrial and developing societies unequal access to health and health care takes on a variety of forms, some of which are concomitant with disadvantages in other spheres of life. The poor, ethnic minorities, the less-educated, the unemployed, the elderly, and women are social categories whose access to social resources, including those of health, is often relatively limited (Annandale and Hunt, 1999; Shuval and Anson, 2000). Differential access to resources is also embedded in the ecological distribution of social goods. Unequal access to health and health care overlaps ecological divisions such as rural-urban, center and periphery, prosperous and disadvantaged neighborhoods (Shuval, 1992; Ross, 2000).

Health inequalities are intertwined with the question of equity. In many welfare states, the emphasis on universal access to social resources allocated to health brings about inequity in the distribution of these resources. Thus, for example, in many Western countries health services are much better developed in terms of quantity, quality, and variety in urban areas than in rural areas. Yet, in terms of health needs, rural dwellers are in greater need of these services. Universal access to health resources is thus often circumscribed by the latent costs associated with services located far from the residential and social environments of those who need them. Similarly, material costs such as time and travel expenses, and socio-psychological costs such as alienation and separation from the social support network, limit the access of persons residing on the periphery to services available in the center.

Some of these issues are addressed in this chapter. We start by looking at the differential access to health and health care resources of individuals in different social categories. Then we examine the degree to which health status and availability of health services vary among villages in different geographical locations and different levels of economic development.

The largest health inequalities in China lie in the gap between urban and rural environments. These have been presented briefly in chapter 2 and are not repeated in this chapter, since the focus of this essay is on rural China. Gender health differences are discussed here, but a comprehensive discussion of women's status and reproductive health are presented in detail in the next chapter, and the special case of the elderly is taken up in chapter 8.

Health Inequalities Between Social Categories

One of the most consistent findings in epidemiology and the sociology of health and illness is the inverse relationship between social class, mortality, health, and illness. No less consistent are gender differences in mortality, morbidity, and utilization of health services, which have been studied intensively in developed countries since the early 1970s.

Communist and socialist governments are ideologically committed to abolishing class- and gender-based inequalities and to eradicate the differential access of particular social groups to valuable social goods and resources. The experience of the former Soviet Union, however, has proved these efforts to be quite futile, unable to overcome unequal access of persons in different social categories to the available resources. In this section, we explore class- and gender-based gradients in access to health and health care.

Social Class

Research in health inequalities usually employs three indicators of social class: education, income, and occupational status (Lahelma, 2001). All three are important general resistance resources positively associated with longer and healthier life (Antonovsky, 1979). The exact mechanisms through which general resistance resources enhance health are still not clear. Higher levels of education and material resources facilitate the acquisition of knowledge and life style which promote health and longevity. The causality, however, is much more complex, and the relative position of individuals and groups in the stratification system appears to have health consequences far beyond access to material resources (Wilkinson, 1992). The ways in which access to health and health care are shaped by social class in rural PRC are presented below.

1. Level of Education

The efforts made by the CCP to expand education and health care resources for the rural population were described in Chapter 1. These efforts have resulted in a dramatic increase in the level of education and in the eradication of illiteracy among the younger generations (Chapter 1, Figure 1.2).

Nevertheless, schooling is not evenly distributed, despite increased access to education. Furthermore, the relationship between level of education and health in rural China takes on a very similar pattern to that observed in other societies, and the least educated farmers are far less healthy than those who complete six or more years of schooling. This pattern clearly emerges in the ways farmers in HeBei Province evaluate their health: a higher proportion of respondents with less than primary school education felt in poorer health than their better educated counterparts: 16.5 percent of the respondents with fewer than six years of schooling evaluated their health as poor or very-poor, compared with 8.4 percent of those who finished primary school and 5.2 percent of those with more than nine years of schooling.

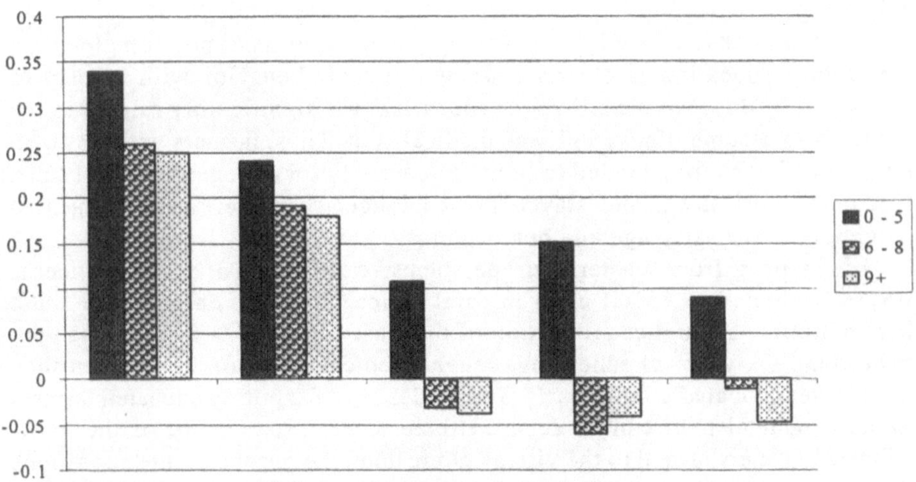

Figure 6.1 Health status and years of schooling, adults (age 15 +), HeBei, 1996–1999 (means adjusted for age and sex)

* A higher score indicates poorer health.

It has been well documented that subjective evaluation of health is the best predictor of longevity (Idler and Benyamini, 1997). A person's perception of his/her own health is a comprehensive summary of general well-being, physical ability, satisfaction with life, mental health, social relations, etc. Indeed, the pattern of association between self-evaluation of health and education is repeated when different dimensions of health status are examined (Figure 6.1). Thus, persons over the age of 15 who never finish primary school education are burdened with more chronic conditions and long term functional limitations and acute health problems, difficulties in fulfilling their regular roles due to physical and/or mental problems, and poorer mental health (note that Figure 6.1 presents mean scores after accounting for age and sex).

Another, less frequently used indicator of health status is oral health (Hunter and Arbona, 1995; Kressin et al, 1996). Consistent with previous studies in developed countries, oral health in rural China is also associated with social class: on the average, persons with less than primary school education were missing between 5 and 6 teeth. This compares with less than one tooth among persons of the same age who attained nine or more years of schooling.

The poor sense of well being among people who have not completed an elementary education is clearly reflected in their behavior with respect to illness. In HeBei Province, level of education was significantly related to the tendency to assume illness and seek medical help. Thus, farmers with less than six years of schooling tended to limit their activity for a longer period of time, lost more work days, and stayed in bed longer than their better educated neighbors of the same age and health status.

As in reports from Western Europe, intensive utilization of health services is inversely related to social class in rural China. For both chronic and acute health problems a higher proportion of the least educated farmers, those with fewer than six years of schooling, sought medical attention more often than their better educated counterparts. The tendency of the poorly educated farmers to seek medical help can be seen on three levels: First, more of the least-educated farmers turned to the village clinic upon the onset of acute conditions than the better- educated peasants of the same age; Second, the mean number of doctor visits per health condition decreased inversely with the number of years of schooling completed by the respondent; Finally, the better educated were prescribed with fewer medications.

The association between educational achievement and these three indicators of illness behavior suggests that in rural HeBei higher education enabled farmers to better distinguish between acute health episodes and chronic conditions. In the case of the former, education increased the farmers' confidence in their own capacity for self care, decreasing their dependence on health services. As a result, better-educated farmers were less likely to seek a doctor's help when ill and used fewer drugs for acute illness. When chronically ill, they used over-the-counter medication more often than the poorly-educated. These patterns of behavior resulted in higher medical expenses for the better-educated. On the average, health-related expenditures of persons who complete more than middle school education are 34.8 percent higher than those of the less-educated respondents of the same age and health status. The difference was due entirely to the cost of medicines.

Nevertheless, level of education did not affect access to preventive care. The World Health Organization recommends that doctors perform a blood test once a year and check blood pressure at each visit for all persons 45 years of age and older, regardless of the purpose of the visit. This practice was relatively rare in rural HeBei: just 7.8 percent of our sample had had a blood test during the year before they were interviewed and blood-pressure was taken in 17.1 percent of the respondents aged 45 and older. Level of education, however, did nor increase or decreased one's odds to undergo these procedures.

2. Income

Before the economic reforms of 1979, variability in income was much more dependent on the village and county level of economic development and natural resources than on individual success. During the decollectivization period, special attention was paid to allocating land according to household size, providing equal opportunities for generation of income (Chapter 1). The income of a household, then, is dependent on three major factors: First, the quality of the available economic resources, which varies considerably with the geographic location of the village; Second, the ability of the local authorities to develop successful local rural industry and services and thus offer households the opportunity to generate additional, non-farming income; Finally, individual households vary in their ability to utilize the resources available to them, for example, to develop and market sideline production (e.g. develop a small business, producing handcraft or raising animals for sail). The variability in household per-capita income is reflected in its members' access to health resources.

Unlike education, income had a direct bearing on the ability of members of the household to enjoy better living conditions and a higher standard of living. Some of these conditions, such as living density, the availability of sanitary services, and refrigerator ownership are directly related to health. In rural HeBei an average of 1.9 rooms was available for each member in households whose per-capita annual income exceeded 2,667 Yuan, compared with 1.5 in households whose per-capita annual income was lower than 1,500 Yuan. The proportion of the wealthier households with indoor toilets was double that of the poorer households (11.4 percent and 4.7 percent, respectively) and bathrooms were six times more common in the better off households than in the poor (36.3 percent compared with 6.6 percent). Similarly, while two in five well-to-do homes own a refrigerator, fewer than one in ten of the poorest households do. At the end of the working day, almost all of the households in the upper quartile are able to enjoy TV programs, 77.0 percent of them in color; among the poorest, only 25.8 percent of the households own a color TV set and 10.4 percent have not got a TV set at all.

Relative access to material resources clearly mirrors access to health. Twice as many persons whose annual per-capita income fell below 1,000 Yuan as those who earn 2,667 Yuan or more evaluated their health as very poor or poor. By contrast, while 41.6 percent of the poorest persons evaluated their health as good or very good, 64.5 percent of the persons in the highest income group did so. Similarly, the poor were burdened with more chronic and acute morbidity, disability, difficulties in performing their usual activity, and poorer mental health (Figure 6.2). Oral health was also negatively associated with income: persons in the lowest income quartile reported a mean of close to four missing teeth, while farmers of the same age in the highest income groups were missing one tooth, on the average.

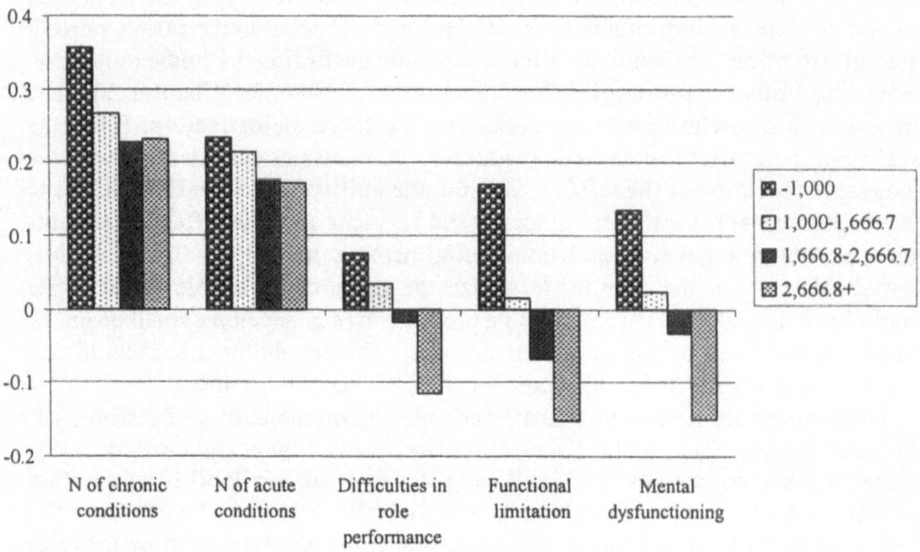

Figure 6.2 Health indicators by income, HeBei, 1996–1999 (means adjusted for age and sex)

* A higher score indicates poorer health.

The association between annual per-capita income and different dimensions of health is almost linear, except for chronic and acute health problems. Following the post-economic reforms in rural HeBei, material prosperity enhanced the sense of well-being far beyond the prevalence and the incidence of diagnosed health conditions. Economic success augments the sense of competent role fulfillment, ability, and emotional well-being.

The tendency to assume the sick-role is considered to reflect the way in which individuals perceive their health and well being and is thus associated with social class position. Per-capita income was inversely related to the all aspects of sick-role behavior. Poorer persons of the same age, education, and health status were more likely to lose working days, restrict their usual activity, and stay in bed because of poor health.

Material resources, however, are not associated with illness behavior, and income was unrelated to access to or the utilization of health services. The behavior of rich and poor when seeking help is very similar, once chronic and acute morbidity are taken into account. Regardless of income, one in four persons burdened with a chronic health problem did not see a doctor during the month prior to the interview, while 17.3 percent paid one visit to the doctor. Both rich and poor people with an illnesses that had appeared recently paid, on the average, 2.1 visits to a doctor over a two-week period, one-third of them to a village doctor. Higher income did not increase access to preventive care or dental health.

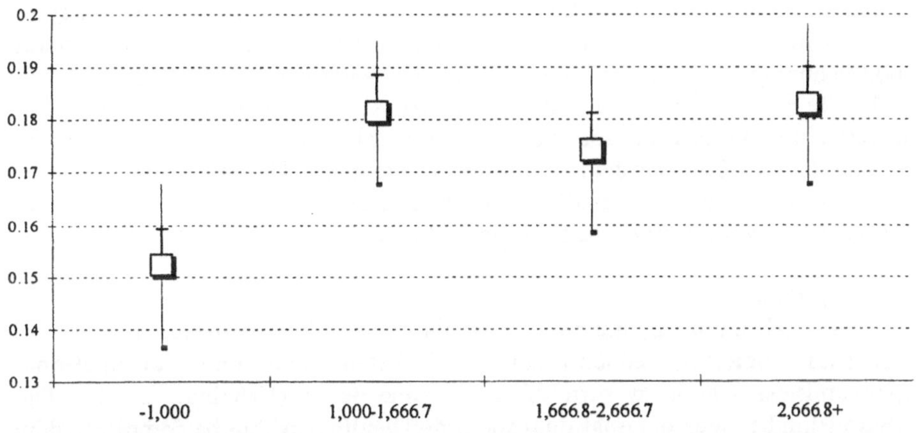

Figure 6.3 Annual health expenditures by per-capita income (Log transformation), HeBei, 1996–1999 (means adjusted for age, sex, and health)

Nonetheless, despite similarities in the behavior of those seeking help, income is associated with health expenditures. The poor, whose annual per-capita income was less than 1,000 Yuan, spent much less on their health than the better-off farmers (Figure 6.3). On the average, a poor person spent almost half the amount of money spent on health by a person the same age, sex, and health status whose annual per-capita income exceeded 1,000 Yuan during the year before the interview: 8.3 Yuan compared with 15.7 Yuan. A rich person of the same age and sex and a similar number of chronic and acute health problems spent, on the average, 18.4 Yuan on health that year. Most of the difference was due to higher expenditures for medication. As observed in other parts of the PRC, though the same number of drugs are prescribed to rich and the poor alike for a given condition, those who are better able to pay and those who are covered by a third party are more likely to receive more expensive treatment (Dong et al, 1999a, 1999c).

The differences in health expenditures between the poorer and the richer rural populations in HeBei Province are particularly pronounced among the elderly, whose health needs are naturally greater than those of younger persons. Elderly people whose income is 1,000 or less spent, on the average, 14.2 Yuan during the year prior to the interview. Seniors in a comparable health status with a per-capita income above 2,667 Yuan spent an average of 80.7 Yuan.

The differences in health expenditures of the richer and the poorer elderly are related to differences in patterns of consumption of health services. Similar to the younger rural population, income level was not related to behavior patterns among those seeking help, in terms of the number of visits to a doctor and the number of different drugs consumed. Nonetheless, elderly people with higher income who were burdened with chronic or acute conditions tended to utilize more county-level services (30.7 percent of the highest income group, compared with 20.1 percent in the entire sample). This tendency involved traveling costs and often resulted in increased expenditures for registration at the tertiary-level facility, medication and treatment.

3. Occupation

Occupational status is another commonly used indicator of social class. In industrial societies, educational level often determines occupational opportunities, which in turn affect income level (Lahelma, 2001). The relationship between occupational status and health may thus be complicated by the effect of education and income on health. However, occupations vary in their non-material rewards as well as in demands by the individual (Siegrist, 2001). While prestige can enhance a sense of well-being, work-related stress may have negative health consequences.

Four main occupational groups could be identified among respondents of working age, that is between 15 and 60, in rural HeBei: farmers (73.0 percent of the sample), white-collar employees (11.6 percent employed in services, teaching, and administration), manual workers (8.0 percent), and 7.5 percent in other occupations. The farmers in HeBei Province had completed the fewest years of schooling, some 7 years of schooling on the average, and their families had the lowest per-capita income – a mean of 2,000 Yuan a year. Those in white-collar occupations had attained the highest educational level, slightly more than eight years on the average, of 8.26 years of schooling, and their average per-capita annual income was 3,020 Yuan. The educational and income of manual workers fell only slightly behind that of rural white-collar workers. Those in other occupations enjoyed the highest annual income, 3,250 Yuan per-capita on the average, though their mean level of education fell significantly below that of the white- and blue-collar employees.

Nevertheless, unlike reports from Western Europe, by most of the health indicators we used the farmers and manual workers did not appear to be in poorest health. The poorest health status was reported by the members of the residual category of "other occupations". Thus, after adjusting for age, sex, educational level, and per-capita income farmers reported the lowest number of chronic and acute conditions and, together with manual workers, had the lowest scores of disability and functional limitations. Those in the "other occupation" category on the other hand reported the highest number of acute and chronic health conditions, more disability, and the poorest mental health. At the same time, the four occupational groups did not differ in the way their occupants evaluated their general health status and role performance.

The picture that emerged, then, is, that holding a middle-class white-collar position in the labor market does not facilitate access to good health in rural HeBei. Rather, it seems that occupation is a function of the ways in which families allocate their resources in the countryside of HeBei Province. The better educated opt for non-farming occupations and their contribution assures a higher standard of living for all the members of their households. The less able persons, among whom there is a relatively high prevalence of chronic illness and a higher tendency to fall sick, are employed in residual types of work, at the cost of their psychological well-being. The higher per-capita household income of this occupational group, which suggests that some of them come from better-off families and some generate reasonable income by themselves, does not alleviate the negative health consequences caused by the stress involved in non-conventional occupations.

It may be concluded, then, that there is a clear relationship between social class and access to health. Both educational level and per-capita income are significantly and positively associated with all indicators of health status. At the same time, social class is not related to access to health care. As seen in the previous chapter, perceived acute health need is the major determinant of seeking help. With few exceptions, the privatization of the rural health services has not affected the level of the utilization of these resources.

Gender Health Differences

During the past three decades, gender health differences have been well documented and extensively studied in North America and Western Europe. In these societies, mortality rates of men are higher than those of women at all ages (Waldron, 1993), while women's morbidity rates are higher than those of men, except during infancy and childhood (Kroenke and Spitzer, 1998; Gijsbers van Wijk et al, 1992; Gissler et al, 1999; van den Bosch et al, 1999; Verbrugge, 1985). Gender mortality and morbidity gaps generally expand during adolescence, reach a peak during the productive and reproductive stage of the life cycle, and tend to converge somewhat thereafter, though higher male mortality and rates disability among women persist during old age. In this section, we explore the degree to which gender health differences in the rural PRC follow this pattern.

There is no single, comprehensive explanation for gender health inequalities. It is accepted that these are the result of some combination of biological predisposition, acquired risks, psychological well-being, and coping resources (Anson et al, 1993a; Anson et al, 1998; Verbrugge, 1985, 1989). Biological differences, mainly those embedded in genetic and hormonal make up, are believed to contribute to women's greater resistance to mortality and proclivity to gender-specific illness. Acquired risks are relate to gender differences in health behavior, self care, and behavior in seeking help. As seen in Chapter 5, Chinese women are less likely behave in ways that may risk their health and generally tend to seek medical help more often, as they do in industrial societies (Henderson et al, 1995).

Women report poorer mental health, self esteem, and more psychological distress than men in most Western societies, which accounts for much of the gender health gradient. These are believed to be the result of their lower social position, expressed in gender segregation in the labor force, lower earnings, and responsibility for housework and child care. Finally, women generally have fewer personal coping resources than men. Their occupational status and earnings fall short of those of men and women generally score lower on tests of coping resources such as the sense of coherence (Anson et al, 1993b). Poverty and lack of social support are particularly prevalent among older groups, because fewer women participate in the labor force and also lose their financial support upon widowhood. Many women who do not work outside their home are dependent on their husbands' medical insurance which become unavailable for them upon marriage dissolution.

The social status of rural Chinese women is discussed at length in Chapter 7, which is devoted to issues in reproductive health. Here, suffice it to mention that the many aspects of the social position of women in rural China resemble those found in post industrial societies. At the same time, the communist regime has taken several legislative actions that, together with expansion of education, change in family structure, economic reforms, and the entry of men into rural industry, have provided women with new opportunities to accumulate resources. As a result, the status of women in the PRC has changed dramatically since the CCP came to power in 1949, with important implications for their health (Anson and Sun, 2002).

In industrial societies, preschool and school-age girls are generally healthier than boys of the same age, as measured by probability of survival and utilization of health services (Gijsbers et al, 1992; Waldron, 1983). By contrast, fertility surveys in the PRC indicate that the odds for survival of Chinese rural female infants and girls during early childhood are less favorable than those for male infants and preschool children, especially for second or higher parity girls with no male siblings (Ren, 1995; Xu et al, 1994; Banister et al, 2000). Often, such patterns are interpreted in terms of cultural preference for sons, which legitimizes the neglect of female infants and children in terms of feeding and the provision of health care. In the health survey conducted in rural HeBei between 1996 and 1999, however, there were no indications of such neglect. The health of preschool and school children as reported by their mothers or primary care takers did not vary by the child's sex, nor did we find any signs for gender differences in seeking medical help. Seeking help for children was the result of perceived need, as we have seen in the previous chapter. The only indication of possible discrimination against young girls was that school boys were kept in bed longer when sick.

In Western societies, gender health inequalities start to emerge during adolescence, the result of the interaction between hormonal changes associated with puberty and social transitions experienced at this stage of the life cycle, when children become aware of their future adult roles and expected adult behavior. Moreover, considerable gender differences in mental health emerge at this age and more teenage girls than boys report poorer psychological well being, the result of lower self esteem (Watkins et al, 1997).

These patterns did not emerge in our study in rural HeBei (Table 6.1). The analyses of the data collected from young adults, 15–24 years of age, did not reveal gender differences in any of the dimensions of health status, including psychological well-being. Nor was gender related to sick-role or illness behavior. The lack of a gender health gradient can be the result of the relative access to social resources of these young women and men. A similar proportion of men and women of this age had acquired an education; only a minority had never gone to school (5.8 percent and 5.9 percent, respectively). Moreover, the average length of schooling completed by women and men was almost identical – eight years. Labor force participation patterns of the young adults of both sexes were very similar: close to 20 percent of men and women had not yet entered the labor force and 8.4 percent of both sexes were working in service occupations. A slightly lower proportion of men than women were in agriculture (41.4 percent vs. 43.7 percent), as somewhat more men entered manual labor (14.9 percent vs. 10.6 percent).

Most of the sociological explanations for the peak in gender health inequalities during the productive and reproductive stage of the life cycle have been developed in reference to the social construction of gender in the West. As mentioned above, the experiences of rural Chinese men and women both resemble and differ from those of North Americans and West Europeans. In rural HeBei, gender differences in labor market experience and in the accumulation of general coping resources emerged among the 25–44 years old respondents. Many more women than men, 84.6 percent and 67.6 percent, worked in agriculture, and non-farmers experienced occupational segregation: 46.1 percent of the men, but just 19.6 percent of the women, did manual work; 57.7 percent of the women were engaged in "feminine" occupations such as services and teaching, as compared with 34.2 percent of the non-farming men. It should be noted, however, that women whose husbands left agricultural work often managed the family farm, supported and empowered by the government, and practically all – except three men and four women – of the respondents of this age were members of the labor force. Both of these phenomena are rare in industrial societies.

Table 6.1 The health of adolescents and young adults (age 15–24) by gender, HeBei, 1996–1999 (means [a] adjusted for age, education, and household income and ANCOVA statistics)

	Men	Women	F
Number of chronic conditions	0.004	0.003	0.202
Disability	0.004	0.006	1.246
Number of acute conditions	0.005	0.005	0.004
Difficulties in role performance	-0.239	-0.235	0.065
Functional limitation	-0.39	-0.382	0.348
Mental dysfunctioning	-0.245	-0.257	0.182

[a] A higher score indicates poorer health except for mental health, where a higher score indicates better health.

The older cohort of the 25–44 age group was born just after the Communist revolution and the introduction of mandatory elementary education. Women of this generation had somewhat fewer chances to acquire this important resource. A higher proportion of women than men never went to school (6.7 percent and

1.4 percent, respectively) and women, on the average, left school a year earlier than men. On the other hand, familial support was readily available for women. The great majority of the participants of this age were married, only 5.8 percent and 2.7 percent, respectively, never married and less than 1 percent of both sexes were formerly married.

Table 6.2 The health of older adults (age 45–59) by gender, HeBei, 1996–1999 (means [a] adjusted for age, education, and household income and ANCOVA statistics)

	Men	Women	F
Number of chronic conditions	0.373	0.475	6.593**
Long-term disability	0.724	0.942	10.317***
Number of acute conditions	0.246	0.32	9.052**
Recent interference with daily activity	0.053	0.184	8.335**
Long-term health evaluation	0.075	0.215	12.191***
Mental health	0.064	0.124	3.502

[a] A higher score indicates poorer health except for mental health, where a higher score indicates better health.
* p<.05;
** p<.01;
*** p<.001

Indeed, gender health differences started to emerge among the adults (ages 25–44) in rural HeBei, though on a much smaller scale than usually reported for post-industrial societies. Women in this age group reported more acute conditions and difficulties in performing their regular roles. Yet, there were no differences between the mental health, disability, and daily functioning of men and women, contrary to the documentation in many developed countries for this age.

Such gender differences were observed among older adults, between 45 and 59 years of age (Table 6.2). Among the older adults, women scored lower than men on all indicators, except mental health. In this age group, larger differences in the level of education and the occupational status of men and women were also found. The younger people in this group were of school age at the time the Communist revolution took place and had little opportunity to enjoy the changes introduced by the CCP. In our data this was reflected by a generally low level of educational achievement and in a significant gender gap. Almost one-quarter of the women (24.1 percent) had never gone to school, compared with 5.7 percent of the men of the same age; among those who had attended school, women had completed an average of 4.3 years of formal education, while men had completed an average of 6.5 years.

Lack of formal education seemed to hamper the chances of women in the labor force, keeping them from entering non-farming occupations. Thus, although all except four of the women were members of the labor force, 90.3 percent of them were in agriculture; of the men interviewed, 36 were retired and 69.5 percent were farmers. The occupational distribution of those not in agriculture was highly gender- segregated and similar to the pattern observed in the 25–44 age group. The most striking observation was that four times as many non-farming men as women were employed in white-collar administrative jobs that bear considerable economic benefits, power, and prestige (Meng and Miller, 1995).

As with reports for North America and Western Europe, the health differences among the elderly (over 60 years old) seemed to have narrowed relative to the younger age group, and elderly women in rural HeBei were significantly more handicapped than men. Yet, again, there were no gender differences in the mental health of elderly men and women.

The lack of gender differences in mental well-being in all age groups is of particular interest. We would like to stress that this finding is not the result of methodological faults. It has been argued that Chinese culture discourages any overt expression of depression and emotional difficulties (Cheng and Hamid, 1996; Lai, 1995). However, as Lai (1995) concluded, Chinese people are perfectly capable of expressing negative emotions and these can be detected using research tools developed in the West. Moreover, the results obtained with Chinese respondents show a distribution quite similar to that obtained in the USA. Also, variation in mental health among women in rural HeBei has recently been reported by Anson and Haanappel (1999). In their analysis, mental health varied with the degree of intra-family power and responsibility. Elderly women residing in their son's household and enjoying traditionally embedded power within the family reported the best mental health. The association between mental health and the three indicators of social class presented above took on the well-documented, universal patterns of negative relationship and lent further validity to the unique findings reported in this section.

The lack of gender health differences, particularly in mental health, is probably the result of the improved social status of rural women, their increased access to general coping resources, and their new economic strength and power within the family structure. Studies of the changing patterns of mortality in the PRC have also documented considerable improvement in the life expectancy of women, and evidence of the disappearance of discrimination against women was already apparent in the 1973–1975 mortality survey (Banister et al, 1997, 2000). Since then, the life expectancy of women has continued to improve relative to that of men, providing further evidence of the improved status of women in the PRC.

There is another factor to consider regarding the unique pattern of gender health inequalities in rural China. One of the health risks encountered by women in North America is a shortage of material resources. More women than men live in poverty, fewer women have access to health insurance, old age pensions, and social support as a result of changing marriage patterns (Meyer and Pavalko, 1996). Some half of the divorced women and widows in Western society fall into poverty, particularly if they become single mothers. Shortage of financial resources does not seem to be gendered in the same way in rural China. Universal marriage and low divorce rates, and single person households, which prevail in Western societies, comprise only 6 percent of all households in the PRC (China Yearbook, 1999). Single person households are even scarcer in rural China, as the widowed and the divorced tend to remain integrated within an extended family household. Patrilocal living arrangements provide both men and women with emotional and instrumental support in old age, while their Western counterparts are at greater risk of poverty and social isolation (Chapter 8). Thus, poverty is a family or household rather than individual condition, though the degree to which household resources are equally or equitably allocated is unknown.

Similarly, in the USA fewer women than men have access to medical care, because they are less likely to have medical insurance. As described in the first two chapters of this volume, the cooperative medical scheme collapsed after the transition to the 'socialist market economy', but men and women lost entitlement to an equal extent. In rural HeBei, women and men had similar access to health services, and equally visited the doctor when the need arose (Anson and Sun, 2002).

Health Inequalities Between Villages

China being the size of a continent, there is large-scale variation in the level of economic development between the different provinces, counties within each province, and between townships within each county. Thus, the average annual per-capita income in the nine counties surveyed in HeBei Province during 1996–1999 ranged from 1,600 Yuan to 3,740 Yuan.

The poorest county in our sample was Ping Shan, located in the mountains. More than one third of its 713 villages are comprised of fewer than 50 households. The main natural resources in Ping Shan county are marble and water, including hot water springs around which tourism and an entertainment industry have been developed. The main industries in the county are a power station and iron mining, but most of the villages live on marketing fruits and nuts. The topography of the county leads to considerable variation in standard of living in the villages. The per-capita annual income in the 32 villages sampled for our study varied from 400 Yuan in Bai Shu Wan to 3,320 Yuan in Xi Shui Niang. Bai Shu Wan is a small mountain village with 240 residents who live on agriculture 45 Km from the county administrative center. Xi Shui Niang is located in the foothills, just 3 Km from the county center and its population (832 residents at the time of the survey) is engaged in industry and services in addition to agriculture. The richest county in our survey was San He City, a suburb of Beijing. The mean per-capita annual income in this county, 3,740 Yuan in 1999, also masks a large range, from 300 Yuan in the poorest village, to 5,000 Yuan in the better of one.

Much of the variation in the mean annual per-capita income within each county was related to the geographical location of the villages within the county. Luan Nan County is one example. The poorest village sampled in this county is located in the mountains and its 1,128 inhabitants had an average annual per-capita income of 1,200 Yuan in 1999. During the same year, the 703 households of Han Se village, located close to the capital Beijing, had an average annual per-capita income of 3,430 Yuan. Between these two extremes were 12 villages in North-East HeBei, with an average per-capita income of 2,200 Yuan a year, and 17 coastal and lowland villages whose average annual per-capita income was 2,400 Yuan.

It has been well established that poor areas are characterized by greater health needs. As mentioned in the introduction to the chapter, the health services in many societies are not distributed according to the population needs. Equity is hardly achieved even in societies where health is highly valued and ideological commitment to health care for all has led to universal health insurance (Annandale, 1998; Shuval and Anson, 2000). Specialists and primary care doctors tend to seek support from the sophisticated facilities that are mainly located in hospitals, and to avoid professional as well as social isolation in remote geographical areas (Connor et al, 1995). Fee-for-service health care delivery systems run the risk that the care providers, especially physicians, will congregate in areas that are economically better off and thus offer better economic opportunities.

These two issues are the focus of this section of the chapter. First, we examine the extent to which the level of economic development of a village eases or limits access to health resources. Then we look at the equity in the distribution of health services according to location of the villages.

Economic Development and Health Resources

There is very little variation in income within the population of a given village (Lee and Xiao, 1998; Secondi, 1997). The social class health gradient described above on the bases of individual level class indicators thus largely present the health needs in villages of different levels of economic development. This association is farther supported by the hospital utilization indicators, showing a greater use of hospitals in lower-income villages. Annual hospital discharge rates, for example, are three times higher in the lower than in the upper income quintile: 3.3 per 1,000 populations in poorest villages, 1.2 per 1,000 populations in the richest villages. Beyond the greater health needs, the poorer villages find it particularly difficult to provide for their populations. The dismantling of the collective with the economic reforms of 1979 deeply affected the financial basis of the village and seriously hindered the ability of the local administration to invest in local services for its inhabitants (Chapter 1).

These processes, which started a decade and a half before our exploration of health and health care in rural HeBei, were clearly reflected in the village-level public investment in health. The local administrations of three-quarters of the 288 villages we studied did not contribute financially to the health delivery system in any way, and public investment was closely related to the average annual per-capita income in the village. After dividing the villages into income quintiles, we found that the village administration invested in health in twice as many villages of the highest quintile than in those of the lowest quintile. This contribution, however, was rather limited, regardless of to the average per-capita income of the village. Whether poor or reach, the village administration invested in health between 1.00 Yuan and 1.04 Yuan per-capita.

The ability of the village authorities to invest in infrastructure such as sanitation also varied according to the level of economic development of the village. As mentioned in Chapter 3, closed sewage systems are extremely rare in rural China; the great majority of the rural sewage systems are open channels to which households and public facilities are connected, and ditches where waste is collected for agricultural use. The existence of such systems, however, and the proportion of the households connected to them, varied according to the economic development of the village. Most of the poorest villages in our sample (81.2 percent), where the average annual per-capita income did not exceed 1,800 Yuan, had no sewage system at all. Such system was more common in the more affluent villages, and 58.9 percent of villages with annual per-capita income of 3,200 Yuan and over had sewage system. Farther, while in one in five of the highest per-capita income quintile all houses were connected to the sewage system, all household were connected to the system just in 7.3 percent of the lowest income quintile villages.

The primary health services in rural China are allocated to villages according to their population size (Chapter 4). Indeed, our data for rural HeBei show that the number of residents accounted for half of the variation in the number of clinics in the villages and the number of the doctors in a village. Nevertheless, the size of the village is not completely detached from its economic opportunities. Small villages are less able to develop and support rural industry and/or services and are often dependent on agriculture alone for their income; some geographical locations are more difficult to develop and sustain a large population. In HeBei Province, the mean size of the villages in the lowest annual per-capita income quintile (average of less than 1,800 Yuan) was 1,033 inhabitants, ranging from 140 to 3,656; the mean size of the richest villages, where the average per-capita annual income was equal to or above 3,200 Yuan, was 1,505, ranging from 540 to 7,847 residents.

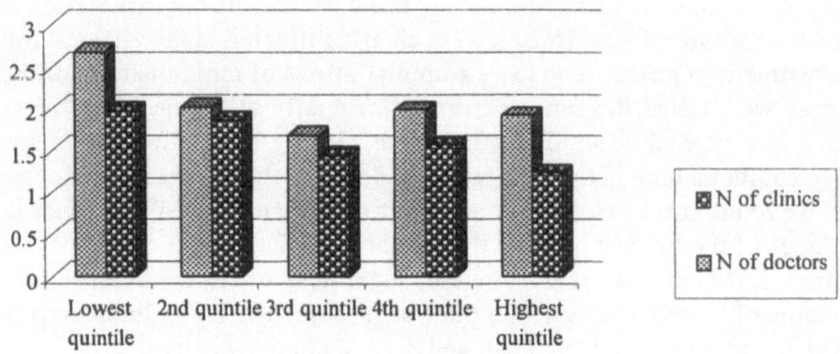

Figure 6.4 Number of clinics and doctors per 1,000 population by village's per-capita income, HeBei, 1996–1999

Given the formal regulation of clinics per population size and the differences in size between villages of different levels of economic development, it was not surprising to find that more of the poorest villages have no clinic at all. One in eight of the poorest villages did not have a local clinic and had to seek help at a neighboring village or in a township health center, compared with 1.8 percent of the other villages. Nonetheless, considering the services available in neighboring villages and township health centers, poorer villages were equipped with more clinics per 1,000 populations (Figure 6.4). In the poorest villages where, as we have seen in the first part of this chapter, the health needs were greater, an average of 2.0 clinics per 1,000 populations were operating; in the richest the average was 1.2 clinics.

Moreover, these clinics were not remnants of the cultural revolution, an era during which the rural health services flourished. Most clinics were staffed and active. In fact, the doctor/population ratio in the poorest villages was far higher than in those that are better-off: 2.7 village doctors per 1,000 populations in the lowest per-capita income quintile, compared with 1.9 in villages of the two upper income quintiles.

These figures are consistent with China's commitment to meet the health needs of its population. The equity in distribution of health facilities and personnel had been recorded in the past, in a study conducted during the late 1980s, some years after decollectivization and privatization of half of the primary rural health services (Henderson et al, 1995). Such equity, however, cannot be achieved by market forces alone. As demonstrated in Figure 6.5, the poorer villages were least able to sustain collective-supported health services; the poorest were also unable to attract enough from private practice to meet the health needs of the population. Where neither collective nor sufficient privately owned health services were available, the government stepped in, encouraging publicly financed hospitals to open outpatient branches and provide services for the population.

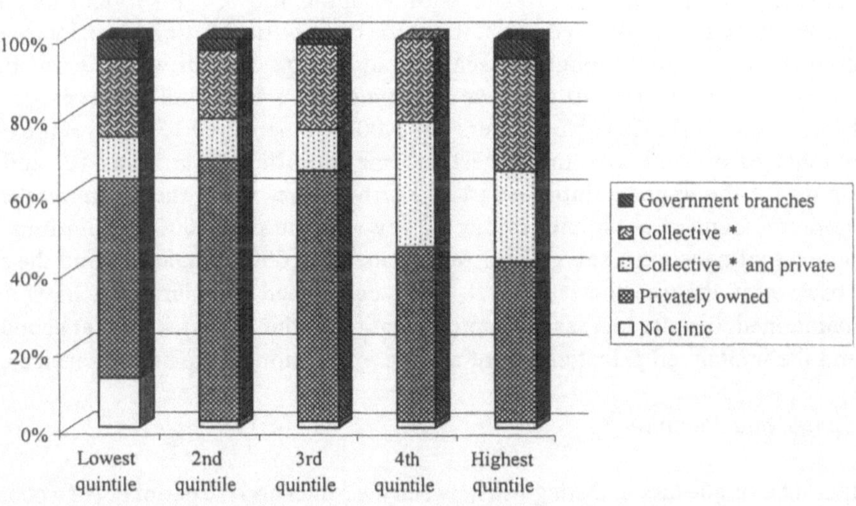

Figure 6.5 Type of clinic by village's per-capita income (percent)

*Fully or partially supported by the village authorities/collective.

Interestingly, however, a similar proportion (5.4 percent) of the richest villages also enjoyed the services of government hospital branches, although wealthy villages were capable of supporting – fully or in part – collectively financed clinics (see Chapter 1). In HeBei Province, more than half of the villages in the two upper income quintiles had retained the collective clinics almost two decades after the economic reforms, though often alongside privately owned clinics. They have nonetheless also attracted hospitals with primary care facilities.

It appears that health needs, service demands, and income-generating opportunities jointly determine the availability of health services in rural HeBei. In the poorer villages, the greater needs, and therefore the higher demand for services, compensated for the relative inability of the population to pay high fees. Medical practitioners could thus make a living by providing a larger quantity of low-fee services. The richer villages, on the other hand, offered opportunities for profit by providing expensive services to a relatively healthy population. As we have seen in the previous section, the health expenditures of the well to do farmers far exceeded those of their poorer counterparts. These opportunities attracted private practitioners as well as hospitals under pressure to raise by themselves an increasing part of their budget.

Despite the concerns voiced by critics of the privatization of rural health services in the PRC (Chapter 1), other health services were also distributed according to need in rural HeBei. Mother and Child health services and anti-epidemic stations followed much the same distribution pattern as primary care clinics and doctors, though the scale of advantage of poor villages was much smaller. Thus, in the villages we surveyed there were, on the average, 1.8 Mother and Child Health providers per 1,000 women aged 15–60; yet the mean number of providers in the lowest income quintile villages was 1.9 and the figure for the upper quintile was 1.6. Furthermore, while the mean number of epidemic control personnel in our survey was 0.8 per 1,000 populations, the poorest villages were served by 1.0 persons per 1,000 populations and the ratio observed in the wealthiest was 0.9. Thus, equity had been largely achieved and maintained, despite increasing implementation of the 'socialist market economy' and the unplanned privatization of a large proportion of the health services.

Center and Periphery

It is not a simple task to distinguish between the center and the periphery of a country, even when the country is geographically small (Anson, 1998). The social meaning of "center" is not necessarily based on physical geography. Rather, the social meaning of "center" is often derived from the power to control, or at least influence, the allocation of social goods. Such power is embedded in the politico-economic structure of a given society, in the actual or symbolic proximity to the decision making social agencies.

As shown in Chapter 2, the cities, in which the smaller urban population lives, were more successful in the competition for health resources than the counties, which represent the majority rural population. This was demonstrated by the relative investment in health and health resources during the greater part of the five decades of the PRC. Urban China enjoyed a more rapid development of health institutions (hospitals, for example) and a higher proportion of urbanites enjoy one of the three forms of medical insurance coverage. In this section, we explore the degree to which peripheral villages have differential access to health and health care.

In order to study this question, we considered as "central" the 59 villages located within a radius of less than 35 Km from the nearest urban center (20.6 percent of the villages we studied); those located farther than 80 Km from the nearest urban center were defined as "peripheral" (57 villages, 19.9 percent of the villages we studied). The economic development of central and peripheral villages in terms of the average per-capita income in the village was not significantly different. On the average, the annual per-capita income of central villages was just 172.5 Yuan higher than that of the villages located on the periphery. The small income advantage of "central" villages, however, masks a considerable variation (Figure 6.6).

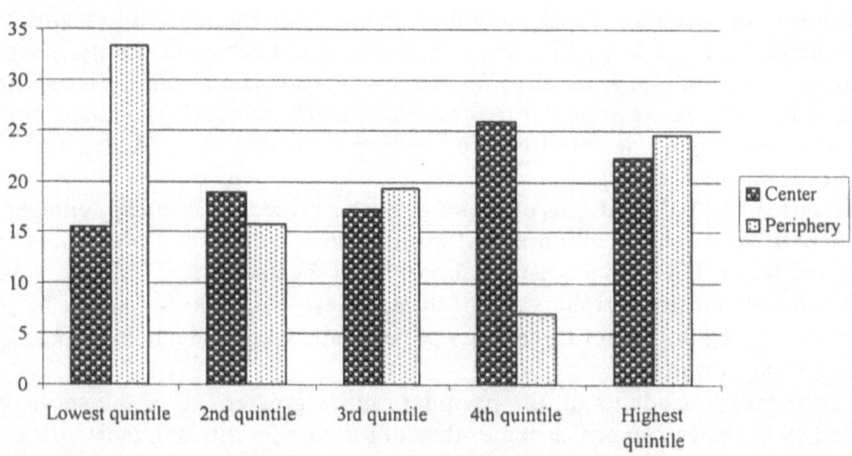

Figure 6.6 Annual per-capita income by village location, HeBei, 1996–1999

Twice as many peripheral as central villages were in the lowest income quintile and their average annual per-capita income fell below 1,800 Yuan. Most of these, 13 out of 19, are located in the mountains. At the same time, 14 of the peripheral villages belong to the wealthiest villages, 5 are located on the prosperous sea-shore, and 9 are close to a county administrative center. These 14 peripheral villages are significantly better off than central villages, enjoying, on the average, 400 Yuan more per-capita income annually than central villages in the same income quintile.

Peripheral villages, however, are smaller in size. The mean number of households in the central villages in our study was 596.5 and the mean number of residents 1,680.7; the respective figures for the villages on the periphery were 310.0 and 1,267.1. These were important determinants of access to health, health care, and local investment in health.

Unlike the social class health gradient, no clear, consistent pattern of health differences that cut across all health measures emerged when center and periphery were compared (Figure 6.7). Nevertheless, farmers in peripheral villages reported more difficulties in fulfilling their daily roles and poorer mental health than inhabitants of the same age, sex, education, and income in villages located closer to urban centers. Symbolic marginality appears to take its toll in China as it does in other societies.

Subjective evaluation of health, of the ability to perform one's daily duties, and self evaluation of mental state may very well be interrelated. It is commonly accepted that the Chinese culture discourages overt expression of depression (Cheng and Hamid, 1996). The cultural emphasis on harmonic relationship between mind and body thus results in an inclination to manifest unfavorable feelings in bodily, somatic symptoms. Living on the periphery geographically and symbolically, far from where decision making is taking place, enhances a sense of powerlessness and impairs the sense of control, both of which are important resources for coping with distress and depression (Turner and Lloyd, 1999).

Congruent with the patterns of seeking help described in Chapter 5, villagers on the periphery consumed more health services than did those who reside in central villages. This was evident in almost all of the health care indicators we used. Farmers on the periphery who felt sick were more likely to seek help, typically visiting the doctor three times per episode, while the modal number in central villages was two.

Furthermore, residents on the periphery made greater use of the services offered by the township health center than of the care facilities in their village. While 38.0 percent of the villagers close to an urban center went to the village and 12.5 percent traveled to the township health center, the corresponding figures on the periphery were 28.5 percent and 20.5 percent, respectively.

Health conditions and dis-eases evoked or intensified by poor mental well-being of the patient are not easily cured, and the cultural constraints on unreserved discussion of negative mood and uncomfortable feelings probably further impede treatment. Patients may find it easier to confide such emotions away from the village, in the more anonymous setting of the township health center. Moreover, a village clinic offers little privacy. As described in Chapter

4, the waiting room in a typical clinic is just the other end of the doctor's office, and not a separate unit. The doctor-patient conversation may take place in the presence of others waiting for their turn. Appointments are rare and when made there is no guarantee that an unscheduled patient or patients will not drop by. Care providers, on the other hand, whose professional training regarding psychosomatic conditions is limited, tend to encourage patients with psychologically etiological health problems to seek help elsewhere.

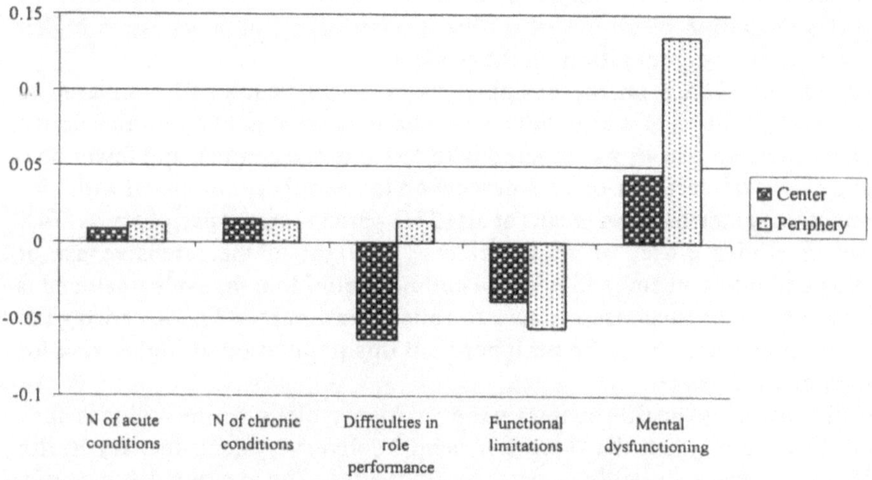

Figure 6.7 Health indicators by village location, HeBei, 1996–1999 (means [a] adjusted for age, sex, education and per-capita income)

[a] A higher score indicates poorer health.

The health services available on the periphery add to the understanding of the differential pattern of consumption of health services in the center and the periphery. Unlike reports from some developing countries and other developed countries, primary health services were more available in the central and the peripheral villages. The mean number of village doctors per 1,000 populations was slightly higher on the periphery: 2.2, compared with 1.9 in the villages located closer to an urban center; the average number of clinics per 1,000 populations was similar in both locations, 1.6 on the periphery and 1.5 in the center. However, given the relatively higher proportion of small villages in remote areas, a higher proportion of villages on the periphery had no health services of their own (12.3 percent compared with 3.4 percent), and were served by clinics located in close-by villages or by the township health facility.

Moreover, the choice of primary clinics in the peripheral villages was more limited than in the center, a result of both their relatively small size and geographical location. In close to half of the central villages, farmers could choose between two or more local clinics, while only some third of the farmers in peripheral villages had such choice. Moreover, twice as many central as peripheral villages were served by more than one type of local clinic: 14 and 7 villages, respectively. Given the differences in the quality of equipment and personnel available in the different facilities as presented in Chapter 4, the unequal distribution of clinics of different ownership limits access to higher quality care for the population on the periphery.

Indeed, the clinics on the periphery were poorly equipped compared to clinics located closer to a city. Fewer medications were held by clinics on the periphery (a mean of 146.9 compared with 195.6 in the center), and fewer held electric means of sterilization (3.3 percent on the periphery compared with 38.2 percent) or any sterilization means at all (28.3 percent on the periphery vs. 74.1 percent in clinics closer to urban centers). In light of the intensive use of injection and infusion embedded in the cultural belief that invasive treatment is the most efficient procedure for cure or relief (see Chapter 4), the shortage in sterilization equipment on the periphery put this population at higher risk for communicable diseases.

While township health centers were relatively close to the villages they served, in keeping with the three-tier health delivery system, tertiary health services were less accessible to peripheral villages. The average distance of a township health center from the villages in HeBei was about 2.1 Km, whether the village was located in the center or on the periphery. However, inhabitants of peripheral villages had to travel twice as far as farmers residing in the center to reach the nearest county hospital. On the average, central villages were located 15.1 Km from the nearest county hospital, while the mean distance of a peripheral village from a county hospital was 29.7 Km.

The village doctors serving the periphery seemed to adapt their practice to the absence of professional support, tending to refrain from referring patients to upper-level health facilities. While village doctors in the center referred more of their patients to township health centers, county hospitals, and city hospitals than village doctors on the periphery.

Summary

In this chapter we examine health inequalities and the equity of the distribution of health services more closely. Focusing on the third purpose of the book, we look at the degree to which health and health care are accessible to all. Following the debate in developed societies, the question of health inequalities and the equity of the distribution of health services is addressed on two levels: individual social class and gender characteristics, and the village economic development and proximity to the center.

As in other developed as well as developing societies, a clear social class gradient of health is present in rural China. Educational achievement and income are both associated with better health status, that is, with less morbidity, disability, and better mental and oral health. The largest health differentials were observed between the least educated and the rest of the rural population. Health status, however, had an almost direct line relationship to annual per-capita income. It appears that in rural China under the 'system of household responsibility', economic prosperity has added to the sense of well-being, far beyond what could be attributed to the prevalence and incidence of health problems.

Despite mass privatization of the health services, social class was not related to access to health care when health status held constant. When in need, the behavior of the poor and the rich, the least- and the better- educated in seeking help was very similar. Similarly, social class did not inhibit or facilitate access to preventive or dental care. There were, however, two exceptions. First, the better-educated were less dependent on health services in general and were more likely to rely on self-care. Second, the rich spent twice as much on their health as did the poor of the same age, sex, and comparable health status. These higher expenses were not the result of differential utilization of health services, but mainly the consequence of using more expensive medication. The elderly stood out in their tendency to take advantage of their higher income in both seeking help in higher level facilities and in the medication they consumed.

Gender health differences took on a different pattern from that commonly observed in post-industrial societies. In North America and Western Europe gender health inequities emerge with adolescence and peak during the productive and reproductive stage of the life-cycle. In rural HeBei, on the other hand, slight gender differences started to appear at age 25–44 and peaked at ages 45–59. Of particular interest is the lack of differences in mental well-being, which is believed to play a significant role in the poor general health of Western women in comparison with men.

Before the economic reforms, China had achieved a relatively high level of equity in the distribution of health services. However, removal of the financial base of the village local authorities following the implementation of the rural reforms in 1979 limited their ability to invest in health and health services. Sanitary conditions and public finances allocated to health, for example, vary according to the economic development of the village, and the poorest villages were less able to support collectively-owned health services or to attract private practitioners. In many of these villages the provincial government has stepped in to ensure that the health needs of these poorer villages are met and hospitals have begun to provide outpatient primary health services. In HeBei Province, for example, the poorest villages enjoyed the highest ratio of clinics and doctors per 1,000 populations. The provision of public health, that is, epidemic control and Mother and Child Health, took on a very similar pattern.

Official regulations stipulate that primary health services be distributed in proportion to the size of the village population. However, our data point to three other basic factors that, apart from population size, determine the distribution of primary health services in rural HeBei: health needs, service demand, and profit-generating opportunities. Thus, the wealthiest villages also enjoyed the services of hospital branch clinics, though they had fewer health needs and were able both to attract private practices and maintain collectively supported health services.

There were more barriers to the provision of health care in city and county hospitals for the population of the periphery, but equal access to primary and township health services. The village doctors seemed to adjust their practice to the distance from a higher level facility, at least with respect to referrals. Inhabitants of peripheral villages also had poorer mental health and more acute health conditions. Consequently, more health services are consumed on the periphery. Additionally, the cultural preference of somatization and reservation in the expression of negative emotions encourages dwellers of the periphery to seek help in the more anonymous township health centers.

Chapter 7

Women's Health

In all societies, women's health is largely dependent on their relative position in the social structure. It is the status of women in society that determines the extent to which they have the power to control their life style, their life chances or opportunities (Weber 1978), and their access to the available social resources. Thus, within the limitations imposed by other social categories, such as social class or ethnicity, women's social status hinders or facilitates the acquisition of individual social resources such as education and property. In a similar way, women's position in the social structure determines the degree to which women may legitimately use all available resources for their own needs. Health and health care are among the important social resources to which women's access is limited in comparison with men in most industrially developed and developing societies (Shuval and Anson, 2000; Arber and Thomas, 2001; Carpenter, 2000).

One mechanism through which the position of women in a society is perpetuated is the process of socialization (Bernandez, 1984; Verbrugge, 1985). During this process, younger generations of both males and females absorb stereotypical attributes of men and women, the "appropriate" behavior, roles, and social standing of each sex. "Atypical" behavior or expectations are likely to be socially defined as deviant and calling for social control, not only by the immediate social environment of the woman in question but by herself as well. Illness is one form of social deviance and medical care is a form of social control. Social attitudes that portray women as inferior to men often result in low self-esteem among women and in legitimate gender discrimination. Both of these, as has been consistently documented, have detrimental health consequences (Anson et al, 1998; Kessler et al, 1999).

These issues are discussed in this chapter. The first section is devoted to the status of women in China. In line with the general structure of this volume, we focus on the changes in the status of rural women during the communist era in general, with special attention to the economic transition of 1979. We then turn to fertility policies, which have very important implications for women's health. The third section of the chapter focuses on reproductive health. The degree to which the access to health and health care of Chinese women, as compared with those of Chinese men, are in concordance with or diverge from those observed in Western societies has been discussed in Chapter 6 as part of the general consideration of health inequalities among social categories.

The Status of Women in Rural China

What is considered today to be the Confucian tradition regarding women's place can be traced to four books written and published between the first century and 1624 (Zhan, 1996). All four were written by women: the earliest book, *Women's Precepts*, was written by Ban Zhao; *Analects for Women* by the sisters Ruoshin and Ruozhao Song (780 – 804); *Instructions for Inner Courts* by the Empress Ren Xiao (1362 – 1418); and *Short Records of Exemplary Women* by Wan Xiang's mother in 1624. That year the four books, published in a single volume, became the leading teachings for women and were incorporated into the Confucian tradition regarding women's status, behavior, and roles. Although all five women were well educated, had considerable accomplishments to their credit, and were highly regarded in the court of their times, they accepted women's inferior position to men and the inferiority of younger women to the older women. In their writings they instructed women to honor the principle of 'triple obedience' – to parents, parents-in-law, and husband – and to abide by the four virtues of women – chastity, manner of speaking, maintenance of proper appearance, and occupations of a woman.

Three of the books were composed for ordinary women as well as for the nobility. The books were written in rhyme and illiterate women could memorize their contents and recite them by heart to their daughters. Well into the 20th century, generations of women were socialized in accordance with these four books. When all-girl schools were established during the second half of the 19th century, the collection was included in the regular curriculum (Zhan, 1996). Folk stories praising women for complying with the virtuous behavior were distributed by the state, further socializing women to accept their patriarchal obligations and sacrifice themselves for their families and society. Moreover, in the absence of a legal code based on concepts of equality before the law prior to the late Qing Dynasty (1644–1912; Rigdon, 1996), the instructions in these books were often referred to as legal obligations of women.

The combination of universal marriage for women, patriclocal living arrangements, and marriage at young age meant that both the productive and the reproductive capability of any daughter would be exploited by her husband's family. Indeed, daughters were considered 'goods on which one loses' in the Confucian tradition (Pearson, 1995; 1996). Daughters could be legitimately sold or exchanged; marriages were arranged; women could initiate divorce only under extreme circumstances (such as rape by male in-law) and could not remarry when widowed.

The emancipation of women from the 'four mountains', that is feudalism, capitalism, colonialism, and male superiority, was an important objective of the Communist revolution (Pearson, 1995; Anson and Haanappel, 1999). The liberation of women from traditional barriers would have served the dual goal of eradicating the Confucian social and cultural order on the one hand and achieving greater social equality on the other. Thus, article 48 of the Constitution of the People's Republic of China provides women with equal rights in all spheres of life, that is political, economic, cultural, social, and within the family. Almost immediately after the 1949 revolution, the first Marriage Law was passed. The law banned concubinage, polygamy, arranged marriages, sale of children, and interference with the remarriage of widows. It set the minimum age for marriage at 18, ensured women of equal rights with respect to employment, equal pay for equal work, ownership of property, inheritance, and divorce.

Yet, the Confucian tradition was slow to disappear, especially in rural areas, where the great majority of the population still resides (Beaver et al., 1995; Johnson, 1985; Shek, 1995; Wolf, 1985). The young revolutionary government did not take active steps to enforce the marriage law. Under the slogan 'women hold up half the sky', it was expected that the patriarchal values, the 'remnants of feudalism', would be dissolved through women's education, paid employment and participation in political life. The patrilocal living arrangements that persisted in rural China further inhibited social change (Benjamin and Brandt, 1995; Weisha, 1998).

Women and Work

Paradoxically, some of the economic policies pursued by the CCP over the years even strengthened the traditional patriarchal system. The process of intensive collectivization at the end of the 1950s is an outstanding example of such measures. The establishment of public dining halls indeed freed women from an important part of the housework, but the already existing patrilineal and patrilocal kin groups were converted into working teams in order to smooth the transition to collectivized rural production. Since the Marriage Law was not systematically enforced, many brigades assigned women to less profitable jobs than men and granted them fewer work points than men, even for the same economic contribution (Entwisle, et al, 1995; Meng and Miller, 1995). Moreover, the work points earned by women were paid to their husband or the male head of the household. In other words, men maintained their superior status and women hardly had more control over the income they generated than before the revolution.

The transition to a socialist market economy in 1979, particularly the 'system of household responsibility' and the rapid development of rural industry, brought about new opportunities for men and women. However, the new opportunities were also accompanied by some of the old ills of traditionalism as well as new ills characteristic of a free market. The development of the rural industry, particularly the township-village enterprises, gave new power to local cadres: job assignment. While wages were decided by company management, most positions were allocated by the local administrators. This new power enabled traditional gender attitudes and stereotypes to affect women's position in the labor force. In some places, women were excluded from the labor force and local leaders played an important part in emphasizing the role of women as supporters, creating a good working environment for their husbands (Beaver et al, 1995). In other regions of rural China, the economic reforms offered women opportunities many were eager to take.

Relatively few women entered rural industry, where they encounter the glass ceiling. They tend to concentrate in the low prestige positions of ordinary workers and are under-represented in the more rewarding positions of administration and management, as is frequently the case with women in industrial societies (Meng and Miller, 1995). Like those of their Western counterparts, women's salaries, on the average, are lower than those of men. In a study conducted by Meng and Miller (1995) in four counties of four provinces in 1985, job segregation accounted for 2–3 percent of the differences in men's and women's wages, but intra-job discrimination accounted for 22.2 percent of the wage differentials. Thomas and Aiping (2000) reported in their 1991 study of two counties that women's income was 23–31 percent lower than that of their husbands.

Evidence of a segregated labor market was also observed among the village doctors who participated in our study in rural HeBei. Relatively few women (21.1 percent) practiced privately; 48.3 percent were salaried employees in clinics owned by government hospitals. The income from their medical practice was also lower than that of their male colleagues – 3926.7 Yuan compared with 4838.4 Yuan of male doctor. Women village doctors earned less than men in each type of practice, though the average annual income gap between male and female doctors varied from 961.7 Yuan in group practice and 896.3 Yuan for private practitioners to 728.3 Yuan for salaried employees.

Gender inequality in the economic sphere led the government to amend the Marriage Law and to pass the Law for Protection of Women's Rights and Interests in 1992 (Pearson, 1995). An intensive campaign aimed at educating women about their rights followed this legislation, yet the degree to which the legislation brought about social change and enhanced gender equality in the work place is an open question.

As men entered the developing rural industry women became the primary farmers, supported by the central and local government. Since 1989, for example, campaigns titled 'double learning', that is learning general knowledge and specific skills, and 'double competitions' of achievements and contributions have been promoted in rural China (Yu, 1996). By 1995, 120 million women took part in at least one of these campaigns. 90 million were trained in agriculture techniques and more than one million households, managed primarily by women, were recognized as 'scientific and technological demonstration households'.

Taking advantage of the vocational training offered to them, many women combined farming with side-lines, such as greenhouse agriculture and horticulture, with significantly enhanced family income as the result. Furthermore, women's specialization in agriculture affected the division of economic decision making in the household (Zhang, 1998). Women whose husbands left agriculture for services or industry made most decisions related to farming, from what and how to cultivate to where and when to market the farm products, etc. The patrilocal living arrangement enabled women to share farm work, housework, and child care and to gain more control over their work schedule.

Education

The CCP took special measures to eradicate illiteracy and provide education for all (Chapter 1). It has been suggested that under the 'system of household responsibility' children's productive capacity once again became economically important and that girls were more likely than boys to be deprived of education (Pearson, 1996). Moreover, with a lack of nursery schools and the emerging pattern of neolocal living arrangements (see Chapter 8), daughters were more likely to be engaged in child care, attending their younger siblings (Wang et al, 1996). These arguments are often supported by the higher prevalence of illiteracy among women than among men. In 1998, women comprised 71.3 percent of all the illiterate in the PRC and 22.6 percent of the women aged 15 and above were illiterate or semi-illiterate, compared with 9.0 percent of the men of the same age (China Yearbook, 1999).

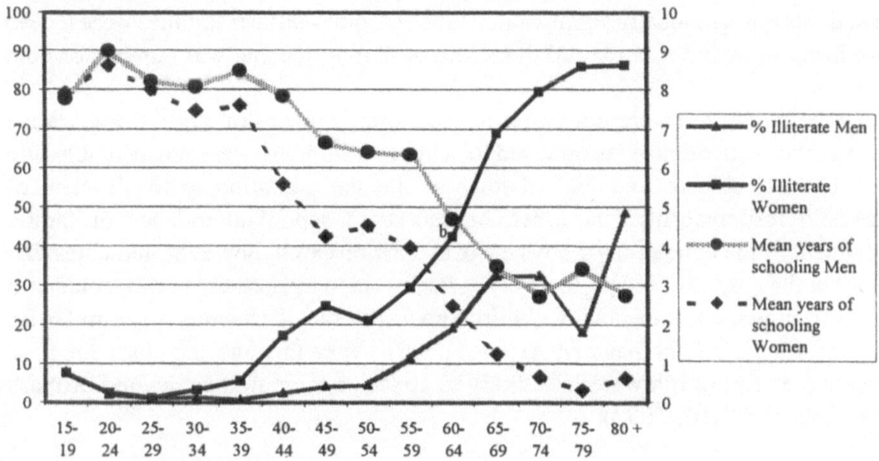

Figure 7.1 Illiteracy and mean years of schooling by age and sex, HeBei, 1996–1999

At the same time, according to the official statistics, primary school enrollment in the late 1990s reached 100 percent for boys and girls and the proportion of females in primary education increased from 44.6 percent in 1980 to 47.6 percent in 1998, parallel to the relative proportion of females in the population (China Yearbook, 1999; The World Bank, 2000). Furthermore, during the same years the proportion of women in regular secondary schools increased from 39.6 percent to 45.5 percent and from 23.4 percent to 37.3 percent in institutions of higher education.

The data, however, do not differentiate between rural and urban residents, nor do they consider the cohort effect. Our survey in HeBei Province showed that the high rate of illiteracy among women is a product of the aging of the population and the higher proportion of women among the elderly. As shown in Figure 7.1, more than 70 percent of the women aged 65 and older, women who were in their late teens at the time the PRC was established, never went to school, compared with 32 percent of men of the same age. Furthermore, the average number of years of schooling was similar for men and women aged 15–25, but diverged consistently with age thereafter. Our data survey, however, was not designed to detect whether or not children, boys or girls, were taken out of school during the intensive agriculture season.

Nonetheless, in the 288 villages we surveyed, school attendance by children was far lower than the officially declared 100 percent enrollment. In our study, 19.4 percent of the boys and 21.4 percent of the girls between 7 and 15 years of age, the age of compulsory education, did not attend school. The proportion of children of both sexes not attending school declined significantly with age, from three in five of the 7 year old children to one in ten of the 15 years old. At all ages, the 0.5–2.5 percent more girls than boys did not attend school, though the difference was not consistent by age and was not statistically significant. Children from wealthier families were indeed more likely to attend school, and the effect on family income was similar for both sexes.

All these children were born after the economic reforms of 1979. Comparative data on school attendance, as opposed to school enrollment, were not available. We were thus not able to examine whether or not the transition to the 'system of household responsibility' increased or decreased school attendance or family investment in the education of boys or girls. Past research, however, indicates that this is not the case. According to an estimate provided by mothers in two counties in 1987, the annual costs of raising children up to the age of 15 were very similar for boys and for girls (Thomas and Aiping, 2000). After this age the costs for boys increased, as rural girls were less likely to continue their studies beyond primary school (Yu and Sarri, 1997).

Women in Politics

Woman's participation in the political life of the PRC has increased dramatically since the liberation in 1949. Nevertheless, as in many industrial countries and the former Soviet Union, the part played by women in all political institutions is far smaller than their proportion of the population. The share of women in the National People's Congress increased from 12.0 percent in the first congress of 1954 to 22.6 percent in the fourth congress (1975), but then stagnated at 21–22 percent. In the Ninth National People's Congress of 1998 women comprised just 21.8 percent (China Yearbook, 1999). Furthermore, In the first half of the 1990s, women comprised only 14.1 percent of the total membership of the Chinese Communist Party, while just 13.5 percent of the participants in the Eighth and the Ninth Chinese People's Political Consultative Conference were women.

Political executive functions were also largely dominated by men. In 1991, 6.5 percent of the ministers and vice ministers were women and a similar proportion of women was to be found among governors or deputy governors on the provincial level. As in many Western countries, women have a larger share in local political institutions (Herzog, 1994). It has been estimated that women's share among the local cadres is close to one-third (Pearson, 1995).

Today, Chinese women are organized in the All Women Federation. Every village and urban work unit has a woman representing the federation. Local representatives take part in decisions regarding the distribution of the birth quota (see below), job assignments, women's education and training, and mass mobilization during specific campaigns.

Women in the Family

As described in the introduction to this chapter, the Marriage Law of 1950 was intended to liberate women from the burden of the Confucian traditional patriarchalism within the family. Traditionally, uxorilocal marriages were arranged, the woman married at a young age (usually upon the advent of puberty) and joined her spouse's family in her village according the patrilocal rules. The degree to which the Communist regime brought about social change in the relationships within the family has been subject to considerable debate (Pearson, 1995, 1996). Most scientific evidence, however, is to be found in studies of the fertility changes in China. While this body of research will be discussed in the next section, its findings regarding family relations are presented here.

The patterns of age at marriage have changed steadily for women and men since the revolution (Riley and Gardner, 1997). The average age of women at marriage has increased by 0.7 years per decade since 1940 and reached a mean of 19.8 in 1960. In 1980, the mean age of marriage for women was 23.1, a result of the population control policy which banned marriages before the age of 23. However, after the relaxation of this policy, the old patterns of teenage marriages for women were not restored. During the late 1980s, women married between the ages of 21 and 23 and, like patterns observed in industrial societies, the age of marriage of recent cohorts is related to the socio-demographic characteristics of women. Thus, rural women tend to marry at a younger age than urbanites, the better educated later than those with less education, and farmers earlier than those employed in non-farming occupations. According to the data collected in rural HeBei in 1996–1999, only one in five women was married at age 20–24, but by the age of 25–29, 92.8 percent of the women were married.

The age of men at marriage also changed. Before liberation, not only did men marry at an older age than women, but the range of ages at marriage was considerably larger for men than for women. After independence, the ages at marriage of men and women converged, particularly with regard to the range. Indeed, in rural HeBei, 86.8 percent of the men married between the age of 25 to 29.

The current age of men and women at marriage seems to reflect a more profound social transition than the mere fertility-related policy. First, arranged marriages have been on the decline at least since the massive collectivization during the 'great leap forward' in the late 1950s (Thomas and Aiping, 2000). The abolition of local free markets, along with brothels and gambling houses, has eliminated the traditional meeting places of adult men. This, in combination with strict migration policy, has led to a decline in inter-village communication, limiting the opportunities for arranged marriages of offspring. A 1991 survey (Yu, 1996) showed that at that time most young persons chose their spouses by themselves, though this pattern was slower to develop in the countryside than in the cities. In both cases it took root faster among men than among women. Nearly all urban respondents (95.6 percent of the men and 94.7 percent of the women) made their own marriage decisions, compared with 79.0 percent of rural men and 70.9 percent of rural women.

Closely associated with the limited inter-village communication was the erosion of the taboo on village endogamy and the pattern of uxorilocal marriages (Thomas and Aiping, 2000). Although patrilocal living arrangements persisted, they took on a different form. The husband's family provided the new couple with a house, often built in the same yard as his parents' house. The new bride was thus not detached from social support networks, that is, her own family and friends who, like her and her spouse, are now more likely to stay in their birth-village.

Moreover, the prevalence of stem families is declining (Ming et al, 1995; Zhao, 2000). As will be illustrated in Chapter 8, the data we collected in rural HeBei suggested that both the elderly and the young couples preferred independent living and stuck to this arrangement whenever possible. Some half of the young married couples in our sample, 45.3 percent of the 20–24 age group, started their life together by living in the household with the husband's parents, but once their own living unit was completed they moved out. By the age of 25–29, only one in four couples was living in a stem family household.

Findings from several studies suggest that mothers-in-law still enjoy considerable power over their daughters-in-law (Holroyd et al, 1997; Anson and Haanappel, 1999). Studies of fertility patterns have consistently found that women living with their in-laws tend to comply with the traditional preference for sons and progress to higher parity significantly more often than women in neolocal households (Larsen, 1990; Cooney et al, 1991, 1994; Li, 1995).

Yet, these same studies also suggested that communication within the marital dyad has been improving steadily (Riley and Gardner, 1997). One indicator to such improvement is the fact that the great majority of women gave birth to their first child during the first year of marriage. The 1991 study reported by Yu (1996) provided a more direct measure of dyadic relationships as it explored how decisions are made in several spheres of family life. In their study, most decisions were made jointly by husbands and wives: joint decisions regarding fertility were made by 79.1 percent of the urban respondents and 82.9 percent of their rural counterparts; joint monetary decisions were made by 81.0 percent of the rural couples and by 76.3 percent of urbanites.

As with the patterns observed in industrial societies, the division of housework and child care in China is highly gendered (Lai, 1995). However, it appears that inequality in family work was not related to distress and poor mental health among Chines women, unlike their Western counterparts (Lai, 1995; Anson and Sun, 2002). In the countryside, household chores and child care were integrated into the farming routine and specialization by women in farming work allowed them to regulate and control their work schedules.

There is little doubt that the status of adult women in the PRC has improved, although equality has not yet been reached (Ren, 1994, 1996). It is the status of widows and female infants and children that remains unclear. Despite the legal prohibition on interference with remarriages, widows are not likely to change their marital status (Li, 1998; Jiang, 1995). According to the 1990 census, 60 percent of the old-old men (that is, more than 75 years of age) were married, but only one in ten of the women of that age were. Although these findings also reflected the greater longevity of women as compared with men and consequently a limited marriage market, the possibility exists that traditional attitudes toward remarriage encouraged women to retain their status as widows.

An unusual sex ratio at all ages has been observed in the PRC since the one-child policy was implemented in 1979 (Riley and Gardner, 1997). This phenomenon, which has been labeled 'the missing girls' phenomenon (Ren, 1995; Riley, 1996; Xu et al, 1994), seems to imply that daughters are still considered 'goods on which one loses'. Analyses of the fertility surveys conducted in China throughout the 1980s, together with the census of 1990, demonstrated higher male-to-female ratios than those in other societies, both industrial and developing, including Asian societies. Particularly alarming was the high sex ratio at birth, especially in higher birth orders, and its increase during the 1980s (Table 7.1).

Table 7.1 Reported sex ratio at birth in china, selected years 1982–1989*

Year	1st	2nd	3rd	4th	All births
1982	106.5	105.0	109.4	111.9	107.2
1983	107.5	107.2	108.2	109.3	107.7
1984	102.1	113.6	112.6	122.2	108.3
1985	106.1	116.1	114.3	121.5	111.2
1986	105.2	116.8	123.2	124.7	112.1
1987	106.7	112.6	118.9	121.2	110.8
1989	104.9	120.9	124.6	131.7	113.8

**Source*: Zeng et al, 1993.

While the sex ratio observed for first-born children was comparable to that reported elsewhere in the world, higher parities had an exceptional proportion of boys, resulting in a high male/female ratio for all births (Zeng et al, 1993; Anderson and Silver, 1995). Moreover, in second parity a higher than expected proportion of boys has been born since 1984, when the one-child policy was relaxed and allowance made for a second child under particular conditions (a detailed history of the population policy will be discussed in the next section).

These findings were interpreted in light of the traditional preference for sons, particularly in the rural areas. Sons are needed to carry on the family name and, as will be presented in Chapter 8, are the main source of support for the elderly in the countryside. The Confucian tradition emphasizes the responsibility of sons to support their aging parents, and the scarcity of an old age pension in rural China compels seniors to depend on their offspring. The obligation of children to provide for their elderly parents was further strengthened by a series of laws, including the Marriage Law of 1980 and the Inheritance Law of 1985. While these laws apply to all children, male and female, biological and adopted, and the decline in uxorilocal marriages enables daughters as well as sons to accept this responsibility, only sons assure the continuation of the family name.

The findings of the fertility studies and the 'missing girls' seemed to support the argument for preference for sons. Several studies have shown that the one-child policy was more likely to be violated when the first-born was a girl, though the sex of the sibling(s) was not the strongest predictor (Larsen, 1990; Cooney and Li, 1994). The stronger influence on fertility decisions was the degree to which the couple was under official social control and thus ran a greater risk of being penalized for an unauthorized birth (Li and Cooney, 1993; Cooney and Li, 1994). It came to be generally accepted that when freed from social control, couples would choose to continue to produce children until they had at least one male offspring.

However, studies conducted throughout the 1990s showed that having a son was not necessarily the ultimate fertility goal and that Chinese couples are interested in having girls too. First, there were indications that the ideal family size in the early 1990s was considered to be two children, one of each sex (Greenhalgh et al, 1994; Riley and Gardner, 1997). Second, Li (1995) found that not only mothers of daughters were inclined to give another birth; mothers of two sons were also more likely to progress to a third parity than women who had children of both sexes. Although Li concludes that these couples desired a large family, it is very possible that they simply wanted to have a girl as well as boys.

This suggestion was further supported by the findings reported by two other studies. In their two-counties study, Thomas and Aiping (2000) found a very weak, if any at all, preference for sons, mainly because of the high cost of marriage for sons and the favourable economic prospects of daughters. Greenhalgh et al (1994), who returned to the three villages six years after the fertility study of 1987, found that a considerable change in family attitudes had taken place since then. In 1987, the vast majority indeed wanted two children, one of each sex, but would settle for two sons. Six years later, they still wanted two children; however, two sons, or three children were considered too costly to raise and marry.

Still, the sex ratio registered in the PRC and reported by participants in the fertility surveys revealed a social process which resulted in a shortage of girls running into the millions, though the real number is still under debate (Banister, 1994). So is the question of what happened to the girls that are missing. Observers of Chinese fertility provided four plausible explanations, but none of them can account for all of the missing girls and all are subject to severe criticism. The first explanation is the practice of sex-specific abortion, similar to those observed in India and South Korea (Anderson and Silver, 1995).

It is doubtful, however, that selective abortions could account for many of the missing girls. In order to achieve the sex ratio of 106 observed in most societies and among first born children in China, more than half of the female fetuses would have to have been deliberately aborted (Wen, 1993). Most township health centers (those more accessible to the rural population) are not equipped with the technology to detect the sex of the fetus (Hesketh and Zhu, 1997a) and in any case sex detection is forbidden by law, as are sex-selective abortions. Most important, an unusually high sex ratio at birth was not observed among urbanites and the better educated social groups that have greater access to modern technology (Anderson and Silver, 1995). Finally, because more than 80 percent of rural second and higher order births were unauthorized (Cooney et al, 1991), it is hard to believe that women sought ultrasonic services that would have exposed their condition and submitted them to pressure to terminate the pregnancy. Although coercive abortions have been abandoned in recent years, women carrying an unauthorized baby experience considerable pressure to terminate the pregnancy even beyond the first trimester (Hesketh, and Zhu, 1997b; Rigdon, 1996). If having a son was indeed a primary goal of childbearing, it would have been much more reasonable to take such action during the first pregnancy.

The second explanation offered for the 'missing girls' phenomenon is illegal adoption (Riley and Gardner, 1997). The number of legally adopted girls is much higher than that for boys and is believed to be even higher among those not officially adopted. It has been estimated that twice as many girls as boys were given up for adoption, but the data available to date do not allow a valid analysis (Wen, 1993). Informal adoption may thus provide some answers to where the missing girls are (Anderson and Silver, 1995), although it may be assumed that childless families are also likely to prefer boys to girls.

Direct and indirect female infanticide has been suggested to account for the missing girls. Infanticide was practiced before the revolution, as is evident from the sex ratio of higher than 110 males per 100 females in the 1930 and 1940 cohorts observed in the 1990 census (Xu et al, 1994). The practice was legally banned by the CCP and largely ceased during the 1950s. The 1953 and 1964 census records indicated a 'normal' sex ratio of 104.9 and 103.8 respectively. The increased sex ratios during the 1980s, a period of strict population control, were interpreted by some as a revival of ancient practices through deprivation and neglect of female infants and children.

During this period, infant and child mortality declined dramatically, but the decline in boys 'mortality was greater than in girls' mortality. According to the analyses of Xu et al (1994), infant mortality declined by 26.4 percent for males but only by 9.5

percent for females. Based on the in-depth fertility surveys of 1985 and 1987, Ren (1995) found that the curve tracing a girl's chances of surviving infancy and childhood flattened after 1979, while that for boys continued to rise. He concluded that female infants were neglected in comparison with male infants. Moreover, in the 1990s, male and female infant mortality rates started to converge, which, judging by modal life tables, is not expected to happen before infant mortality declines to 20–27 deaths per 1,000 live births (Banister et al, 2000).

The decline in childhood mortality was similar for both sexes, 41.3 percent for boys and 44.1 percent for girls in the 1980s. Analyzing the childhood mortality reported by the Two per Thousand Survey of Fertility and Birth Control 1988, Choe et al (1995) found evidence that discrimination against daughters seemed to have taken place in the second or later birth in families with only daughters. Banister et al (2000) found indications of female discrimination at ages 0–2 in the 1990s, but thereafter girls were treated better than ever before. The proportion of 'missing girls' resulting from neglect, however, is unknown.

Finally, it has been suggested that the overwhelming majority of the 'missing girls' are not missing at all, but were not officially registered and, more significantly, not reported in the fertility history provided by mothers (Bogg, 1998). Bogg (1998) conducted a household survey in six counties in the fall of 1995 and compared the number of female children in the households with both the official registrar and the fertility history provided by the mothers interviewed. In five of the six counties, the sex ratio of children under 18 years of age derived from the household survey was lower than the sex ratio calculated from the official data. Indeed, the size of the household observed during the interviews was larger than the average household size officially registered in these counties. Moreover, the number of girls living in the household exceeded the number provided by the mothers in their fertility history by more than 22 percent. No such discrepancy was found with regard to the number of boys.

In our opinion, the atypically high sex ratio at birth observed in rural China is due in great part to under-registration and under-reporting in fertility surveys. Since parents are responsible for the registration of their newborn they might have avoided registration of a second daughter in order to keep their options open for a third or higher parity. There were no direct benefits to registration, failing to do so did not involve any immediate penalty. It is also possible that the village authorities and local cadres subtly approved of such practice. Not only did they sympathize with the desires of their fellow farmers for larger families, but any violation of the population planning policy in their village might have subjected them to criticism by officials or placed them at risk of material penalty. The omission of female births from the pregnancy history provided by mothers could have been the result of their suspicion that, despite reassurance by the researcher, details about unauthorized pregnancies would reach the authorities.

Nevertheless, the cost of education and immunizations was higher for unregistered children than for the registered ones (Bogg, 1998). The inclination to avoid registering second and higher birth order girls rather than boys could indicate that parents were more concerned about the health and the education of male offspring than of females. The life chances of girls missing from the official records, in the Weberian sense, might thus have been seriously hampered.

In summary, there is evidence that the status of adult women in China has been improving ever since the Communists came to power in 1949 (Ren, 1994, 1996). Women have gained access to education, which has positively affected their health and that of their children. The decline in arranged, uxorilocal marriages and the increase in the number of nuclear families has improved their status within the family. While most rural women were economically active far before the CCP came into power, including the operation of 'sidelines' such as raising animals and selling handicrafts, the economic reforms and the developing rural industry that followed have given women extensive control of the family farm (Entwisle, et al, 1995). The mortality gains of adult women (Banister et al, 2000) and the unique pattern of gender health equality in rural China (Anson and Sun, 2002) clearly reflects women's access to general coping resources.

However, like women in many post industrial societies, full equality is still far ahead. Like Western women, Chinese women experience job segregation, encounter the glass ceiling, and are paid less than men for their work. Labor force segregation is accompanied by gendered division of family work, with women performing most of the housework and child care. The gender gap seemed to be particularly large during infancy and childhood on the one hand and at old age on the other. We now turn to explore whether the transition in women's status was related to reproductive health and health-related behavior of rural women.

Reproductive Health

Family Planning

In all societies, decisions concerning reproduction are influenced by cultural attitudes, religious beliefs, and social and political institutions (Shuval and Anson, 2000). The effect of cultural attitudes toward the ideal composition of the family on reproductive behavior in the PRC, and the consequences for life chances that this behavior had for girls, presented above, are just one example. Moreover, all societies attempt to influence decisions concerning the fertility of men and women, often using the political power of the state or that of a particular elite. In some industrial societies, France, Israel, and Sweden for example, social benefits policies are employed in order to encourage fertility. The orthodox Jewish and Catholic establishments are social institutions which use the power of local spiritual leaders to maximize fertility in their communities. Abortions are regulated in the Jewish and Christian religions as well as by civil law in most Western societies. In some developing countries social resources are allocated to control population growth. The PRC, which had over one-fifth of the world's population in 1998 in a territory the size of the USA is no exception.

Let us present a brief history of the population policies implemented in the PRC since liberation. Upon establishment, most leaders of the CCP believed that a large population was necessary to augment China's strength, boost economic growth, and ensure its defensive power. Contraceptives were rare and abortions, though legal since 1953, were made available only to women at health risk or those women whose birth spacing might hamper breast-feeding of both children (Rigdon, 1996). Health professionals were instructed to turn down applications for pregnancy termination by couples with fewer than four children and contemporary propaganda emphasized the 'health, work, and study' risks of abortions.

With the cessation of war following the success of the revolution, increased agriculture production, and the decline in mortality the PRC indeed experienced accelerated population growth. Natural growth rates increased from 1.6 percent in 1949 to 2.5 percent in 1954 (China Population Yearbook, 1997). However, the slowing down of the economy in the mid 1950s brought some central leaders in the CCP to reconsider the population policy (Larsen, 1990). The first effort to restrain the natural growth of the population was initiated in 1956 and lasted for two years, until the beginning of 'the great leap forward'. The effectiveness of this early program was inhibited by lack of a political consensus on the one hand and limited resources, including reliable contraceptives, on the other. The economic hardship and the famine that followed 'the great leap forward' restrained the annual growth of the population, up to a negative growth of 0.5 percent in 1960. When the crisis was over, however, natural population growth rates started to increase rapidly, exceeding the pre-famine rates.

A second attempt to limit the growth of the population was launched in 1962 (Riley and Gardner, 1997). The government called on the people to postpone marriage, to increase the interval between births, and to have fewer children. Contraceptives and abortions were made available to all but the health services in rural China were not equipped to apply the program nationwide. The government was thus forced to concentrate its efforts among the smaller urban sector of the population. The program was interrupted by the political and social unrest of the Cultural Revolution, to be relaunched in 1971 under the slogan 'wan, xi, shao' – marriage (later), births (more widely spaced), fewer (children).

The health personnel, physical facilities, and birth-control technological resources available in 1971 permitted a more successful program. The expansion of the health services deep into rural China during the Cultural Revolution (Chapter 1), allowed the government to reach almost all of the population. Health education programs introduced the concept of 'birth planning' and the need to limit population growth below or close to replacement level in order to increase the standard of living, eradicate poverty, and advance the status of women (Yu, 1996). Age at marriage was set at 23 for women and the people were encouraged to avoid more than two children with the slogan 'one is best, at most two, never a third'.

Although these measures seemed to be quite successful, as the average number of children born to each woman fell from 5.9 in 1949 to 2.7 in 1979 (Hethketh and Zhu,

1997b), the level was still too high for the social, economic, and political agenda of Deng Xiao Ping's regime (White, 1994). They wished to take China through the 'four modernizations', that is, modernization of agriculture, science and technology, industry, and national defense, promising the people economic prosperity by the year 2000. Most leaders of the CCP believed that it was a feasible goal if the population did not exceed 1.2 billion. But the baby boomers born after the 'great leap forward' and the famine were entering childbearing age and stricter control was necessary. The one-child policy was launched in 1979.

In 1980, the new Marriage Law increased the legal age for marriage by two years for both men and women, although, interestingly, the new legal age was set at 20 for women and 22 for men, three years below the 1971 regulation (Zeng, 1996). The law required every couple to practice birth control and a birth quota system was put into effect (Cooney and Li 1994; Li, 1995). Each year, the State Family Planning Commission set the annual national population target and limited the number of babies to be born in the different provinces, municipalities, and autonomous regions. These quotas were further applied downwards along administrative lines to reach the leaders of work units in cities and heads of the villages in the countryside. In collaboration with the family planning cadres the local officials were responsible for selecting the families who would be permitted to have a child that year and to ensure that 'remedial measures' were implemented to terminate unauthorized pregnancies.

To increase compliance, a 'one-child certificate' was issued upon request to women who committed themselves to the one-child policy (Cooney and Li, 1994; Larsen, 1990). Urban certificate holders were generally granted some financial assistance while the child was growing up (up to the age of 14 or 15), priority in job assignment and housing allocation, and favorable treatment for the child in the education and health systems. Much smaller benefits were granted to rural certificate holders, who were entitled to a greater portion of the collectives' grains, and/or a private plot of land. Not surprisingly, the one-child certificate was much more popular in the cities than in the countryside. In HeBei Province, for example, 4.3 times more urban than rural women accepted the certificate (Table 7.2). Rural acceptance rates decreased further after the implementation of the 'system of household responsibility'. Decollectivation left the local cadres with few resources to distribute among certificate holders. Their ability to do so depended on the level of the economic development of the village and the industrial job opportunities it had to offer (Greenhalgh et al, 1994).

Since 1980, unauthorized births are also penalized. Again, there is great regional variation in the implementation of the policy but, taking HeBei Province as an example, the families of some half of the women who violated the one-child policy have been fined, 15.3 percent of them more than once (Li, 1995). The fines are relatively heavy, with the average fine mounting to about one-quarter of the mean annual family income in the province. The well to do farmers can, of course, bear the costs, but many families have been in debt for years and some have had to sell belongings or had their property confiscated.

The local cadres were also under pressure to meet the quota dictated by the central government. They were rewarded when successful in preventing births in excess of the quota, but sanctioned when failed. Penalties varied by region, ranging from criticism to fines and sometimes loss of jobs (Greenhalgh et al, 1994; Li, 1995).

Table 7.2 Changes in certificate acceptance and second live birth for Hebei Province before and after 1984*

	Rural	Urban	Total
Initial acceptance rate (%)			
1979 – 1983	16.2	69.8	26.0
1984 – 1988	5.8	49.6	11.3
Of initial acceptors – % having second live birth			
1979 – 1983	15.5	3.6	9.7
1984 – 1988	23.7	4.3	13.3
Of all women at risk – % having second live birth			
1979 – 1983	41.8	16.8	37.3
1984 – 1988	46.7	15.4	40.0
Of certificate holders with a second live birth % who received permission			
1979 – 1983	11.2	36.4	15.8
1984 – 1988	51.1	53.8	51.5
Of all women with a second live birth % who received permission			
1979 – 1983	7.5	16.1	8.2
1984 – 1988	15.1	25.1	15.9

**Source*: Cooney et al, 1991

The one-child policy encountered enormous resistance, especially from rural families (Cooney et al, 1991; Cooney and Li, 1994; White, 1994). Estimates based on the fertility surveys of the 1980s show that some half of the rural women had an unauthorized birth. The one-child certificate mainly decreased the odds of a second birth in the cities, where the leaders of the work units had more power and control than the rural cadres. In 1983 the government started to require the sterilization of couples with two or more children and abortions for women carrying an unauthorized embryo (Larsen, 1990). In the two counties studied by Thomas and Aiping (2000) in 1993, the prevalence of sterilization was low among mothers of one child (14 percent for mothers of a girl and 22 percent for mothers of a boy), 71–90 percent for mothers of two children, and 100 percent for mothers of three. In most places, mothers of one child were provided with reversible contraceptives, primarily intra-uterine devices, realizing that the policy, which was declared to be a temporary measure, might change.

Public resistance and noncompliance led the government to publish Document 7 in 1984. This document was meant 'to open a small hole in order to close a large one' and allowed two children under certain conditions. The most important were allowing ethnic minorities fertility levels that would maintain the current size of their population and a second child in rural 'daughter only' families, under the condition of a mandatory four-year interval between births. In the absence of old age pensions (see Chapter 8), families who had lost their only child and families whose first born was severely handicapped were also permitted a second birth. Several entitlements in the document represent the government's acquiescence in the matter of the traditional desire to carry on the name of the family (Li, 1995). For example, a couple could receive permission for a second birth if there were no male offspring among the husband's brothers.

The document regenerated considerable debate among Western women's movements. The main argument was that by allowing one-daughter families a second chance to bear a male child the Chinese Communist government actually institutionalized the lower value traditionally attributed to women (Cooney and Li, 1994). Paradoxically, similar arguments were voiced by conservatives in industrial societies in opposition to laws and regulations intended to ensure equal opportunity to socially disadvantaged groups, such as women and minorities.

Fertility

The changes in the permissible fertility level in the PRC reflect the social, economic and political processes it has undergone since the 1949 revolution. Fertility rates did not increase after the establishment of the PRC, despite the pro-fertility policy and, with some fluctuations, have declined with relative consistency since then. As described in Chapter 1, the process was slower among rural women than among their urban counterparts and in 1982 the total number of children per woman was 2.9 and 1.5, respectively (Larsen, 1990). The degree to which the decline was a result of the policies carried out over the years, particularly the one-child policy, has raised considerable debate among demographers (for a thorough presentation of this debate see Riley and Gardner, 1997).

A detailed assessment of the one-child policy is beyond the scope of this volume. Let us just say that there is sufficient evidence that the policy was successful in the cities, where the work units are the main agencies of social control (Li and Cooney, 1993). The level of success in rural families is still an unsettled question. The magnitude of unregistered and unreported daughters presented by Bogg (1998), and the analysis of the 1988 Two Per Thousand National Fertility Survey of HeBei Province raise serious doubts regarding the effectiveness of these programs (Cooney et al, 1991; Cooney and Li, 1994; Li and Cooney, 1993; Li, 1995). As presented in Table

7.2, nearly half of the rural women of reproductive age had had a second live birth, but only a small minority of them with the approval of the authorities. The difference in the number of women who progressed to a second parity did not change much between 1979–1983, the period of a strict one-child policy, and after the implementation of Document 7 in 1984: 41.8 percent progressed to a second birth in the earlier period, 46.7 percent in the later. The percentage of authorized progression did in fact double, but still remained extremely low – 15.1 percent.

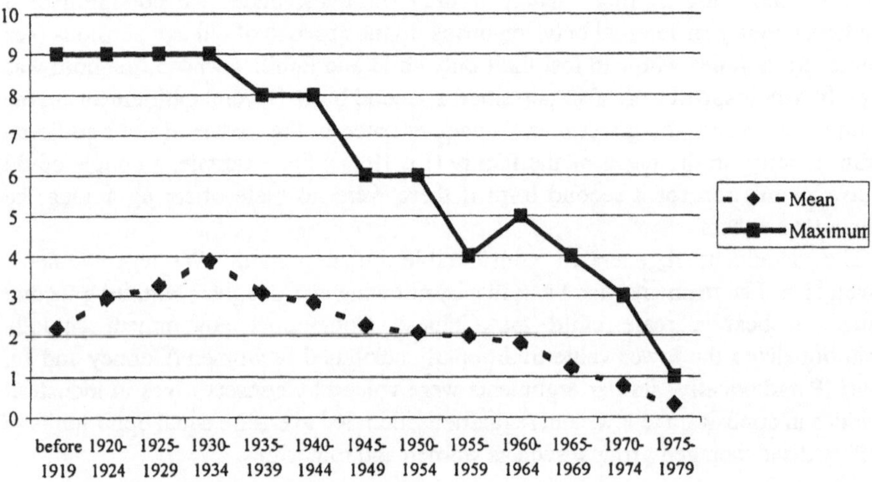

Figure 7.2 Mean and maximum number of children ever born by mother's year of birth, HeBei, 1996–1999

Yet, there is no doubt that fertility declined in both rural and urban settings, even if the rate of decline in the cities was greater (see Table 1.6). This was clearly observed in the data we collected in rural HeBei (Figure 7.2): an increase in the mean number of children born among all women of reproductive age between 1925 and 1929, following the revolution, but a steady decline thereafter. It was not just the mean number of births that declined, but the absolute number as well. Women who at the time of the research were 45–49 years old had given birth to an average of 2.26 children, as compared with women of their mothers' generation, the 70–74 year olds, who had each given birth to 4.38 children on the average. The maximum parity was six and nine births, respectively. The trend is not unique to rural HeBei, and very similar figures were reported by Schultz and Zeng (1995). In our data, fertility declined with no specific dip around the implementation of new policy(ies), a fact noted by other observers as well.

Other social processes were at work, similar to those which contributed to the increase in the minimum permissible age for marriage. One such process was the opportunity for women to accumulate resources, that is, obtain education and enter non-farming occupations (Larsen, 1990). In rural HeBei, literate women of all ages gave birth to fewer children, women in non-agricultural occupations had fewer children than women farmers of the same age.

Change in the status of women within the family also contributed to the decline in fertility. The transition from stem family to neolocality freed women from the control of the extended family, allowing them to make their own fertility and health decisions (Cooney and Li, 1994; Yu, 1996; Cooney et al, 1991; Ren, 1996; Larsen, 1990). All analyses of the fertility surveys conducted in the 1980s consistently indicated that women who lived with parents-in-law for long periods of time progressed to second and third birth more often than women who lived with their husbands only.

Modernization, and the modernization of agriculture in particular, not only decrease the need for child labor but also increased the value of children's education (Greenhalgh et al, 1994). Farmers realized that greater income is generated through modern technology than through intensive agricultural labor. Education became important not only because it increased the child's chances for opting out of agriculture but also because it enabled him or her to become a more efficient farmer. Furthermore, in many villages the amount of arable land available began to decrease, either because of the need to allocate land to newly-wed youngsters or because of development programs. Under these conditions, propaganda for fewer but 'better quality' children and against the risk of over-exploitation of resources resulting from a high rate of fertility became prominent and serious.

Maternal Care

As described in Chapter 1, the CCP was committed to improving the health of the population by investing considerable resources in public health, with particular emphasis on Mother and Child Health (MCH). Indeed, maternal mortality declined below the level generally observed in developing countries (Chapter 2). Despite the urban/rural discrepancy and the gap between rich and poor regions, Hesketh and Zhu (1997a) conclude that "perhaps no other country in the world has achieved so much, so quickly, for the health of women and children" (p. 1898).

Much of the decline in maternal mortality was the result of the increase in the standard of living, particularly improved nutrition, personal hygiene, safe water supply, and the decline in infectious diseases. Some of the decline was due to improved access to health care. The three-tier system was applied to MCH, providing prenatal, postpartum, neonatal care and family planning services in most villages. Village level health providers were instructed and supervised by township health centers, whose work was overseen by county hospitals. Most township health services were equipped with a small surgical facility that enabled them to perform safe deliveries and caesarian sections, if necessary. Qualified obstetricians and gynecologists practiced in city hospitals and were responsible for the vocational training and supervision of lower level practitioners. Until the 'socialist market economy' reached the health sector, qualified obstetricians spent one-third of their time in rural facilities.

The competition introduced by the economic reforms of 1979 led hospitals to upgrade their equipment and services. Yet this process occurred mainly in urban centers with more than one hospital, while the specialists' rotation in lower level rural facilities seems to have been somewhat neglected. Furthermore, the number of specialized MCH practitioners in the villages declined. In close to half (47.7 percent) of the 288 villages surveyed in HeBei Province between 1996 and 1999 there were no MCH services. As stated in Chapter 6, affluent villages were more likely to enjoy such services than poorer ones. Moreover, the quality of MCH services varied considerably, according to the availability of government hospital branches in the village.

Comparative data on pre- and post-neonatal care are not available, so it is not possible to explore the interconnecting effect of the economic reforms, privatization, and the one-child policy on maternal health behavior. Nevertheless, according to our study 45.3 percent of the mothers in rural HeBei had no prenatal care at all in their most recent pregnancy. The most important predictor of utilization of prenatal care was the age of the respondent. As presented in Figure 7.3, the proportion of women who received prenatal care increased almost linearly with age, without any dip or peak among women who reached their reproductive age upon the shift to market economy or as a consequence of population policies.

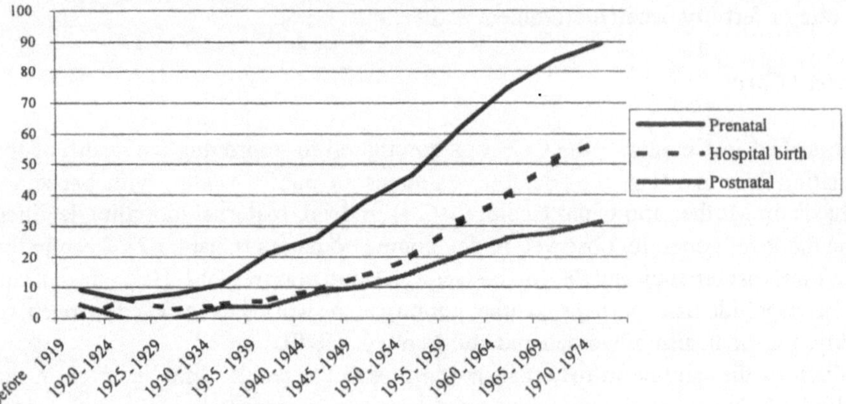

Figure 7.3 Utilization of Mother and Child Health services by mother's year of birth, HeBei, 1996–1999 (percent)

Further, multivariate, analysis showed that, beyond the effect of age, better educated women were more likely to use prenatal services and income was not related to utilization. At the same time, availability of the service in the village increased the odds for prenatal care by 23.2 percent, while each birth decreased the inclination of mothers to use the service by 14.6 percent. The degree to which these mothers abstained from prenatal care because they were reluctant to reveal an unauthorized pregnancy cannot be determined by our data.

Of all the mothers in our sample, 71.5 percent had given birth most recently at home. This figure is lower than the number reported by Wen (1993) for 1975–1984 (somewhat over 90 percent), but it is far from satisfactory, given the association between home birth and maternal mortality (Chapter 2). Like prenatal care, hospital births are more common among younger women, but 44.3 percent of 25–29 year old women respondents in rural HeBei had delivered their most recent child at home at the time of the survey.

Hospitals on the county or city level seemed to be increasingly utilized by rural women for child birth. Some half of 25–29 year old women gave birth in such hospitals, in comparison with 4.3 percent of women aged 55–59, their mothers' generation. Township health centers, on the other hand, have never appealed to rural women as a place for childbirth. Of all the mothers surveyed, only 2.6 percent had delivered their youngest in such a facility. Similar to the utilization of prenatal care, family income was not related to home delivery. The educated and those in non-farming occupations were more likely to give birth in a hospital, while farmers, higher parity mothers, and women living a long distance from a hospital (over 75Km) were more likely to give birth at home.

The proportion of women who received postnatal care was even lower (Figure 7.3). The inclination to use postnatal services had increased over time, but even among the youngest mothers in our sample, fewer than one in three had had a postnatal checkup. Again, apart from age, education, occupation, the total number of children born, and the availability of MCH services in the village, but not family income, emerged as important factors affecting the utilization of postnatal care.

The PRC government was not indifferent to the absence of MCH in so many villages, nor to the under-utilization of the available services. Committed to the health of women and children, it issued the Law on Infant and Maternal Health, which took effect on June 1st, 1995. The law states that each pregnant woman is entitled to pre- and postnatal care, including comprehensive maternal and child health education. She is to be instructed about adequate nutrition during pregnancy and infancy, about the endemic health risks prevalent in her neighborhood (such as the iodine deficiency disorders discussed in Chapter 3), proper hygiene, normal child growth and development and child psychology. The law obliges local governments to give priority to MCH when allocating resources, to ensure the professional competence of MCH care providers, and to make MCH services affordable to all. The remote, poor, and needy areas are specifically addressed in this law.

At the same time, the Law on Infant and Maternal Health was also introduced to cope with the high social and economic burden of disability. All couples applying for a marriage license were obliged to undergo medical examinations and delay marriage until treated, if either member was found to be seriously ill. Couples burdened by genetic disease or defects that 'make childbearing inappropriate' were required to use long-term contraceptive methods, usually sterilization. Termination of pregnancy was to be advised in cases where the fetus had a serious defect or the mother's life was at risk.

In the PRC, the 1995 Law on Infant and Maternal Health was considered a major step forward in MCH. In the West, however, the articles aimed at limiting the burden of disease were seriously criticized (Hesketh and Zhu, (1997a). Linking a marriage license to health status and disability was criticized as a violation of the basic human right to family formation, although it had been practiced in China for years before the introduction of this legislation. Denying parenthood for genetic reasons and the sweeping recommendation that fetuses with serious defects be aborted, indeed the very notion of an 'inappropriate child', seemed eugenic to Western eyes.

State intervention in private life is ideologically unacceptable in many post industrial societies. Yet, most Western countries do just that in many areas. Euthanasia, for example, is illegal in the West and has to be socially approved by the agency of social control, the courts. The legal status of induced abortions has been a major issue in every recent presidential election in the democratic United States. The Israeli Ministry of Health bears the costs of terminating a pregnancy for women under 17 or over 40, for pregnancies resulting from extramarital or incestuous relationships, and in pregnancies where the mother's health is at risk, or if the fetus has a serious defect. Similar regulations prevail in other industrial countries, with no more detailed specification than the PRC 1995 law. Amniocentesis, a technology developed and constantly refined at considerable cost, is recommended for all pregnant women over 30 or 35, mainly to avoid the birth of viable though often severely disabled and highly costly Down's syndrome children.

These articles in the Law on Infant and Maternal Health should be evaluated in the context of the PRC. As Potter and Potter (1990) observed, the Chinese concept of privacy and invasion of privacy are very different from those of the West. Most persons accept that the state, being responsible for meeting the needs of all citizens, has a legitimate right to regulate and balance the 'two types of production', procreation and material output.

The effect of the different population policies on women's reproductive health cannot be easily assessed. The decline in fertility has no doubt freed women from the risks associated with frequent pregnancies and childbirth in a country which still has a high maternal mortality rate in comparison with industrial societies. It is very possible that the remarkable decline in maternal mortality has been achieved by reducing these risks, creating fewer but 'better quality' pregnancies along with fewer but 'better quality' children. Safe contraceptives and legal abortions have freed women from traditional, often unsafe, methods of terminating pregnancy (Riley and Gardner, 1997).

In some places, particularly where the policy encountered persistent resistance and a high rate of noncompliance, semiannual gynecological examinations were introduced (Greenhalgh et al, 1994). These took place in the fall and spring, during the agricultural slack season, and became a part of the annual cycle of village life. Diseases of reproductive organs detected in these routine examinations were treated along with IUD insertion and detection of unplanned pregnancies. It thus combined family planning with high quality reproductive health services. Women willingly utilized the new services, partly because the terminology used by health professionals led many to confuse early detection with prevention (Hoeman et al, 1996).

At the same time, family planning in China was exclusively aimed at women and sometimes placed them at some health risk (Wang et al, 1998). As mentioned above, mothers of an only child were provided with an intra-uterine device, while sterilization was proposed to parents of more than one child. The number of women sterilized during the early 1980s and 1990s was 5–6 times higher than the number of men, although a tubal legation is a more complicated, riskier, and more costly procedure than vasectomy (Pearson, 1996).

Another method of birth control used was the termination of unauthorized pregnancies. Official data regarding legal abortions are not available. Estimates based on population census and fertility surveys suggest that approximately 400 induced abortions were performed per 1,000 live births in 1982, 760 in 1984, and 530 in 1986, similar to the levels reported in Western societies (Rigdon, 1996). By law, all abortions have to be performed by trained personnel in a health facility. During the first trimester abortions generally do not involve health risks, especially when performed by vacuum aspiration, as is done in China. Yet, small-scale surveys indicated that between 1980 and 1983, from one-quarter to one-third of the terminations were performed in the second and the third trimester, mainly to prevent the birth of a third child (Rigdon, 1996). These abortions were risky for the mothers as well as more expensive and required highly trained professionals and advanced technology. As a result, local cadres were pressed to reduce the prevalence of late-pregnancy induced abortions and were subject to penalties if they failed to do so.

The degree to which abortions adversely affected women's health is not clear. It has been suggested that the use of traditional methods in rural China may have been revived after the reforms and the privatization of health services (Rigdon, 1996). Similarly, some argued that unauthorized births led women to hide their pregnancies, forgoing medical help in general and prenatal care and professional birth assistance in particular. The data collected in rural HeBei (see above) indicate that the latter concern seems to be largely invalid, as the utilization of MCH services continued to increase after 1979.

Summary

The Chinese Communist Party has strongly advocated the emancipation of women and sought to achieve complete gender equality. These principles are specified in the constitution and in a series of laws protecting the rights of women in all spheres of life. There is no doubt that the status of women in China has improved dramatically, both in the rural and the urban areas since the revolution. Women have gained access to education, although in rural China they are still less likely than men to continue studying beyond primary school. Arranged, uxorilocal marriages have largely disappeared and the minimum permissible age for marriage as well as the formation of nuclear families have both increased. These processes could be the result of migration, collectivization, and fertility policies, but some more fundamental changes seem to have taken place. Dyadic communication and joint decision-making are gradually becoming normative, and women's specialization in farming as a result of the rapid development of rural industry following the economic reforms of 1979 has enhanced their power and status within the family.

However, as for women in post industrial societies, full equality still lies in the future. Both Western and Chinese women experience job segregation, encounter a glass ceiling in the workplace, and earn less than men for similar work. Labor force segregation reflects and strengthen gender division of household labor and family work, with women performing most of the housework and child care. Gender inequality seems to be particularly serious at both ends of the life cycle. Although the marriage laws forbid any interference with the remarriage of widows, such remarriage remains extremely rare.

Analysts of census data and data collected in fertility surveys conducted during the 1980s have suggested that there is discrimination against females during infancy and early childhood. It is believed that the population control policy of 1979 worsened the life chance of female children, particularly second or third children in a family with only daughters. Millions of girls are missing from official records and survey data, the result of selective abortions, informal adoption, indirect infanticide, and under-reporting. After reviewing the extensive literature available on the subject, we believe that under-reporting accounts for the overwhelming majority of the missing girls. However, because rearing an unregistered child involves higher costs, the well-being and the educational opportunities of these girls could be jeopardized.

Like many other industrial and developing societies, China has established an official population policy. The policy has changed over time, varying according to economic and political changes since the 1949 revolution, from the pro-natal policy of the early years of the PRC to the one-child policy. The one-child policy has been quite successful in the cities, where work units are an efficient mechanism of social control. It has been far less successful among rural women, whose fertility rates have remained higher than among urbanites. Yet, rural fertility has also declined dramatically, the result of the same social processes which have improved the status of women. The most important of these appear to be education, occupational opportunities, decline in the prevalence of stem families, and modernization.

China's achievements in reducing maternal and infant mortality are unique, particularly in light of its limited resources. The CCP is committed to improving Mother and Child Health and these services have grown in parallel with the development of the rural three-tier care delivery system. Currently, however, in about half of the villages such services are not available locally, possibly the result of the massive privatization of the health services since the 1979 economic reforms. Nevertheless, in rural HeBei, the great majority of women under 30 have received prenatal care during their most recent pregnancy. Only half of the women of that age, however, have given birth in a hospital or other health facility, and less than one-third have received any postnatal care.

The same factors that are associated with limited fertility are also associated with the utilization of maternal health care: younger age, education, occupation, and the availability of the service in the village. In rural HeBei there was no evidence that either the costs of the service or the fear of exposing one's unauthorized pregnancy affected utilization. Usage rates for all three services increased monotonically with age, regardless of family income and parity.

Committed to Mother and Child Health, the CCP passed the Law on Infant and Maternal Health in 1995. The law ensures the right of women to pre- and post-natal care, safe delivery, and health education that includes a wide range of health issues. It requires local authorities to assure access to Mother and Child Health services for all women, particularly those living in remote and poor regions, as well as the quality of the services. While the law has been welcomed in China as a progressive milestone, the articles which are aimed at reducing the burden of disability have been heavily criticized in the West. These critiques relate to issues of human rights and eugenic policy. We discuss these articles in the Chinese context and point to similar laws and regulations, some of which are indeed under constant debate, in post industrial societies.

It is difficult to assess how the population policies have affected the health of women. Reducing the frequency of pregnancy and birth under conditions of relatively high maternal mortality and the expansion of gynecological services has undoubtedly enhanced the health of women. On the other hand, female sterilization and induced abortions during the second and the third trimesters of a pregnancy involve health risks. The case of third trimester abortions has been addressed by the health authorities through pressure on local cadres whose regions are characterized by a high rate of late abortions.

Chapter 8

The Elderly

Old age is highly valued in Chinese society. In the Confucian heritage the elderly are regarded as a source of wisdom and younger members of Chinese society are admonished to respect the elderly and obey their instructions. Chinese cultural tradition emphasizes the duty of sons to support their elderly parents and to fulfill their wishes (Jernigan and Jernigan, 1992).

The leaders of the communist revolution sought to eradicate feudalism along with the Confucian tradition that for centuries had been exploited to legitimize the feudalistic social order. The Marriage Law described in the previous chapter, for example, altered the Confucian expectation for total obedience of children to their parents. In that chapter, we also showed how, paradoxically, patriarchalism had been strengthened during the extended collectivization period. The Confucian obligation for children to support and provide for heir elderly parents, by contrast, was overtly adopted by the CCP.

Nevertheless, like their counterparts in many industrial and developing societies, the senior citizens of the PRC run a high risk of financial hardship and experience deterioration of health status and disability, both of which increase their propensity to fall into poverty. The sociodemographic processes which affect the likelihood of the rural elderly in China to enjoy the social support required for their overall well-being are the focus of the current chapter.

China, Yet Another Aging Society

In all societies, the proportion of the elderly in the population depends on the fertility rate and survivorship, especially of infants and children (Jiang, 1995). The PRC is no exception. The dramatic decline in fertility and the changes in mortality in China have already been described in Chapters 1, 2, and 7. As in other societies, these processes resulted in an increase in the proportion of the elderly in Chinese society.

The pace of the increase is not easily determined, because official statistics do not use a consistent definition and details of age distribution are mostly unavailable. The China Yearbook of 1999, for example, reported the number of persons past working age in the 1953, 1964, 1982, and 1990 census. During this period, the proportion of women over 55 and men aged 60 or above increased from 8.9 percent of the total population to 10.3 percent. Many of the persons included in this definition are at least five years younger than the accepted criteria in Western societies, where retirement age is commonly 60 years for women and 65 for men. Still, these figures offer some insight into the volume of economic resources, if not necessarily health resources, needed to provide for persons past employment age. The dependency ratio of that group, that is, the number of persons above the official working age divided by the working age population, was 17.2 per hundred populations in 1953. It subsequently declined to 15.8:100 in 1964, but climbed back to 17.2 per hundred populations in 1990.

Using the more common definition of senior citizen, a person 65 years of age or over, enables us to compare the process of aging in the PRC with that of neighboring societies. Examining changes in the proportion of the elderly in the total populations of the eight societies selected for comparison reflects not only the demographic transition but also the vulnerability of the elders. Above and beyond the effect of the decline in fertility and mortality, the proportion of the elderly in China was affected by famine, social unrest, and war. The famine of the early 1960s, for example, brought about a decline in the proportion of the elderly in the PRC, despite the stagnation in birth rates during this period. No similar fall in the proportion of the elderly can be observed in Mongolia and the Republic of Korea, which also experienced shortages of food during this period.

The proportion of the aged in the PRC continued to decline until 1970, during the years of economic and social upheaval, although fertility had started to decline some five years before (Figure 8.1). A steady increase in the proportion of seniors aged 65 years and older in the population of the PRC has been observable since 1975, mainly due to a decline in fertility. Since 1980, the average proportion of the elderly in the population has increased by 3.2 percent annually, reaching 6.7 percent of the total population in 1998, and is expected to reach 8.9 percent by 2015 (The World Bank, 2000). Consequently, the dependency ratio of the elders has increased since the early 1970s, reaching almost 10 percent by 1998. According to a World Bank estimate, by 2015 there will be one senior citizen aged 65 years or over for every eight persons of working age.

Often, the PRC's governmental efforts to control population growth and related policies are blamed for the rapid increase in the proportion of the elderly (Leung, 1997). Our doubts regarding the role of these policies in the declining fertility rates were discussed in detail in the previous chapter. These doubts are further strengthened when we compare the pace of the aging in Chinese society with that in other Asian societies. The annual average growth in the proportion of the elderly from 1980 to 1998, that is, after the 'later, longer, fewer' campaign and the implementation of the 'one-child policy', was slower in the PRC than in six of the eight societies selected for comparison. While the elderly Chinese population increased annually by a mean of 3.2 percent the elderly population increased by 4.1 percent in Mongolia, by 3.9

percent in the Republic of Korea, by 3.8 percent in Thailand, by 3.6 percent in Singapore and Japan, and by 3.4 percent in Sri-Lanka. None of these countries had a population control policy. The relatively slow increase in the proportion of the elderly in the Chinese population could have been a result of the relatively slow decline in adult mortality (Chapter 2). Until the late 1980s, the mortality of elderly men was stable, while that of women declined only moderately (Banister et al, 1997). The trend of old-age mortality during the 1990s is unclear, though some data suggest that the rate is on the decline (Banister et al, 2000).

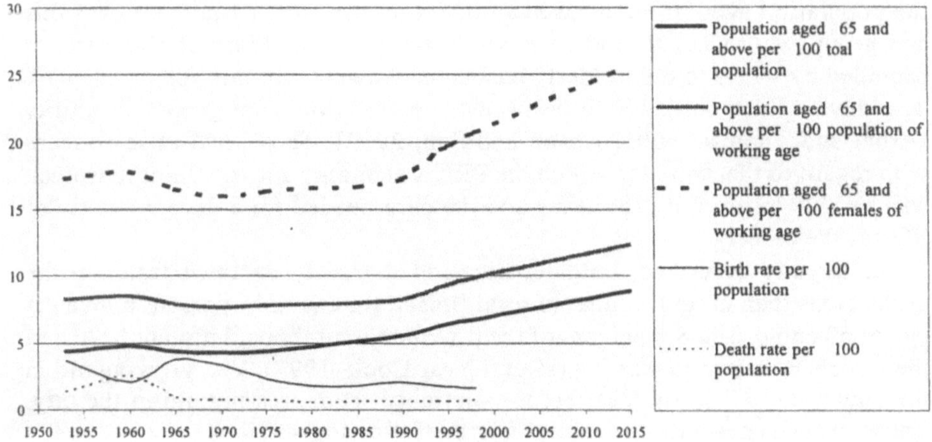

Figure 8.1 Elderly, dependency, births, and deaths rates, China, 1953–2015
Source: World Development Indicators, 2000.

The dependency ratio mainly reflects the load of a given social group on the economy of a society. Often, however, social groups that are not economically active also require special care and nurturing. In all societies, the care for minors, seniors, and the disabled is perceived as a natural role for women. Wives, mothers, daughters and daughters-in-law are expected to care for the frail members of the family (Avgar, 1997). The dependency ratio of the elderly on women of working age, that is, daughters and daughters-in-law who often provide care for senior family members, is also presented in Figure 8.1. The population projections of the World

Bank for the PRC enable us to compare the economic dependency rate of the elderly with the expected care-load on women. The comparison suggests that the care-load that women of working age will experience in the future is likely to increase faster than the economic load.

Moreover, as mortality declines, the proportion of the old-old in the elderly population tends to increase. In the PRC, seniors aged 80 or more comprised 0.33 percent of the total population in 1953, a proportion which more then doubled by 1995, when the old-old population reached 0.81 percent of the total population. During the same period, the increase in the proportion of the elderly (65 years of age and over) was much more modest, from 4.4 percent to 6.2 percent. Naturally, the old-old became increasingly visible among the elderly population. Between 1953 and 1995 the proportion of the old-old within the population aged 65+ increased from 7.4 percent to 13.1 percent. It is this age group whose health and care needs are greatest. Most of this care, is provided by wives to their elderly husbands. However, at this age, women are as likely as their husbands to be in poor health, with even greater disability (Arber and Thomas, 2001; Anson and Sun, 2002). These data raise concern with regard to the degree to which the PRC's economy and the Chinese women will be able to provide the means and the care needed for a decent quality of life for the elderly.

As already described, both fertility and mortality declined faster in the urban areas than in rural China. In rural HeBei, for example, persons above the age of 60 comprised 8.6 percent of the province's rural population in 1996 and their dependency ratio was 9.4 (HeBei Year Book, 1997). Yet, growing old in the countryside is quite a different experience from growing old in the city. These experiences will be discussed in the following sections.

Social Support for the Elderly

Formal Support

In line with its socialist ideology, the CCP saw care for the poor, the sick, and the elderly as the responsibility of the state. A comprehensive social security system was initiated to ensure retirees with housing, health care, and an old-age pension. Those entitled to benefits under these programs, however, were salaried state employees working in industry, service jobs, and government administration. In other words, the system covered mainly the urban population, which accounted for 12.5 percent of the total population in 1952, 19.4 percent in 1978 on the verge of the economic reforms, and 30.4 percent in 1998 (China Yearbook, 1999).

Senior citizens living in rural China are constitutionally entitled to housing, food, clothing, health care, and burial, which are the five basic rights (the 'five guarantees') of all citizens of the People's Republic of China. However, as described in the first chapter of this book, the economic development of the PRC was unable to sustain universal welfare subsidies for all individuals, especially not for the large rural population. The government's efforts were, and still are, concentrated on providing for the very poor villages. Villages faced by persistent poverty or temporary hazards are provided with food (mainly grains), an emergency action taken to prevent starvation. Longer-term counseling and assistance are given to poverty-stricken villages in order to improve production to achieve economic self-sufficiency and help them to escape constant poverty (Tang et al, 1994).

Unable to live up to its ideological commitment to provide all citizens with at least the 'five guarantees', the CCP was led to rely on local communities and the family as the main source of support for the old and the needy. Such a policy, which strengthened the family and local authorities, was not only incompatible with socialist ideology, but had also the potential to bring about social fragmentation, reinforce local loyalties, and fortify the patriarchal Confucian value system. Yet, the dangers inherent in strengthening counter-revolutionary ideology not withstanding, the obligation of children to support their elderly kin was enshrined in the constitution as well as in a series of later laws that were enforced by local governments and communities (Tang et al, 1994).

Since 1979, the obligation of adult children to provide for their elderly parents has been embedded in the criminal law, with criminal detention the punishment for those who fail to comply with the law. A year later, the obligation for parental support was expanded to include adopted children, under the revised Marriage Law. The Inheritance Law of 1985 permitted the disinheritance of children who abandon their parents in their old age, while providing caring children with a larger proportion of the property of the deceased parent.

The most recent law augmenting the legal obligation of children to support their elderly parents was passed by the Legislative Affairs Commission of the Standing Committee of the National Congress of the PRC in August 1996. The "Law of the People's Republic of China for Protection of the Right in the Interest of the Elderly" re-emphasizes the duty of family members to provide for the elderly and support them, to assure them of food, clothing, a roof overhead, and medical expenses. In the countryside, family members are required to cultivate the lands of the elderly, to husband their livestock, and to transfer to them the income generated.

Naturally, some elderly people cannot be supported by their kin. Childless seniors with no other dependable relatives, no source of income, and unable to work and provide for themselves – the 'three nos' – are entitled to the 'five guarantees'. These elderly are dependent on the village and are provided for by its authorities. Before the dismantling of the collective and the implementation of the 'system of household responsibility', the 'three nos' elderly could rely on the village welfare safety network fund. The work points deducted from the work brigade were used to provide basic needs and health care to lone and frail seniors. The economic reforms, however, jeopardized the ability of many villages to maintain this provision (Leung, 1997; Li and Tracy, 1999).

It was not only those who were lone and elderly who were affected by the economic reforms. The introduction of the socialist market economy and the massive decollectivization that followed revitalized the family as an economic unit responsible for fulfilling the needs of all of its members, while the village welfare safety net was considerably weakened or disappeared altogether. Most elderly farmers were not entitled to an old-age pension, because in most cases they were neither government employees nor employed in a public sector that entitled them to an old age pension. According to some estimates, some 11 percent of the elderly men (aged 60 years or older) and 1 percent of the retired women in rural China received an old age pension, compared with 94 percent and 53 percent, respectively, of the urban elderly (Lee and Xiao, 1998).

The most important question raised by the data above is the degree to which the rural family could be relied upon to provide financial support and care for its aged members, considering the demographic processes taking place in China. Two such processes are most relevant to this issue, the decline of fertility and the increase in urbanization. Some of the consequences for the family of the rapid decline in fertility have already been discussed in Chapter 1. We described the transformation of the kinship system and the gradual disappearance of traditionally meaningful relationships, such as those with older brothers and paternal uncles that had been most important sources of informational, emotional, and tangible support in the past. The present steady decline in fertility is increasing the probability that the rural population will grow old without the culturally-preferred support of an adult son.

The process of urbanization is also increasing the risk that the rural population will grow old without the support and care of their children. The urban population of the PRC has doubled since the introduction of the population control policy and the economic reforms. Between 1979 and 1998, the proportion of urbanites in the total population increased by 63.0 percent, while the population grew by only 26.8 percent (China Yearbook, 1999). As implementation of the one-child policy was more efficient in the cities, rural to urban migration accounts for most of this increase. As in many developed and developing societies, those most likely to migrate are people who have the means to initiate and adjust to the exigencies of the transition (Browning and Feindt, 1969; Landale et al, 2000). They are usually younger, more highly educated, healthier, and better equipped to handle the hardships than non-migrants and thus potentially more dependable in providing for their old parent.

It is possible that the extensive legislation aimed at protecting the rights of the elderly and ensuring filial piety was, at least in part, the government's reaction to these demographic processes. The experience of post-industrial societies shows that in the long run industrialization and urbanization are associated with a decline of traditional family structure and changes in norms of family commitment. The low divorce rate in the PRC, however, less than one percent in 1998, seems to indicate that no similar processes are taking place there. Yet, formal support services for the elderly are scarce and as long as such services are unavailable in rural China legislation is one, uncostly, mechanism which protects them from abandon.

Institutionalization of elderly people is very rare in China. Less than one percent of the elderly stayed in long-term care institutions in 1994 and only 503 such institutions were operating in 1998 (Leing, 1997; China Yearbook, 1999). Institutional care, however, is not a strange concept in the PRC. One consequence of the civil war was homelessness and many elderly were found adrift in the cities after the revolution. The government made every effort to unite these elderly people with their families and those with no kin were resettled in their villages to be cared for by the collective (Ineichen, 1998).

During the collectivization and the 'great leap forward', old age homes started to emerge, established and supported by the commune. Yet, with the fall of the collective kitchen in the early 1960s most institutionalized elderly were returned to the community to be cared for by their families if possible and by the working brigade if they were eligible for 'the five guarantees'. After the economic reforms of 1979 and the subsequent abolishment of the collectives, institutions for the seniors started to appear again, though the number of long-term care beds still falls far behind that of industrial societies. Each township is expected to develop at least one such institution, yet the degree to which this expectation is actually implemented varies considerably between regions.

In recent years, the government has encouraged the development of community-based services for senior citizens, including the provision of home assistance, meals, and emotional support. The target population was the single elderly, mainly those living alone. Yet, the development and operation of such services was provided mainly in the cities by the Street Offices, each of which covers a neighborhood of 30,000 – 50,000 residents. Moreover, the provision of services for the elderly largely depends on the ability of the Street Office to generate the necessary funds, so that the extent and quality of the services vary greatly. Such services are even more scarce in rural China and the elderly still rely heavily on the family for support.

Informal Support

As mentioned above, in most societies female kin are entrusted with the care of the elderly, sick and disabled family members. Wives support their husbands in their later years, though they are often old, sick, and disabled themselves (Medjuck et al, 1992; Chen et al, 1995). Daughters and daughters-in-law are expected to care for parents and in-laws. In the PRC, these expectations are augmented by the Confucian tradition on the one hand and by the legal system on the other.

The availability of a spouse varies significantly with age and gender in all societies as a consequence of mortality patterns and the normative marriage age for each sex. This was clearly apparent in our representative sample of rural households in HeBei Province, in which 881 senior citizens 65 years old and above were interviewed. Almost half (45.0 percent) of our elderly respondents were young-old, and 101 (12.8 percent) old-old, that is, over 80 years of age. The oldest respondent was a woman aged 97. The ratio of women to men increased with age, the result of higher male mortality rates. In our study, like in previous reports from the PRC, there were 80 women per 100 men among the young-old, but 144 women per 100 men among the old-old.

The majority of the elderly were married, 79.1 percent of the men and 71.3 percent of the women interviewed in rural HeBei, yet the proportion of married people varied with age. Among both young-old men and women, those between 65 and 69, 86.5% were married and few, 10.5 percent men and 12.8 percent women, were widowed. However, among the old-old, those 80 or older, 62.7 percent of the women had already lost their husbands, but only half the proportion, 34.1 percent, of men of the same age were widowed. Thus, many more men than women could rely on support provided by their spouses when they were old, findings very similar to the gender differences observed in industrial societies.

Nevertheless, familial support is more readily available for the elderly in the PRC than for those in Western societies, because of the prevailing pattern of patrilocal living arrangements and multi-generation households. A single-person household is quite rare among the Chinese elderly. The census of 1990 reported fewer than five percent of the elderly living alone. Only 6.4 percent of the elderly respondents in rural HeBei were living in a single-person household. All other seniors lived either with their spouses or with one or more of their children, regardless of the latter's marital status, or with other relatives (Li, 1998; Lee and Xiao, 1998; Li and Tracy, 1999).

These living arrangements were consistent with the cultural obligation of the family to support its elderly members. Yet, the status of the elderly within the household seems to have changed from the traditional preference for a multi-generational household headed by an elderly man. Li (1998) suggested that, although current living arrangements for the elderly in the PRC make social support available, the traditional senior position of the elderly has declined over the years.

Basing his claim on the 1990 census data, Li (1998) reasoned that elderly parents have lost their traditional power and respect. This argument was founded on an analysis patterns of living arrangements among the elderly and household headship. Traditionally, the ideal type of living arrangement during the last stage of the life cycle was a multi-generational household, headed by a senior male. This arrangement, however, was not the modal household in 1990, when the prevalent type of household including an elderly member was a family household headed by one of his/her descendants.

More germane to this argument was the relationship between the socioeconomic characteristics of the elderly and the household headship. Age was the most important determinant of living arrangements: the traditional ideal was more prevalent among the young-old, observed among some one-quarter of the elderly aged 65 – 69. It declined to 3 percent among the old-old, those above the age of 80. In other words, as parents grew older and increasingly weaker and more limited, their offspring took over the responsibility for the household, including the symbolic status as head of the household.

Furthermore, the elderly called on extra-familial resources to help them retain their status as head of the household. Education, highly esteemed in the Chinese culture, was one such resource. The traditional preferred living arrangement was more prevalent among elderly who had completed high school. Close to one in three of the educated seniors were heads of multi-generational households. This type of living arrangement was much less frequent among the illiterate, of whom just one in eight headed extended households.

Li's analysis, however, did not consider possible gender differences. Among the old-old as well as among the illiterates, women outnumbered men. In 1998, there were 226 widowed women per 100 widowed men and 2.5 times more illiterate women than men in the PRC (China Yearbook, 1999). The traditionally preferred living arrangement discussed by Li applied to men, while women expected and were expected to live with one of their sons, holding a senior status among the women of the household but not formally heading it (Beaver et al, 1995; Anson and Hanaappel, 1999). Being dependent on an adult son did not, therefore, indicate a loss of status for women, but rather an appropriate, culturally-preferred living arrangement for women who had given birth to a male child. Indeed, Anson and Hanaappel (1999) showed that mothers of a head of household enjoyed considerable power in a rural family. They had the power to determine their own work load and their proportion of the household tasks, perceiving themselves as healthy and more able than younger women, despite their physical limitations and chronic morbidity. In this study, the culturally-preferred living arrangement was associated with better mental health. Elderly women who lived in their offspring's household reported significantly better psychological well-being than women who headed their own households, an arrangement which was relatively scarce and culturally deviant.

We conducted a similar analysis of the data of our survey in rural HeBei, considering the relationships between the living arrangements, age, gender, literacy, and marital status of the elderly. The relationship between living arrangements and age in rural HeBei was very similar to that described by Li (1998). The status as head of a multi-generational household indeed decreased inversely with age, declining from 32.8 percent among men aged 65– 69 to 4.9 percent among men of 80 and more (Figure 8.2a). At the same time, being a dependent elderly man in a household headed by a descendant was quite rare among men 65– 69 years old (4.8 percent), but increased to 20.0 percent among men aged 70–79 and became the modal arrangement after 80. In rural HeBei, however, the proportion of men living alone also increased with age, although it remained low compared with most industrial societies: 6.3 percent among men aged 65–69 and 12.2 percent among men over 80. Moreover, more than half of the men below the age of 80 and 30.0 percent of the men above that age lived with their wives in a two-person household.

This last observation may suggest that a new pattern of extended family is emerging in which elderly parents and their adult children maintain independent households in geographical proximity to each other, which facilitates intensive social support when needed, along with independent living for both generations. A very similar transition has been observed among Jews born in Asia and North-Africa who immigrated to Israel with a cultural heritage that encourages extended family households headed by the senior male (Shuval 1992).

The pattern of living arrangements among elderly rural women in HeBei Province is much more sensitive to marital status and social expectations. At all ages, very few elderly women headed their own households. Those few who did tended to be widows under the age of 80 (Figure 8.2b). The higher widowhood rate among women is apparent in the low proportion of women who are the wives of heads of multi-generational households and in the lower proportion of old-old women living with their husbands in two-person households. The relationship between widowhood and dependency on offspring is very clear among women of all ages: even most young-old women became members of a household headed by one of their children when they lost their husbands, while only 1.8 percent of them lived alone.

Our data showed the relationship between education and the living arrangements of the elderly to be weaker than that reported by Li (1998) and statistically significant only for men. Very few of our senior respondents (8.9 percent of the men and 1.8 percent of the women) had more than a primary school education and we had to divide them into two groups, literates and illiterates, in order to have sufficient cases for a meaningful analysis. We observed that literate elderly men were indeed more likely to be heads of multi-generational households and less likely to be dependent (Figure 8.3a). Illiterate men, however, retained the traditionally preferred household less frequently and were more likely to be living alone.

The pattern for women, though not statistically significant, is of particular interest (Figure 8.3b). It suggests that literate women were more inclined to live in an independent household than were illiterate women. More of the literate senior women lived with their husbands in independent households and fewer lived in households headed by their children than did elderly women with no schooling at all.

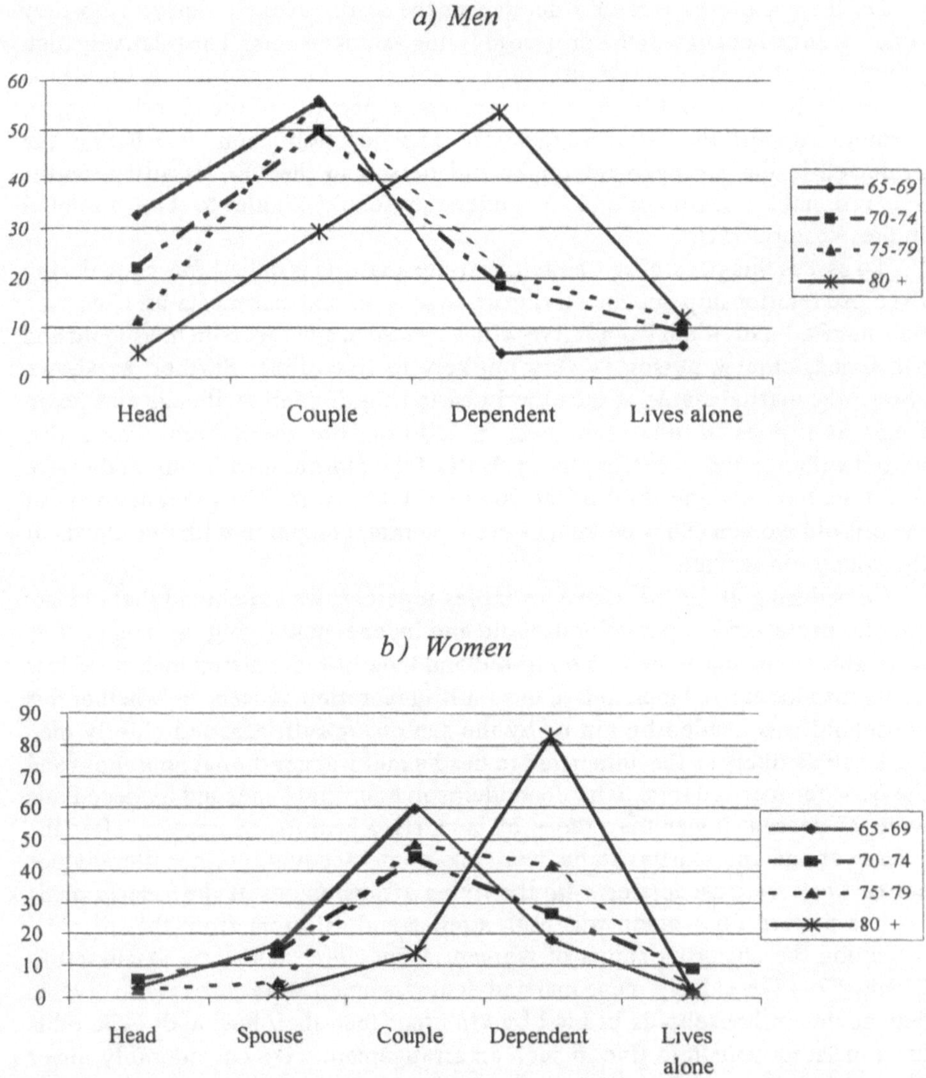

Figure 8.2 Living arrangements of elderly by sex, HeBei, 1996–1999 (percent)

Do these patterns reflect a decline in the status of the elderly or do they reflect a social change in the preferred living arrangements? The relatively high proportion of independent households of elderly couples and the relationships between education and living arrangements, especially of the elderly women, seem to support the latter suggestion. The question, then, is whether the preferred living arrangement for an old person in the PRC is still a multi-generational household or an independent household, similar to those common in the Western world.

To assess this possibility, a multi-variate analysis is called for, considering the close relationship between living arrangements and marital status. Clearly, a non-married individual cannot live with a spouse in a two-person household and a married, elderly person is very unlikely to live alone. Further, as shown above, the marital status of the elderly varied significantly with age and sex in China as it does in other societies. In addition, literacy in rural China also varied with age and sex (Chapter 7). Half of the old-old men in our study were illiterate, but only one-third of the young-old men were. The great majority of the old-old women (86.4 percent) were illiterate, compared with two-thirds of the young-old women.

Considering all of the above variables together, we concluded that elderly couples preferred a separate household and independent living, as long as they were able to maintain them. Young-old and the old-old married men were less likely than unmarried men to live in a multi-generation household, whether this household was headed by kin or by the senior himself. Married elderly men were half as likely as the unmarried to head a multi-generational household and the odds for married men to be dependents in households headed by decedents were 75 percent lower than those of unmarried seniors. Moreover, after the effects of age and marital status were taken into account, neither literacy nor active work were associated with the living arrangements of the elderly men.

The pattern for women was both similar and different from that of men, reflecting the changing status of women in the Chinese society discussed in Chapter 7. Like elderly men, married senior women were unlikely to live as dependents in households headed by kin other than their husbands. The odds for a married woman to live in such an arrangement were considerably lower than those for men and negligible compared with those for an unmarried woman (8:100). More important, however: women who were still working in agriculture, that is, the healthier and physically more able women, were 4.5 times more likely to live in an independent household and half as likely to live in a household headed by a child, regardless of their age and marital status. Elderly women who were able to carry out agricultural work seemed to be reluctant to accept the traditional role of mother-in-law and preferred independence even at the cost of losing traditional power. As long as they were capable of independent living, they preferred to maintain their own households.

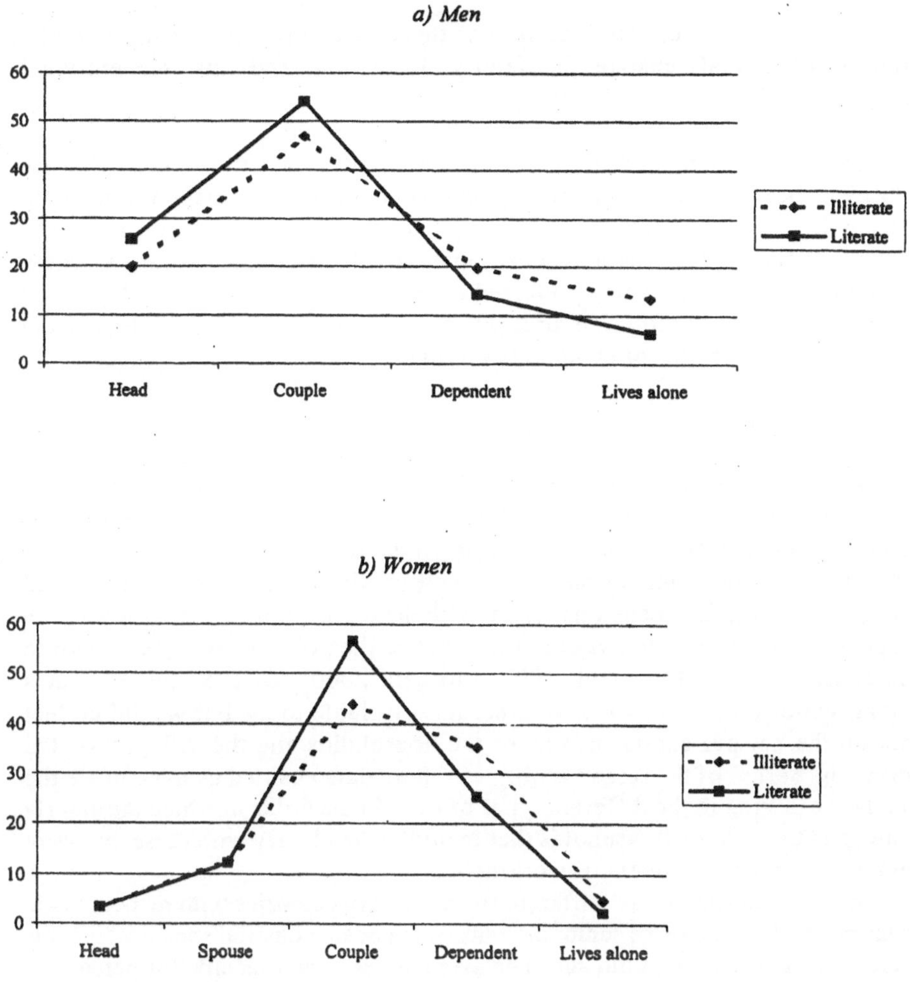

Figure 8.3 Illiteracy and living arrangement of elderly by sex, HeBei, 1996–1999 (percent)

The findings of our study, as well as those of other studies, suggest that a process of social change in family formation and inter-generational relationships is taking place both in rural and urban China (Ming and Huang, 1995). Co-residence in a multi-generation household has ceased to be the preferred living arrangement in China. Married men and women who are relatively healthy and economically independent tend to maintain separate households. Such preference is not unique to rural China. Transformations in traditional family patterns have been observed, for example, in Japan, where independent living is clearly preferred by elderly women (Izuhara, 2000). As we show in the next section, in rural HeBei this pattern of living is rather costly for the elderly in terms of standard of living.

Financial Support

In many industrial countries, the elderly constitute one of the social groups which run a high risk of poverty (Shuval, 1992; World Health Organization, 1995; Turner, 1997). Moreover, poverty tends to be more widespread among elderly women than among men, the result of differential work patterns and saving toward old-age pensions. Thus, with the dissolution of the family a high proportion of elderly widows are falling below the poverty level (McLaughlin and Jensen, 1995; McDonald, 1997; Morgan, 2000). Data on poverty rates among senior citizens of the PRC were not available to us, but we did collect data on the net per-capita income of the households and the villages visited during the period of the research project. These data enabled us to estimate the standard of living in the different types of rural households in which the elderly reside and to compare households that included the elderly with those that were composed only of members of working age.

China is both similar and different from Western countries with respect to the economic well-being of its senior citizens. As in post-industrial societies, income decreases significantly in old age. The average per-capita income for persons in their prime years of production, 45–55, was 2,503 Yuan in 1996–1999, while that of a person over 65 years of age was, on the average, 1,351 Yuan, 45 percent lower. Furthermore, the annual income of the average elderly person was 1,041 Yuan lower than the average per-capita income of the village where she/he lived.

At the same time, the gender income differences consistently observed in developed countries were absent in rural HeBei, where widows were no poorer than their married counterparts. In fact, the net per-capita income for households in which elderly married women lived was on the average 20 percent lower than for those that included widowed women. As can be seen in Figure 8.4, the joint living arrangements indeed afforded the elderly, particularly elderly women, a higher standard of living. Pooling family land as well as the labor of the young and the old increased the net per-capita income of the household. As a result, the elderly who lived as dependents in their decedents' household were better-off, while elderly couples who maintained an independent household were the poorest. The one exception was senior men living alone, whose income was similar to the per-capita income of households where a dependent elderly kin lived. These men demonstrated that, as with women of the same age, they preferred independent living to the traditional arrangements.

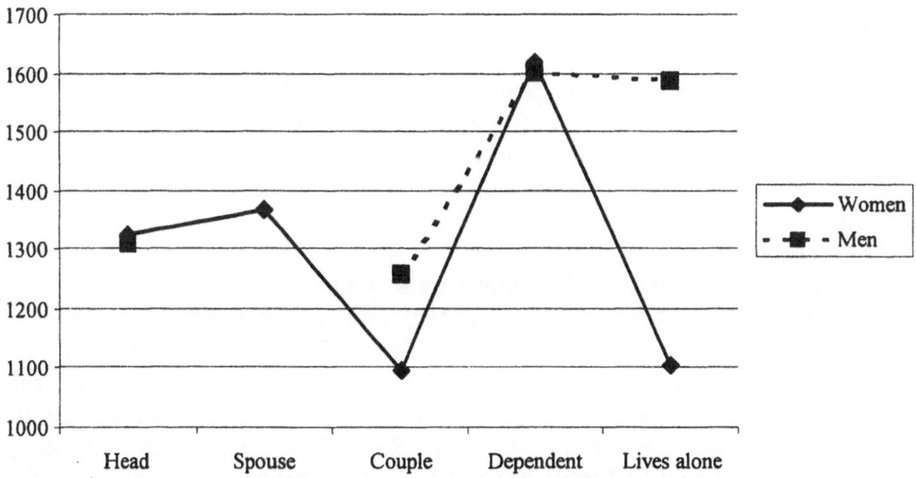

Figure 8.4 Standard of living of elderly people by living arrangements, HeBei, 1996–1999 (net per-capita income, Yuan)

These observations do not necessarily mean that the standard of living of elderly people who maintained an independent household was lower than that of the dependent elderly. Several studies documented that the most common type of intra-familial financial transfers in the current PRC are from adult children to their aging parents (Liu et al, 1995; Secondi, 1997; Lee and Xiao, 1998). The data presented here refer to the per-capita income of rural households in HeBei Province. Inter- generational transfers were not included. Nor were food products raised and consumed by the members of the household or goods transferred by kin counted as income. Yet the most important finding is that the rural Chinese family was indeed the major source of social support and economical welfare of its elderly members.

Age, Gender and Health

Health, unfortunately, deteriorates with age. The purpose of this section is to examine how morbidity and disability changed with aging in rural China and how the elderly perceived their own health. Such an analysis allows us to assess the well-being of the elderly in the countryside, their health needs, and their need for care.

Chronic Morbidity

It appears that, on the average, the elderly in rural HeBei were not burdened by chronic health conditions. Half of them were not aware of any chronic disease at all and the average number of long-term illnesses per person was 0.9. Moreover, there were no differences between elderly men and women, nor did the prevalence of chronic health problems increase with advancing age.

The prevalence of the three chronic conditions which are believed to be associated with the demographic transition was much lower in our sample than generally reported in health surveys in developed countries. Thus, 10.4 percent of the elderly in our sample had a heart condition, 5.5 percent had experienced CVA, and 8 seniors had cancer. Health surveys in Israel and Belgium, for example, yielded almost double that figure for the equivalent age groups in 1996–1997 (Anson, 2000; State of Israel, 1998). Similarly, chronic illnesses, considered as risk factors for cardiovascular and cerebrovascular diseases, were scarce among the elderly in rural HeBei, in comparison with industrial societies. Hypertension was reported by 18.3 percent and diabetes by 3.3 percent of the seniors interviewed.

Are the elderly in rural China healthier than their counterparts in Western countries? There is no direct answer to this question. Several explanations can be proposed, but none can be conclusively tested in the absence of comparative data from both developing and developed societies.

The first and simplest explanation could be genetic. It could be argued that the genetic heritage of the Chinese population offers protection from hypertension and diabetes and thus from cardiovascular and cerebrovascular diseases. Given the role of health behavior in the etiology of these illnesses as well as in cases of cancer, genetic differences cannot explain why the prevalence of chronic morbidity among the elderly in rural HeBei is about half that of societies that have completed the demographic transition.

The second explanation could be natural selection, reaching into old age. In other words, healthier persons survived to old age, while others, who were less healthy, did not. To estimate this explanation we examined the prevalence of chronic illness among adults over the age of 40. A consistent pattern was observed for each of the 11 chronic conditions we studied: the prevalence of each condition increased with age up to 70, but declined thereafter. Natural selection, thus plays a considerable role in the aging process of rural China.

Another possible explanation is related to the stage of epidemiological transition of the PRC. As described in Chapter 2, China is in the midst of such a transition, especially in the rural areas. This argument is supported by examination of the causes of death and a comparison of rural residents with city dwellers. The reader may recall that leading causes of death among the urban population are degenerative diseases, similar to the pattern that is common in post-industrial societies. In rural China, however, infectious diseases are still responsible for a larger proportion of deaths.

There is yet another possibility: chronic health problems are perceived as a part of normal aging and so are not reported or are not diagnosed. This is particularly true for cardiovascular and cerebrovascular risk factors such as diabetes, hypertension, and hypercholesterolemia. The last two conditions are asymptomatic and do not interfere with daily activity or with the performance of normal roles and duties. As we showed in Chapter 5, the utilization of health services in rural HeBei was mainly a reaction to acute health needs, that is, acute illnesses that brought about sudden and sharp decline with daily activity.

Moreover, the modal village clinics were not equipped to perform the laboratory tests necessary for the detection of diabetes and hypercholesterolemia (Chapter 4). Fewer than one in ten of our elderly subjects had had a blood test during the year before the survey and fewer had had a urine test. Even blood pressure was measured in only one of every four elderly people, although all village clinics were equipped with a mercury sphygmomanometer. Outreach programs were no longer feasible after the economic reforms and the massive privatization of the rural health services.

At the same time, subjective evaluations of their own health by the seniors in our sample resembled those of elderly people in developed countries. The majority (73.8 percent) perceived their own health as fair or good, while only 3.6 percent perceived it as very poor. These figures are very similar to those reported in Israel and Belgium (Anson, 2000; Nirel et al, 1996) and in other samples from the PRC (Liu et al, 1995).

Disability

Like the elderly elsewhere around the globe, old people in rural HeBei experienced increasing disability with advancing age. The process was faster for women than for men, particularly after the age of 80 (Figure 8.5). Similar to seniors in industrial societies, those with higher income levels were less disabled.

Only 16.1 percent of the elderly in our study were not limited in any given activity; 8.0 percent were limited in all activities of daily living and important sensory functions. Half of the elderly were severely limited in at least one daily activity, the most common being climbing stairs or a ladder. Least common was difficulty in caring for themselves, that is, dressing or bathing: 18.5 percent needed some help with these activities, while 6.0 percent were unable to bathe or dress themselves.

Sensory function also deteriorated with age. Among the young-old, 59.9 percent were short-sighted. The prevalence of shortsightedness increased to 67.0 percent among the old-old, but only 36.5 percent of those who could not see well used eyeglasses. Hearing loss was less prevalent: 2.9 percent of the young-old reported severe difficulties in hearing, compared with 20.0 percent among the old-old.

Disability impairs quality of life for anybody. A study of urban Chinese elderly people demonstrated that those who perceived their health as good and their income as comfortable evinced greater satisfaction with life, while disability had a significant negative effect on satisfaction with life (Zhang and Yu, 1998). The pattern observed among the rural elderly was very similar. Furthermore, the negative effect of disability on psychological well-being among the elderly was even stronger than that of perceived health. Not only was the mental health of the severely limited hampered, even moderate difficulties in performing daily activities had a negative effect on the mood of elderly people.

In rural China, disability, moderate as well as severe, did not change the odds that older people would be doing agricultural work. The majority of the elderly, 68.3 percent of the men and 69.2 percent of the women, were still engaged in agriculture when interviewed. Disability did, however, constrain independent living. The severely disabled were more likely to be dependents in a household headed by kin than living under any other arrangement.

In the absence of formal services for the elderly, the disabled had to rely on informal, principally family, support. Family members indeed provided most of their care. According to a large scale survey conducted in 1987 (Wang and Xia, 1994), more than 60 percent of the senior citizens needed at least some assistance with activities of daily living (ADL). Wives provided needed care for 48.2 percent of the men in this study, while husbands cared for only 13.5 percent of the disabled elderly women; other family members, mainly daughters and daughters-in-law, cared for 26.2 percent of the senior men and 38.1 percent of the women. Yet, with the demographic process currently taking place in the PRC the question is how long the family will be able to bear the financial and physical strain of support and care.

The Future of Family Support

For the rural elderly, as previously described, the family is often the only source of support (Wang and Xia, 1994; Li and Tracy, 1999; Leung, 1997; Lee and Xiao, 1998). What is the likelihood that these traditional arrangements will continue to exist in the future, in light of declining fertility and increasing migration to the cities?

Several analyses addressed this question (Jiang, 1995; Zhao, 1998, 2000; Zhou, 2000). The most common method employed was a computer simulation in which the prevailing demographic parameters of a society at a given period – levels of fertility, mortality, and marriage norms - were used to calculate the availability for support and care of different types of kin at a given age and time. A thorough description of these methods and their outcomes are beyond the scope of this book. Let us, however, examine the availability of kin support later in life.

The results of these simulations seem to indicate that, despite rapid increase in the proportion of the elderly in the PRC, the availability of kin support will not reach crisis before well into the middle of this century. Zhao (1998) reckoned that the increase in fertility of the early 1960s, after the 'great leap forward' and the famine, which was accompanied by a considerable decline in mortality, ensured the support of elderly men for the next three decades. Some two-thirds of these men will still be married at the age of 70, 40 percent at the age of 80. Under the demographic conditions of the early 1990s, the continuing increase in life expectancy, particularly that of women, suggests that three out of four men 70 years of age, and two out of four at the age of 80, will have a living wife to care for them. Thus, as long as the almost universal marriage and low divorce rates are maintained at the current level, the care needs of most elderly men will be met.

Moreover, the decline in infant and child mortality increases the likelihood that elderly men will have adult children to support them. Even when the sharp decline in fertility is taken into consideration, only about 10 percent of the men over the age of 60 will be childless. Most men (62.6 percent) will have at least one married child well into their 70s, while only 2.4 percent will have neither child nor spouse to provide support.

The future seems similar for elderly women (Jiang, 1995). Although gender differential mortality will result in a larger proportion of spouseless elderly women than men, marital status has only limited support implication for women, particularly in the countryside. As described earlier in this chapter, only a few rural Chinese women are economically dependent on their partners, because most men in rural China are not entitled to an old age pension. Furthermore, elderly women are better able to care for themselves and can do so for a longer period of time than can elderly men. Moreover, Chinese men, like their counterparts in developed countries, are less likely to provide their wives with support in daily living activities than vice versa. Even in the presence of a spouse, disabled women are mainly dependent on their daughters and daughters-in-law for assistance in fulfilling their daily care needs.

According to the simulation conducted by Jiang (1995), there will be no shortage of children to support elderly women born during the 'baby boom' of the 1960s, those who will be senior citizens by the year 2030, despite the sharp decline in the fertility of their own generation. The results of her analysis indicate that the decline in fertility is likely to be counterbalanced by a decline in mortality. Rural women aged 65 can expect to have an average of 1.21 sons, 75 year old women will have an average of 1.40 sons. Just 2.0 percent of the senior women will have no surviving son by 2030, compared with 8.1 percent in 1990. The norm of patrilocal living and the associated traditional responsibility of sons to support their elderly parents led Jiang to focus her analysis on sons, but one can assume that most women will also have a greater number of surviving daughters, an unknown number of whom will live nearby.

At the same time, the very same demographic transition will place an increasing burden of support on the children of the surviving elderly. The steady decline in fertility will result in fewer offspring to share the load and the decline in mortality will mean longer periods of parental support. In 2030, a 45 year old rural person will have, on the average, 1.2 parents to support and at the age of 60, on the verge of retirement, 0.3 parents. For comparison, the corresponding figures for 1990 were 0.7 and 0.1 parent.

Adult children will not only have to support more elderly parents in 2030 than in 1990, they will have to do so for longer periods of time. At the age of 45, a rural person can expect another 10.47 years of coexistence with parents, an increase of 63 percent from 1990; at the age of 60, coexistence with parents will last another 1.27 years, compared with 0.43 in 1990. When the declining number of siblings is considered, the burden of elderly support in 2030 on a 40 year old son or daughter will be 2.3 times heavier than the burden carried by a 40 year old son or daughter in 1990.

Thus, while the demographic transition increased the availability of spouse support for men and did not restrict the availability of support by descendants for both sexes, it brought about a mounting burden on adult children, a load which can be expected to grow in the future. Furthermore, none of these analyses referred to the possible effect of rural to urban migration, which is on the increase, as shown above. Under these new circumstances, then, having surviving children can not necessarily be translate into support. While money transfers do not require residential proximity, nearness is essential for the provision of daily care and, to a large degree, for emotional support.

Under these circumstances, the elderly may have to turn to other kin for daily care. Increased survival ensures the availability of siblings, and both men and women will be able to rely on their younger siblings for help. The experience of Shanghai shows that the young-old can easily be recruited to support the old-old, those who are more likely to be disabled and dependent on assistance for daily living. Jiang (1995) reckoned that, when siblings are taken into consideration, the number of available supporters will increase, assuming that they are willing to divide the care and emotional support among them. When siblings are considered, people aged 65–69 can expect that 5.2 caretakers will be available for them in the year 2030, when the care-load is expected to reach its peak, compared with an average of 4.7 in 1990.

Although the culturally-preferred source of support is an adult son and his family, relying on siblings and other relatives is not unknown in Chinese society. Historical research into patterns of household composition and family formation clearly indicated that the traditional ideal of a multi-generational household was rarely possible before the demographic transition. In a simulation of the fertility, mortality, and nuptiality rates of 1930, Zhao (2000) calculated that 26.2 percent of the 60 year olds lived in a one-generation household, that is with their spouses or siblings, and 22.2 percent in two-generation households, that is, with children. According to his estimates, half of the 70 year olds lived in three-generation households, but the proportion of elderly of this age who lived in a one-generation household increased by 50 percent and reached 33.9 percent.

The ideal of at least one son to provide care in old age was also not attained in 1930: 33.3 percent of the 60 year olds and 37.7 percent of the 70 year olds had no surviving sons at all. On the other hand, 47.1 percent and 27.3 percent, respectively, had a surviving brother. Relatively high numbers of never-married men was another factor which encouraged sibling dependency. If this ancient filial support pattern is revived, the rural Chinese elderly will be able to rely on their offspring at least for financial support and on other kin for daily care. These arrangements will be able to meet the needs of the elderly as long as their families do not encounter economic crisis, often associated either with the unemployment of children or with heavy medical expenses, and as long as filial willingness to provide support persists.

Summary

We start the chapter by describing the aging process in the PRC. After the famine of the early 1960s and the social disorganization of the Cultural Revolution, the proportion of the elderly in China started to increase, the result of a decline in both fertility and mortality. Elderly dependency ratios have increased and are expected to reach 12.4 percent in the year 2015, when the elderly will comprise 8.9 percent of the population.

Formal support for the rural elderly population heavily relies on the family and has been the subject of extensive legislation. The decline in fertility and increased rural-urban migration endanger the welfare of the rural seniors. Most are not entitled to old-age pensions and welfare benefits (the 'five guarantees') are granted only to those who have no dependable kin or income and are unable to work ('the three nos'). In the absence of long-term care institutions and formal community services for the elderly, the rural family is responsible for the financial, emotional, and daily support of its elderly members.

Informal social support, however, is readily available for the rural elderly. Very few men and even fewer women live alone in the countryside. The most common arrangement up to the age of 80 is a two-person household, where husbands and wives live together. Our data suggest that the elderly of all ages prefer this type of household to the traditional multi-generation household headed by an elderly man. Furthermore, our analyses showed that women prefer this independent living arrangement, as long as they are capable of working in the fields, to the traditional role of a mother-in-law in their son's household.

Similar to the experience of the elderly in many industrial societies, the income of the elderly in rural HeBei falls considerably below that of persons of working age. Nonetheless, poverty is not gendered as it frequently is among the elderly in Western countries, and senior men and women in rural HeBei have a comparable standard of living. Furthermore, the widows we interviewed were better off than their married counterparts, especially if they complied with the social norms and joined the household of one of their offspring. The example of HeBei Province clearly demonstrates that the rural family provides a welfare safety net for its elderly members.

The prevalence of chronic health problems, such as cancer, cardiovascular and cerebrovascular diseases, hypertension, and diabetes, is lower than that usually observed in industrial societies. While this is consistent with the belief that China is in the midst of an epidemiological transition and that the transition is slower in the countryside than in the cities, it is possible that these conditions are under-diagnosed. Disability rates among elderly rural Chinese resemble those reported in health surveys of developed countries. Similar to these reports, disability increased with age and was more prevalent among the poor and among women. Disability considerably impairs the psychological well-being of the elderly, but not their participation in agriculture work. Disability, however, affects independent living: the seriously disabled tended to live with families headed by other kin. Thus, in rural HeBei families do meet the daily needs of their elderly members for care, on top of their financial needs.

Familial support will continue to be available for the elderly in rural China in the foreseeable future, despite the policy of population control. Examination of the demographic transition reveals that the decline in fertility has been counterbalanced by increased survivorship and by 2030, when the proportion of the elderly in the population is expected to peak, the number of potential care providers may be greater than it was in 1990. Rural-to-urban migration may constrain the feasibility of provision of social support by offspring, but revive the ancient pattern of reliance on kin other than married sons.

Chapter 9

Summary and Conclusions

In this volume, we examine the access to health, broadly defined, and health care of the rural population of the People's Republic of China. In each of the previous chapters we approached the subject through a detailed inquiry into one specific issue of health and health care, addressing universal health issues those under debate in developing as well as in post-industrial societies. In this chapter, the findings of our research in rural HeBei, secondary sources, and past research are discussed in light of the three central aims of this volume: the role of ideology, politics, and economy in shaping the access of rural population of the PRC to health and health care; pattern of lay and professional behavior; and patterns of health inequalities. Possible lessons for policy makers in developing as well as in developed countries are suggested.

Ideology and Economy

In many societies there seems to be a structural tension between proclaimed government ideology and the health, education, and welfare policies the government actually carries out. Often, the discrepancy between the ideologically based obligation of the state to its citizens and the services provided is rationalized by economic constraints and a shortage of public resources. In some societies, this tension brings about a change in the underlying ideology with respect to state versus individual responsibility for ensuring the citizens' welfare (Shuval and Anson, 2000).

The second half of the 20th century witnessed a dramatic rise in the cost of health brought about by both the aging of the population and the escalating cost of new medical technologies. Major reforms in the health care system took place in most industrially developed and developing societies (Twaddle, 2002). In many societies the containment of these costs became a primary objective (Chernichovsky, 1995; Stevens, 2001), yet there were additional aspects of the political-economic transitions of the health care systems, such as the demand for increased public involvement and patient autonomy in the provision of health care. Patients were no longer willing to accept the traditional paternalistic mode of medical care and insisted on a more egalitarian doctor-patient dyad, one in which their needs, desires, and structural constraints would be taken into account wherever decisions concerning health care were involved.

In some societies, such as the United Kingdom and Israel, these demands took on the form of a formal assertion of patient rights and care providers' duties vis-a-vis their clients (Annandale, 1998; Shuval and Anson, 2000; Anson, 1999). The following sections describe the processes that have taken place in the rural health care system of the PRC since 1979, in light of the main issues concerning health reform in Western Europe during the past two decades.

Ideology

Around 1980, apprehension increased among Western societies related to the expanding costs of the welfare state. Many felt that these costs were incompatible with the economical condition in industrial societies, and could no longer be sustained (Shuval and Anson, 2000). At the same time, a remarkable decline became apparent in the willingness of the wealthier sectors of these societies to continue to contribute the portion of their income necessary to maintain a welfare state. Conservative political movements saw in the private sector a key factor in the economic development of their country. They considered the reduction of taxes on individual and corporate earnings to be an essential condition for boosting economic growth. Actions taken to cut or at least limit the social resources allocated to health and welfare were accompanied by a reexamination of the core values of the welfare state. This ideological debate focused on the appropriate division of responsibilities between the collective and the individual, the state and its citizens. It has been argued that the provision of welfare services by the public sector is inefficient, brings about a waste of resources along with invasion of client autonomy, encourages dependency, and interferes with individual development of coping resources and skills. Privatization and competition became the accepted remedies for efficiency, quality, free choice and development.

While similar measures have been instituted in the People's Republic of China since 1979, they have not been accompanied by the same ideological transition. Since liberation, the CCP has been ideologically committed to equality of access to the 'five guarantees', that is the right of all citizens to housing, food, clothing, health care, and burial. Although lack of resources prevented the PRC from developing a welfare system which would ensure the 'five guarantees' by universal transfer of benefits to individuals, these convictions have persisted throughout the history of modern China, underlying the social, political, and economic transitions that have taken place since independence.

Social mobilization and economic development were perceived as the right paths to the actualization of these goals. The best documented form of social mobilization is the collective environmental action taken to eradicate endemic parasitic infectious diseases. Mass mobilization on different levels, as a mechanism for guaranteeing the welfare of the population, survived the political, economic, and social transitions that took place in modern China.

Economically successful villages provide guidance and assistance to poverty-stricken villages to foster their economic activity and production, while the central government provides these villages with the food they needed to stave off starvation in times of severe crisis.

Unable to sustain old-age pensions for all, the state recruited family support for senior citizens through legislation, while providing the 'five guarantees' to the most needy of them, those without families and income. Mobilizing the family to provide for the elderly was an outstanding example of the persistence of the ideological commitment of the CCP to provide the basic needs of the population. Unable to provide for the elderly, the PRC communist leaders chose to strengthen this element of the old Confucian tradition, a tradition they actually wished to eliminate, and enforce it by the civil law. The one-child policy is in many ways another form of mass mobilization, a measure taken to ensure the standard of living of current and future generations (White, 1990).

The underlying ideology thus emphasized the intertwined roles of education, health and the economy in promoting the welfare of the population, rather than the tension between the welfare needs of the population and economic growth. Moreover, since the early post-revolutionary period, health has been regarded as an economic asset and not as a budgetary liability. The well-being of the population could not be improved without economic growth, which in turn could not be achieved without preserving and developing natural resources. The most important and readily available resource of the PRC was its people, whose productivity was dependent on the condition of its health. Health promotion and economic development have thus been dependent on each other since the establishment of the PRC.

The innovative way in which China coped with infectious diseases in the early years has been described in Chapter 3. The eradication of schistosomiasis was coordinated with infrastructure development, particularly that aimed at more efficient management of water and arable land. The efforts to control other infectious diseases, whether transmitted by environmental or animal factors, took on a similar pattern. All were aimed at improving the health of the population and optimizing its productive potential simultaneously with the development of other resources such as land, water, and livestock.

The different population control policies also reflected the approach that put the human resources of the PRC at the center of its economic development programs, together with the responsibility of the state to balance the 'two types of production' (Riley and Gardner, 1997). Pro-natal policy during the first decade after liberation, when a large population was perceived as an important resource for development, to initial attempts to control the population growth as an economic crisis approached towards the end of the 1950s. With the political change and the transition to the 'socialist market economy', the PRC's leaders came to believe that the 'four modernizations' could not be achieved without strict population control, especially as the large cohorts of the post-famine baby boom (1963–65) approached child-bearing age. The one-child policy was launched in 1979 to prevent over-exploitation of natural resources for the sake of future generations and to ensure the economic growth necessary for consistent increase in the standard of living.

In all societies, there is tension between the interests of the individual, social groups, and the general public. Western societies tend to lend priority to the former, particularly to the social groups which control valuable resources that can be translated into political power. In some respects the PRC is no exception and public servants were able to ensure themselves of a lifelong income and medical care, unavailable to most farmers. However, individualism, a core value in post-industrial societies, does not yet occupy a central position in the value system of the PRC.

It was the emphasis on the public good that enabled the PRC to conduct policies that put the collective's before individual's interests. The direction of all resources to public health, including the eradication of communicable diseases, brought about an admirable improvement in the health of the population, although curative care for the individual was relatively neglected during the early years of the PRC. The shortage of resources, extreme as it was, and the pattern of disease before the epidemiological transition offer only a partial explanation for this compromised meeting of the health needs of individuals whose condition did not present a public health risk. The other side of the story is the priority given to the public good, even if at the expense of individuals.

In many ways population policies, from the pro-natal policy of the early 1950s to the most recent fertility regulations included in the 1995 Law on Infant and Maternal Health, represent the primacy of the collective and the mobilization of individuals, requiring them to sacrifice their desires and needs for the benefit of society as a whole. In the early 1950s, women were denied safe abortions; from the 1980s women were required to use contraceptives and to terminate unauthorized pregnancy even in late gestational age; the 1995 law denies parenthood to unhealthy couples and advises them to abort unhealthy fetuses. All these are in line with the primacy of the public good, as defined by the political regime at any given time, at the expense of the well-being of an unknown number of individuals.

Some of these policies were heavily criticized by Westerners, where the rights of individual citizens are central to the value system. Yet, in many of these societies, access by the poor and the powerless to social goods, including advanced curative medical technologies, is much more limited than that of the wealthy and the powerful. Furthermore, the costs of these technologies, which are designed to cure the individual patient, could have been much more beneficial if invested in public health programs. A human or artificial heart transplant, for instance, is unlikely to reduce mortality from heart disease of an entire society, but a serious investment in smoking control may do so. Similarly, although Western societies do not deny the right to give birth to persons unable to raise their children, some are less reluctant than others to forbid parenthood, using the legal system to enforce adoption against the parents will.

In sum, the ideology of the PRC did not change, but remained committed to the idea that the state is responsible for the welfare of its citizens. For the CCP, welfare and economy are not competing, but complementary values. When the level of economic development interferes with the fulfillment of its welfare commitments, the latter are met by mobilizing the masses, even at the expense of reviving traditional, counterrevolutionary, values. Similarly, as presented in Chapter 1, the privatization of the rural health services was not the result of a change in ideology, but a by-product of the transition to the 'socialist market economy'.

Cost Containment

Like many other societies, China is experiencing a steady rise in the cost of health and health care. In the midst of the epidemiological transition it needs to cope with communicable diseases characteristic of developing countries and the increasing prevalence of chronic health problems typical of industrial societies. In Western countries the rising cost of care is usually attributed to the aging of the population and the constant introduction of new, expensive medical technology. In rural China, where the great majority of the population lives, the share of the elderly in the whole population is still much lower than the average in Western Europe and many East European countries. The increase in health expenditures appears to be the result of an increase in the supply and demand for medical technology since the economic reforms of 1979, which brought about three intertwined processes: First, the rise in disposable income, which increased demand for higher quality health care (Chapters 1 and 5; Liu et al, 1996; Yip et al, 1998); Second, the privatization of over half of the rural primary health services, the emergence of a fee-for-service care delivery system, in which village doctors make a living by selling medication and performing therapeutic procedures (Chapter 4; Zhan et al, 1998); And finally, the decline in public resources allocated to hospitals and increasing pressure on public health facilities to generate their own income (Chapter 4; Chen et al, 1997).

The leaders of the PRC, then, faced the need to contain costs, as did many other governments around the globe. As other governments have done, the PRC forced the health sector to increase efficiency and enable competition between care providers and manufacturers of medical materia. In line with its ideological commitment to health care for all, it regulated the price of hospital care and profit generated from medication in an effort to maintain affordable health care for the entire population.

With the transition of the pharmaceutical industry from a planned economy to a market economy in 1982, hospitals were able to seek cheaper drugs and purchase them on the free market (Dong et al, 1999a), but this avenue for cutting costs became less feasible as the government resumed control over both the price and the quality of medication. In line with the 'health for all' ideology, since the late 1990s, the prices of essential drugs have been reduced, and hospitals have been fined for using less than standard quality medication (Chinese Medical News, 2001a; 2001b).

Increasing pressure on hospitals to generate their own resources was unique to the PRC. It was expected that cuts in government funding and controlling prices at a level below that of operating costs would lead hospitals not only to increase the efficiency of care delivery, but to initiate non-medical economic enterprise. The volume of such non-medical economic involvement is unknown, though anecdotal reports suggest that some hospitals were involved in rural industry and in joint ventures with the pharmaceutical industry. Clearly, however, the most immediate source of income for health care facilities is patient fees. Hospitals thus tend to dispense large quantities of expensive drugs and to invest in and use advanced technology, for which patient fees are not regulated. In outpatient primary services (Chapter 4) we indicated that doctors in hospital-owned primary clinics performed more medical procedures per visit and charged for more activities than did village doctors in private practice. The ways in which health care facilities coped with the declining share of public resources in their budgets were thus unlikely to contribute toward cost containment but, rather, contribute to the rising cost of health.

As described in Chapter 2, pressure applied by the government to increase productivity led to a decline in the actual number of hospital beds, despite population growth. In the mid 1990s the number of general hospital beds had been reduced by close to one-third. Nevertheless, bed occupancy rates did not increase. This process was more intensive in hospitals owned by collectives, which generally served the rural population.

The paradox between the decline in the number of hospital beds and the persistent low occupancy rates can be the result of two processes. It is possible that the number of beds was adjusted to actual needs, but that increased efficiency led to shorter hospital stays and the use of new technology facilitated quicker transition to ambulatory treatment. However, the possibility that with the collapse of the medical cooperation scheme after the economic reforms of 1979 hospital care was beyond the reach of the rural population cannot be overruled.

Some observers (e. g. Chen, 1997; Liu et al, 1999) noted that the high costs led the poor to avoid hospitalization. A recent study conducted by the Chinese Ministry of Health reports that the shortage in money caused half of the urbanites to refrain from seeking help and one in three patients referred to a hospital did not comply (Chinese Medical News, 2001b). In rural HeBei, the anticipated cost of hospitalization accounted for 14.7 percent of the non-compliance with village doctors' hospital referrals.

Cost containment became a policy issue in the PRC during the 1980s, similar to processes observed in developed countries. Much of the increase in health expenditures was the result of the transition from planned economy to market economy, particularly in the health sector. The measures introduced by the PRC to hold costs down were similar in many ways to reforms introduced in the health care systems of Western Europe. The introduction of managed competition, curtailed public resources, and privatization of the health sector, however, boosted health expenditures, instead of constraining them. Similarly, price control, a measure taken to fulfill the ideological commitment to health for all, seems to have contributed to increasing costs rather than constraining them.

Public Involvement

Another major issue in the health care reforms of Western Europe was the growing dissatisfaction with the provision of health care. The organization of medical care in bureaucratic institutions, professional elitism, and disenchantment with medical science led to increasing alienation and frustration among patients (Shuval, 1995; Shuval and Anson, 2000; Stevens, 2001). These processes were related to the emerging culture of consumerism on the one hand and the expanding exposure to scientific knowledge, brought about by a rising level of education and access to information via the print and electronic media and intensified by the processes of globalization. Patients demanded greater involvement in the organization and management of the health services and greater autonomy in the choice of care and care providers.

The situation in rural China was decidedly different. Despite the appreciable achievements in initiating and developing a rural education system available to all, the level of education in the countryside rarely exceeded primary school (Chapters 1 and 7). Furthermore, because of the policy of isolation maintained by the PRC until the 1980s, exposure to foreign mass media was very limited and available primarily to urbanites. Access to the internet, a powerful information tool which increased the demand for the most recently developed medical technologies, is still fairly restricted, the result of shortage in the necessary equipment, knowledge of English, and some governmental control on overseas communication.

These limitations have no doubt restrained the demand for autonomy and choice of health care. Public involvement in health and choice of care providers was, however, an integral part of the CCP health ideology. The most obvious representations of this ideology were the multi-sectorial action and mass mobilization for public health work described in Chapter 3 and the selection of care providers, the 'bare foot doctors', by members of their own work brigades.

Like adult education, public health work became part of the annual agricultural cycle and of the economic, social and political life of the rural population. Elected representatives of the local rural population were involved in planning; during the slack agricultural seasons the entire population participated in public health work. In the cities, public health activities organized by the Street Office focused on cleaning up the immediate environment. Health workers were chosen by their comrades on the basis of education, personal interest in medicine, and personality. The expense of their training was borne by the community they returned to serve. Health became everybody's responsibility.

It has been argued that mass mobilization and involvement in health ceased after the transition to the 'system of household responsibility', and farmers were unwilling to take part in such collective actions, as the village authorities were not able to compensate them for the time devoted to these activities. Nevertheless, we suggest that many of the features of mass involvement in health work did persist even in the era of 'socialist market economy'.

The implementation of the one-child policy mentioned above (Chapter 7) is one example of mass mobilization, not only because it required individual sacrifice, but also because of the way in which families are chosen within the birth quota of the village. The most recent example of mass mobilization was the National Immunization Days described in Chapter 3. Close to 300 million children received Oral Poliovirus Vaccine at four week intervals during the winters of 1991 through 1996. The performance involved multi-sectorial cooperation and volunteers from the Youth League and the Women's Federation who identified and prepared the target population, going from house to house in some locations (Zhang, 1997, 1998). Community programs for the elderly recruited health and able-bodied retirees to provide support for the sick and the disabled.

It appears that it was not the weakening of the public will to fulfill collective health requirements that brought about the decline in mass mobilization and involvement in health promotion, but rather the changing nature of the requirements themselves. The new public health challenges did not lend themselves to mass mobilization in the same way, and could be met by the application of intensive labor. Many of these challenges have to do with environmental pollution, largely caused since 1979 by mushrooming rural industries. The treatment of industrial waste requires a vast investment in technology. Such investment has been increasing since the mid 1990s.

Other environmental health hazards are caused by the intensification of agriculture. Both traditional and modern methods of fertilization are associated with health risks. The first, which makes use of human and animal waste, increases the risk of transmitting infectious diseases and parasites. The use of modern fertilizers and pesticides, on the other hand, increases the risk of poisoning and water contamination. Waste purification technology is needed to reduce the risks involved in the use of organic material. To date, there is no satisfactory solution to pollution caused by chemicals used in agriculture.

Nevertheless, the prevention of work and road accidents can be significantly reduced by large investment in health education and mass mobilization. With the experience acquired in dealing with other aspects of health promotion, which led to extraordinary achievements in reducing infant, child and maternal mortality, increased longevity and improved general health of the population, the PRC can lead a worldwide safety campaign. Work and road safety are examples of human behavior, which, like any other forms of human behavior, are learnt and can be modified in ways similar to the modification in hygiene and nutrition.

In the same manner, health risks associated with the consumption of different substances and unhealthy food products can be reduced. Consumption of cigarettes, alcohol, saturated fat, salt, etc., according to present scientific knowledge, entails considerable health risks. Serious efforts to control this behavior are rare, since in most post-industrial as well as industrially developing countries, governments gain considerable revenue from the tax paid on much of this merchandise. The PRC is no exception, and very little is done to limit the consumption of substances, except for drug abuse. The most common measure taken in industrial societies to limit the consumption of tobacco and alcohol is price control, which has little effect on public behavior, but increases government revenue. The PRC should avoid this path, and develop health programs aimed at controlling this risk-filled behavior, along with the emerging problem of obesity.

Patient Autonomy and Choice

The reform of the health care systems in Western Europe took place in an era of developing consumerism and increasing emphasis on individualism. As mentioned above, patients required to be more involved in decision-making in matters concerning their own health and there was increasing demand for autonomy and choice of both treatment and providers.

The choices available to patients in rural China were fairly limited throughout the history of the PRC, except for the three decades when farmers decided which of them would make the best 'bare foot doctors'. During this period, however, farmers could not seek medical help in a facilities of their choice, without referral from their work brigade's health workers. With the abolishment of the collective, the community ceased to choose its own provider and the regulations which set a fixed number of practitioners per population limited competition among the providers.

Indeed, in most of the villages we visited in HeBei Province there is not much choice among care providers. As described in Chapter 6, only one village doctor practiced in one-third of the villages and two village doctors in an additional one-quarter of the villages. However, there are no formal restrictions on seeking medical help beyond that available within the village.

Like patients elsewhere, the residents of rural HeBei appreciated choice. Satisfaction with the health care provided in the village was associated with the number of different types of clinics available in the village. The demand for high quality health care has already been documented by past research in rural China and was apparent among some, albeit small, social groups in HeBei

Province. On the other hand, while there were no more formal restrictions on seeking medical help beyond that available within the village, seeking help outside the village involved considerable costs.

The choice of treatment regimen has also been limited considerably since the privatization of the primary health services. In line with the principle of 'walking on two legs', primary care providers should be able to provide both Western and traditional Chinese medicine and the choice between the two healing systems should involve the consumer. In order to encourage the use of traditional Chinese medicine, biomedical research programs continually examine traditional therapeutic methods, some traditional drugs are made available in prefabricated tablets, and the mark-up of traditional herbs is twice as high as that of Western medication. However, as presented in Chapter 4, private practitioners, that is half of the primary care providers in rural China, tend to stock a very limited selection of traditional herbs, which consume more space, require more preparation time, and are less profitable, despite the double profit allowed because of their very low initial retail price.

In sum, the rural health care reforms had a contrary effect on patient autonomy. Within the village, the choices of available providers and healing systems became more limited. However, farmers were less dependent on the services offered in their village and could seek help elsewhere, if they possessed the additional resources required.

Health Related Behavior: Providers and Consumers

Access to health and health care may be eased or constrained by the behavior of individuals and groups, that is, the providers of care, lay persons, and the interface of the two. The behavioral patterns of individuals and groups have been presented in detail in Chapters 4 and 5. In this concluding chapter, we expand on some universal issues that are currently in dispute in many societies.

Care Provision

The interest in the behavioral patterns of care providers as individuals and institutions led to the development of a sub-field in the discipline of sociology, the sociology of the professions (Riska, 2001). It was widely accepted in earlier analyses of service professions that one basic characteristic of such a profession is a sense of 'calling', in the Weberian sense of the concept (Weber, 1978). Structural functionalists have argued that this 'calling' orientation dictates professional behavior which puts service before any other interests. This school of thought, however, rarely dealt with the possible paradoxical interpretation of the primacy of service which stems from the Weberian concern with bureaucracy and bureaucratic organizations. The question of whose interests are to be served, those of the organization, the professional group, or of the client, were not raised until the 1970s (Freidson, 1970).

The Parsonian analysis of the profession of medicine elaborated on the 'calling' orientation, although indirectly (Parsons, 1939, 1951). With regard to health professionals, Parsons was particularly concerned with the risk of exploitation inherent in the inequality of knowledge and, thus, unequal power in the doctor-patient relationship. He emphasized the role of professional socialization, during which, he claimed, collective rather than individualistic values are internalized. It is these values that assure the primacy of the patient's interests when conflict arises between the interests of the professional provider or of the organization providing the care and the needs of the patient. Peer control is the mechanism of social control that protects society from professional deviance and the violation of the collective values. The efficiency of the socialization process and peer control, and the implications of professional solidarity for peer control were, again, largely ignored before the pioneering work of Freidson (1970).

Neo-Marxist analysis, conflict theory, and political economy discourse looked into the role of status rewards, that is, profit and power, in the patterns of service delivery (Turner, 1997). The arguments drawn from this line of thought are particularly relevant in the context of recent health service reforms in the developed and the developing worlds, which applied the assumptions of a free market economy to the provision of social services.

The underlying premise of these reforms was that competition, even if regulated, will meet the objectives of managerial efficiency and cost containment and improve quality of service and client satisfaction. Nonetheless, bureaucratic health care organizations, forced to compete with one another on strict budgets, started to issue administrative regulations to ensure cost containing professional behavior. There is evidence that professional practice was modified in reaction to organizational pressure to reduce the costs of treatment in both the public and the private sectors (Annandale, 1998). The quality of care, however, did not improve (Gross and Anson, 2002). Social scientists and activists became increasingly concerned that the introduction of market attributes to social services would lead to increasingly inequitable access to care and distribution of health resources.

This debate, however, paid little attention to the social context in which the doctor-patient social interaction is taking place. The organizational culture and the characteristics of the work setting are no less important in determining professional practice than the process of professional socialization (Shuval, 1980). Indeed, when we examined the data we had collected in HeBei Province, we found that medical practice appeared to reflect a combination of professional orientation, social integration of the practitioner in the milieu in which he served, and the level of social control exercised in the organizational setting in which medicine is practiced.

As described in Chapter 1, the implementation of the 'system of household responsibility' boosted economic productivity and growth and increased the standard of living of a large proportion of the population. Nonetheless, the same transition also undermined the financial basis of the welfare safety net and the cooperative medical scheme which ensured primary health services to farmers in the village. These processes brought about the emergence of three main types of primary care clinics (Chapter 5) operating under different ownership: private, group practice, and government-owned clinics.

The main source of revenue in all clinics is the payment received from prescribing and selling drugs to patients and from fees collected for treatment and diagnostic procedures performed. Yet, the immediacy of the association between practitioners' income and medical practice varies with ownership type. At one end of the continuum are private practitioners, whose income from medical practice is almost completely dependent on patient fees. Some private practitioners were commissioned to perform public health duties, such as Mother and Child Health and water purification work, which increases their income. At the other end of the continuum are the salaried employees of the government or county hospitals. Village doctors in this work receive a fixed salary and an annual bonus, which reflects their productivity. Thus, Rural China offers an opportunity to test hypotheses raised in the sociological debate presented above. In particular, we will focus on the critique and the undesirable consequences of the continuing process of privatization of health services in Western societies.

The picture that emerged from the data collected from 288 villages in 9 HeBei Province counties was far too complicated to justify the simplistic argument that instrumental motives led to inequity in the distribution of health services, to inequality of access to health care, and to revenue-oriented medical practice. Although there is some evidence for inequity and inequality in the access to care in rural HeBei, the data also suggested that the social context of the medical practice was far more important for an understanding of the differential access to care and professional behavior than the income motive.

Reports from post-industrial societies consistently show inequities in the distribution of health services (Chernichovsky and Shirom, 1996; Shuval and Anson, 2000). In many of these societies, fewer health facilities and health personnel are available for rural populations, on the periphery, for the poor, and for other social groups with greater health needs. Free market in the health sector, it is argued, will increase inequity and inequality, as disadvantaged social groups are less likely to attract providers motivated by income or budget considerations. Several observations in rural HeBei lead us to conclude that private and collective health provision systems do not ensure equity in the distribution of health care and that the public (government) system only partially promotes equality.

1. Equity

The accepted definition of equity is that the distribution of health care facilities and personnel parallels the health needs of the population. A system that allocates health care resources equally does not necessarily bring about equity in the distribution of health care. A policy like that of the PRC, which located village clinics according to population size, may thus result in inequity.

This, however, was not the case in rural HeBei (Chapter 6). The best indicator for the availability of a clinic in the village was the number of inhabitants, but the size of a village was not the only determinant of inter-village variability in access to care. The health needs of the population emerged as an important factor in explaining the distribution of health personnel as well as the distribution of village clinics. The poorest villages, where health needs were greater, had the highest ratio of providers per population and were served by slightly more clinics per 1,000 populations than villages whose mean per-capita income was above the average income in our sample.

This equity was indeed achieved by the intervention of the public sector. As suggested by analyses embedded in the conflict theory, the poorest villages, those in the lowest income quintile, were least able to attract and/or sustain private practitioners. This void was filled by the public sector through the creation of outpatient clinics run by government-owned hospitals. Because these clinics were staffed with more health providers than were privately owned clinics and group practices, a higher ratio of providers to population was achieved. Moreover, because these clinics were staffed by better trained personnel and more patient beds, the intervention of the public sector ensured access to higher quality care for the most needy population.

There were, however, two exceptions that should concern policy makers. First, in terms of equity, public intervention was more efficient in villages located closer to urban centers, at a mean radius of 20 Km from the county hospital. Of the nine primary care hospital branches, six operated in villages located 35–79 Km from a city hospital, while only one farther away.

Second, the regulations regarding the clinic-per-population ratio inevitably resulted in a lack of clinics in small villages. Of the 288 villages we visited during our study in rural HeBei, 11 had no clinic in the village itself. Six of these villages were very poor and were located more than 35Km from the nearest county hospital and more than 80 Km from the nearest city hospital. Thus, though a high level of equity in the distribution of health services had been achieved in rural HeBei through public sector interventions, there were still some pockets whose needs were not met by either the public or the private sector (Anson et al, 2003).

2. Equality

Contrary to expectations derived from the Neo-Marxist approach, however, the privatization of a large proportion of the rural primary health services did not diminish equality of access to care, nor did the public sector increase it. This conclusion is based on several observations in rural HeBei.

First, the type of ownership of the clinic(s) in the village was not associated with help-seeking behavior. In cases of acute health problems, farmers sought the help of a village doctor, regardless of the ownership type of the clinic or clinics available in the village. Second, total out-of-pocket health expenditures were unrelated to the ownership of the clinic(s) in the village. Finally, in villages where private practices, group practices, and clinics still supported by the collective were available, the most commonly cited reason for not seeking medical advice in cases of disease was the patient's own evaluation of the severity of his illness. It was in the villages with government owned clinics that instrumental difficulties most often restricted people seeking help.

At the same time, while the public sector contributed to the equitable distribution of health services it also contributed to inequality. While one-third of the hospital branches were found in the poorest villages we studied in HeBei Province, another one-third were found in the richest villages. The distribution pattern of primary care clinics owned by the public sector in rural HeBei indicated that these clinics were introduced to meet both the health needs of the population and the financial needs of the hospitals. Hospital branches were available in villages with greater health needs, but also in rich villages where the population was able to pay higher fees and thus increase the income of the parent hospital. As shown in Chapter 6, the health expenditures of patients in richer villages were higher than those of patients in poorer villages. Moreover, these villages enjoyed a larger variety of health services and twice as many better-off villages were both able to maintain private practitioners and support collective services. The additional contribution of the public sector, then, enhanced their advantage.

3. Medical Practice

With respect to increased involvement of the private sector in the provision of social services, many social scientists argue that private practitioners are more concerned with generating income than are salaried employees. In particular, it has been suggested that preventive and public health activities, the least profitable for the practitioner, will be neglected. The picture that emerged in rural HeBei did not fully support this argument, demonstrating that in rural China vocational education, social context, and instrumental motives can hardly be separated.

In matters of public health, salaried village doctors were more involved with the village administration. Village doctors in other settings, however, preferred to discuss these matters with county administration. The ownership of the village clinic(s) was not related to the number of health practitioners carrying out public health duties. At the same time, about half of the hospital primary care branches were located in villages with greater health needs. It may thus be argued that the volume and the urgency of the population's health needs, together with the type of clinics' ownership brought about greater involvement in public health activity, rather than unwillingness on the part of private doctors to get involved in activities that were less likely to generate profit.

Salaried employees in the public sector provided more cardiovascular risk control for their patients. This differential medical practice, however, could not be explained by economic incentives alone, although private village doctors were less likely than salaried employees to charge their patients for procedures that were not directly curative, such as measuring blood pressure. Village doctors employed in the clinics set by government hospitals were better trained and socialized to pay more attention to the long-term importance of such individual preventive care, beyond immediate curative needs. Hospital branches are also better equipped than other types of village clinics to perform laboratory tests. Professional socialization, work setting, and expected revenues, then, could each account for the differences between public and private sector village doctors.

Private village doctors in rural HeBei did not perform more profit-generating medical procedures and did not prescribe more medication than did doctors in collectively owned facilities or in clinics owned by government hospitals. On the contrary, the latter reported performing more diagnostic tests and prescribed more medication than doctors in privately owned clinics for treating similar conditions. Once again, this can be the result of different professional training, the work setting, and the desire to increase personal income. The pressure on hospitals to increase efficiency and to generate an increasing portion of their budget, and the bonus system introduced by the hospital management to encourage employees to increase productivity, resulted in economic incentive for medical personnel in public facilities. Approximately one-quarter of the annual income from medical practice in the public sector was generated by either patient fees or the bonus redistributed to the employees of hospital branches.

The instrumental incentive, together with the social context of the work setting, can both explain the differences in fees charging behavior reported in Chapter 4. Almost all village doctors employed by government owned clinics charged their patients for each diagnostic test and treatment procedure, except for public health procedures and treatment in traditional Chinese therapeutic methods. For each procedure, fewer village doctors in private clinics charged their patients, while the behavior of doctors in group practice was closer to that of doctors in government owned clinics.

The work setting of private practitioners is most flexible and the individual village doctor could decide under which conditions patient fees should be collected. Doctors in collective and government-owned clinics did not enjoy such freedom and were much more susceptible to mechanisms of social control. In group practices and collectively supported clinics, doctors were subject to peer control; in government owned clinics they were subject to administrative guidelines and control.

There was only one finding that attested to the greater interest in patient fees taken by private practitioners and village doctors in group practices. In these two types of clinic a limited number of traditional Chinese herbs were stocked, suggesting that choices were not made exclusively on the basis of the space available in the clinics. Group practice settings were more spacious than private ones, but supplied fewer traditional herbs. Because auxiliary staff was present mainly in hospital branches, it seemed that the collection of drugs in the clinic also reflected time and income considerations.

The Consumers

1. The definition of health

Health related behavior is closely connected with culture, and the cultural meaning attributed to social behavior can promote or impair good health. Similarly, the consumption of health services is culturally patterned, because of the interpretation of dis-ease as ill health and the level of symptoms that legitimate seeking help are culturally defined (Quah, 2001).

Three observations in rural HeBei were most important in this respect. First, the primacy of role performance in the definition of health. This cultural feature emerged in the early stages of analysis of the health measure used in our study. In Western societies the instrument we used (SF-12) clearly covers six dimensions of health (Ware et al, 1996). It distinguishes between general health perception, the effect of physical and mental health on the respondent's regular work, physical and social functioning, pain, psychological well-being, and a sense of vitality. In rural HeBei, by contrast, only three dimensions of health emerged: work, or the ability to carry out daily responsibilities; long term limitations on functioning; and mental well-being (Anson and Haanappel, 1999). The source of the limitation seemed not to have any importance; it was the outcome that counted, and first and foremost the ability to perform regular work.

Thus, unlike Westerners, our respondents did not differentiate between the unique contributions of physical ill-health, psychological dis-ease, and pain to their difficulties or inability to perform their regular duties. By the same token, there was no differentiation between the long-term chronic functional difficulties in the physical and the social spheres, and the sense of vitality clustered with a bad mood to construct one facet of mental health. However, of these three dimensions of health, role performance was primarily defined within the domain of medicine and medical care.

Our data from rural HeBei strongly suggested that farmers were likely to define the need for medical help when their physical, sensual, or psychological state interfered with their work and normal tasks. A bad mood, lack of energy, and long-standing functional limitations were far less frequently presented to the village doctor. As shown in Chapter 5, acute conditions, that is, a relatively sudden breakdown in ability to carry out usual daily activity, was the main stimulant for visits to a doctor. Chronic conditions and disability, which by their nature are not associated with a precipitate disruption of usual activity, rarely initiated help seeking.

The process by which a sudden decline in ability to work came to be defined under the jurisdiction of the primary care provider cannot be clarified with the data currently available. One possible explanation could be that acute conditions, which appear abruptly, are culturally defined as amendable to short term intervention such as provided by the village doctor. Long-term health problems call either for adjustment or for the intervention of another healing system. This possibility was not explored in our study in HeBei Province or in past research known to us.

Similarly, the degree to which these patterns of help seeking were influenced by the post-revolutionary attitudes that connected health with productivity cannot be determined. As presented above, the CCP regarded good health as an economic asset and the most important national resource. Individual well-being was secondary to economic prosperity, of which all would benefit in due course. Seeking the help of a village doctor to restore the ability to work and perform daily tasks accorded well with this approach, which laid the foundations of the health care provision currently available in the village.

Whatever the cultural attitudes behind the observed pattern of help seeking behavior, chronic health problems were fairly neglected in rural HeBei. As shown, chronic conditions were likely to be attended to upon the occurrence of an acute health problem. In light of the changing pattern of disease in rural China and the increase in the incidence of chronic health conditions typical of industrially developed societies, such patterns of consumption of health services presented considerable public health risks. Untreated chronic conditions might result in premature mortality caused by cardiovascular and cerebrovascular diseases in particular. Health educators should attend to these risks, and develop adequate intervention programs.

2. Health behavior

The cultural meaning of other forms of health behavior also called for intervention by the public health and health education authorities. Some goods, which at our current state of biomedical knowledge are accepted as health risks, appeared to be seen as status symbols. The most obvious examples presented in this volume were the consumption of saturated fat (Chapter 3), cigarettes, and alcohol (Chapter 5). The social distribution of the consumption of these goods indicated that they were culturally valued and symbolized achievement, maturation, and prosperity.

The positive cultural meaning assigned to the consumption of saturated fat, cigarettes, and alcohol implied that mechanisms of social control were not recruited in order to some of the behaviors that entail health risks. In some societies, the family and the primary group, for example, were effective mechanisms of social control over culturally undesirable behavior, such as substance consumption (Anion, 1989; Umberson, 1992; Shuval and Anson, 2000). In China, however, we found that higher income families and urban families consume more saturated fat and provide their children with a fat rich diet. In rural HeBei the consumption of alcohol and tobacco was highly prevalent among men and increased with age and with the transition to adult social roles such as family formation. The consumption of alcohol followed a similar pattern and was also related to level of education and household headship. In other words, social control mechanisms were effective in preventing women and men culturally defined as 'immature' from assuming such 'masculine' and adult behaviors. This cultural interpretation of smoking, drinking, and nutrition will have to be altered in order to reduce the alarming prevalence of this behavior and promote healthier diet.

The Interface

1. The village doctor and professionalism

The process through which an occupation becomes a profession is another debated issue. Early examinations of the special attributes of these occupations that enjoy professional stance suggested that professionals engage in work that is highly valued in society, posses an esoteric body of knowledge obtained during a long period of specialized training, and share a common code of ethics (Hughes, 1958). These characteristics award professionals with power and prestige, which make the status of a professional rather attractive. The social power held by professional groups and individual practitioners over their clients call for each society to develop mechanisms to regulate entry into the professions in order to protect innocent patients and ensure qualified medical treatment.

Later theoretical developments challenged this functional point of view, suggesting that the transmutation of an occupation into a profession is political in nature (Larson, 1977; Starr, 1982). According to this argument, practitioners of bio-medicine succeeded through collective action in ensuring their common interests. Group cohesiveness enabled them to accumulate the resources necessary to convince others of the supremacy of their knowledge and technology over other healing systems. Licensing, according to this approach, protects the profession and the professionals rather than the society and patients. It is a mechanism to ensure the power of the profession to regulate itself, its monopoly over the provision of medical care, and the exclusion of competing health providers from the reward associated with professional status.

The application of these theoretical debates to rural China is extremely intriguing. Care providers in rural China differ considerably from their Western counterparts and the paths of entry into the position of village doctor are substantially different. Until the dismantling of the collective economy in the early 1980s, health providers were chosen by members of their community, rather than by representatives of the profession, and professional training differed in form and content. The training programs were, and most still are, much shorter. In Chapter 2 we indicated that only since 1985 has a level been required that is equivalent to a secondary medical school, that is a high school education with concentration on medicine, for approval of village doctors. Unlike Western programs, this level of medical education does not emphasize scientific knowledge and its rational integration as the basis for medical practice.

The remarkable outcome of mass involvement in public health and care delivered by these health workers – neighbors who completed a short course of training – led to a considerable demystification of medicine. The rapid decline in mortality brought about by collective action and the contribution of lay persons, combined with the care provided by fellow villagers who obtained practical skills during a short period of time, expedited the process of familiarization.

Moreover, the absence of subdivision in health work and the lack of paraprofessionals led to a greater affinity between village doctors and their patients. In industrial societies, the division of health work between doctors and allied health professions, particularly the nursing profession, increases the social distance between doctors and patients. In these societies, the division of medical care and the associated socioeconomic rewards also correspond with gender division of labor and status, which enhances the differential power of the profession of medicine (Davis, 1996). In rural China, village doctors provide all aspects of care themselves, including simple tasks such as bandaging wounds and giving injections, and thus lack such distance-reinforcing mechanisms. In a more elaborate division of health work systems, such tasks are the domain of the nursing profession, physicians perform tasks defined culturally as 'clean', unless engaged in heroic 'life saving' procedures.

As with other workers and occupational groups in the PRC, doctors are organized in a national union. The functions of labor unions in the PRC, however, are rather different from those of unions in industrial societies, and rarely take actions aimed at improving work conditions or the occupational status of their members (Guidotti and Levister, 1995). Indeed, the licensing policy implemented in 1985 was initiated by the state to ensure at least minimal acceptable competence on the part of the care providers. By no means was it the result of a collective political action taken by a cohesive occupational group to endow it with social legitimacy and the superiority of one healing system over others.

The degree to which village doctors in rural China share a code of ethics is not clear. In analyzing the data collected from village doctors in rural HeBei we found evidence that they were highly committed to serving their patients (Chapter 4). Yet, service orientation is but one, albeit central, value in the ethical code of the profession. Similarly, the social prestige of village doctors is not clear. Their expertise does provide them with knowledge-based power, despite its non-Western attributes. However, their modest income, which imposes on them a standard of living very similar to that of their farming neighbors, together with the absence of other social distance engendering mechanisms, would suggest that they do not enjoy the prestige possessed by their Western counterparts.

2. The doctor-patient dyad

Private, fee-for-service, health care systems are believed to have several advantages over public care provision. Attentiveness to the patients' health beliefs and attitudes and responsiveness to their definitions of needs are often mentioned in this respect (Yuen, 1992). It has been suggested that the escalating health expenditure experienced by the PRC during the past two decades, following the market reforms in the health sector, has at least partly been the result of patient demand for medication. This demand, based on a cultural preference for drug treatment, has been observed in several studies in the PRC (Zhan et al, 1998; Dong et al, 1999a).

In rural HeBei, village doctors were sensitive to the structural constraints faced by their patients. Analysis of the pattern of prescriptions and referral to a higher level facility showed that village doctors took into consideration the distance to the nearest clinic or hospital when deciding on the course of treatment. They were more likely to wait for a patient's condition to develop before administrating medication when the patient lived near the clinic; village doctors whose practice was far from the nearest hospital were more likely to refrain from referring patients to an upper level facility than were doctors whose practice was located near a hospital.

Another indication of the sensitivity of doctors to their patients' wishes was the differential medical practice applied to educated and illiterate patients. As with Chinese patients in Singapore, the better educated patients were reluctant to use medication (Chapter 5, Quah, 1985, 1993). In rural HeBei, village doctors generally respected these attitudes of better educated patients and tended to allow them to wait for the health condition to develop or for spontaneous recovery before intervening.

The Distribution of Health

All societies, rich and poor, are faced with limited resources to meet the needs of their members. In all societies the available resources have to be allocated and criteria for allocation must be negotiated. Public debate often deals with issues of equality of access to health and health care and of equity in the distribution of health services. In reality, however, resource allocation is the result of a power struggle between different social groups. It reflects the ideology and the interests of the social group or groups who have the power to impose their particular agendas during the negotiation process (Shuval and Anson, 2000).

In many ways, the People's Republic of China is no exception. As early as 1953, the report produced by the 3rd National Health Work Conference opened by criticizing 'subjectivism, bureaucraticism and dispersionism', which interfered with effectiveness and the efficiency of public health work (Wilenski, 1977). In the succeeding years, cadres were regularly criticized for their lack of cooperation, perceiving themselves as above involvement in mundane health work, etc. This criticism could reflect a process that concealed a hidden power struggle aimed at protecting and advancing group interests. Interest groups were struggling to define and guard their domains of responsibility, to prevent other groups from invading their 'territory', and to force the dependency of other social groups in order to increase and preserve their own power.

In 1958, less than a decade after the revolution, Mao Ze Dong denounced the Ministry of Public Health for focusing on the urban population, which constituted only 15 percent of the total population of the country, while neglecting the needy peasants. He criticized the Ministry of Health for its slowness in establishing the three-tier care system in rural areas. The combination of administrative stagnation, bureaucratization, and the political needs caused by the 'Great Leap Forward' led Mao Ze Dong to launch the Cultural Revolution in 1966. The Ministry of Public Health and other health institutions were severely criticized and the minister of public health with his six vice-ministers was removed from office as early as in 1967.

Although the expansion of health services and the three-tier health care system were completed during the Cultural Revolution, disproportional access of urbanites to the social resources allocated to health and welfare persisted. Full coverage of health expenses and old-age pensions were, and largely still are, available almost exclusively to government employees (Chapter 8). Though in the current stage of the PRC's economic development such coverage for the total population is not feasible, it is difficult to overlook the fact that the beneficiaries are those closer to the centers of political and social power. Neither the Cultural Revolution nor the transition to market economy brought about greater equality or equity in the distribution of social resources allocated to health and welfare.

Similarly, investment in health facilities was not equally distributed. As presented in Chapter 2, throughout the past fifty years a larger share of the investment in hospitals and hospital beds has been allocated to the above-county level. The economic reforms of 1979, followed by the requirement for greater efficiency and operating profit, resulted in a decline in the number of hospital beds. The decline, however, was greater in county level hospitals, those which had and still have lower occupancy rates. While such a decline made sense from a purely economic point of view it raised several questions regarding equality and equity, to which the data available to us provided no clear-cut answers. Why did villagers whose health needs are greater than urbanites avoid hospital care? To what extent was this phenomenon the result of the collapse of the cooperative health system after decollectivization? What was the role of the village doctors, medical practice and referral behavior in lowering the occupancy rates of county hospitals?

Another factor related to equality and equity in access to health and health care is the uneven economic development of rural China. The effect of the economic status of the village on access to sanitation and health care was analyzed in Chapter 6. The picture that emerged was one of a high degree of equity, if not equality. In other words, primary care services were distributed to meet the needs of the population and more services were made available in some of the poorest villages, where health needs were greater. At the same time, some of the richest villages were able to attract a variety of services beyond their health needs. This pattern of access to primary care seems to be the result of a formal policy of equity, equality, and market forces, as we have already demonstrated in discussing the distribution of government-owned clinics.

Driven by a socialist ideology, the PRC sought to abolish all stratification systems. It wished to eradicate differential access to social goods between urbanites and farmers, manual workers and managers, administrators and peasants. Such egalitarian access to the available social resources, including health and health care, had not been achieved during the planned economy period nor after the transition to a 'socialist market economy'. The major distinctions were found between urbanites and farmers and between poor regions and economically developed ones. Moreover, in HeBei Province we observed health inequalities among the farmers themselves, along characteristics often used as indicators of social class in industrial and post industrial societies.

In Western societies, level of education, income, and occupation are the three indicators used most often to measure social class (Lahelma, 2001). An inverse relationship between these indicators, mortality and ill-health has consistently been documented in these societies. Four factors have been suggested for the explanation of health gradients: artifact, social selection, materialist/structural, and cultural/behavioral. The relative emphasis on each of these explanations varies between disciplines, scholars, and historical periods and is the subject of considerable debate among social scientists, socio-biologists, epidemiologists, policy makers and many others (Macintyre, 1997). We briefly review these four explanations, in their "hard" and "soft" versions suggested by Macintyre (1997) to suggest how the findings of our research in rural HeBei can contribute to the debate.

According to the extreme artifact argument, class health differences do not really exist, but reflect the measures which are used to determine social class, health, or both. The debate focuses on the measurement of class and whether the denominators employed in calculating mortality rates, for example, represent the "real" class structure. In the case of health, defined either by specific morbidity or subjective evaluation of health and disability, the measurements of health come under attack. It has been argued that specific, diagnosis-based morbidity rates are dependent on help-seeking behavior; self-reported health is prone to bias originating in differential reporting behavior. The "soft" version of the artefact argument focuses on measurement errors, which are believed to explain some of the *volume* of class health inequalities.

We have at least two reasons to believe that the relationships between education, income, and health – as measured in our study – we observed in rural HeBei lend little support to the artifact argument. First and foremost, the same reasoning has been used to minimize the magnitude of gender health inequalities. In rural HeBei, gender health differences took on quite a different pattern from those observed in industrially developed societies. As described in Chapter 6, the health status of rural Chinese men and women in the reproductive and productive stage of the life cycle were far less noticeable than those reported for Western countries. Second, the association between health, household income, and living arrangements among the elderly (Chapter 8) suggested that elderly people in two-person households were in better health than those in multi-generational households, though the latter enjoyed higher income.

The "hard" version of the social selection argument, or the drift hypothesis, suggests that health status determines the position achieved in the social structure. According to the "soft" version of this proposition, functional ability and physical and mental predisposition play a considerable role in the accumulation of resources that determine the place of the individual in the social stratification system. Ill-health interferes, for example, with obtaining the level of education and training required for the better rewarded occupations; healthier people are more capable of entering the labor force and maintain better paid jobs.

The observed social class health differences in rural HeBei could be interpreted in light of this hypothesis. Respondents in non-farming occupations were better educated and on the average enjoyed higher income than farmers. Education and per-capita income were strongly associated with health (Chapter 6). Moreover, the relationship between years of schooling and health suggested that the completion of primary education was associated with most health benefits, whereas the association between income and health was almost linear. Furthermore, occupation by itself was generally not associated with health, once level of education and earning were accounted for. It is thus possible that ill-health indeed hindered progress in education, work and income-generating ability. Unfortunately, our data were cross-sectional. A critical test of the selection hypothesis requires longitudinal data.

There was, however, an important exception which challenged the selection explanation. Persons in the marginal category of 'other occupations' were characterized by relatively high education and were members of households that enjoyed, on the average, the highest per-capita income. Nevertheless, these people reported the poorest health after the effects of education and income were accounted for. It may be argued that these persons could not fit into one of the three mainstream occupations because of ill-health, although their health status did not hamper their school performance or ability to generate income.

Yet, the most outstanding disadvantage of those engaged in 'other occupations' was related to mental health. It thus appeared that deviating from the mainstream occupational structure had unfavorable psychological consequences, despite possession of valued social resources. These psychological costs lie at the heart of the "soft" version of the third explanatory framework, the materialist/structural approach.

In its "hard" form, the materialist/structural explanation states that health differences among the social classes are the result of differential access to material goods, such as living conditions, nutrition, and health care. The "soft" formulation, in contrast, emphasizes the psychological costs of class position, relative disadvantage, and perception of social marginality. Wilkinson (1992), for example, found evidence for this argument by analyzing the association between average per-capita income, income distribution, and long-term increase in life expectancy in industrial societies. Average per-capita income was not related to life-expectancy, whereas societies characterized by a relatively equal distribution of income, that is, with a low score on the Gini Index, enjoyed higher life expectancy. Beyond the level of income necessary to ensure the minimal material goods and the physical conditions for survival, the psychological costs of relative deprivation and sense of marginality take over in determining the life chances of the population. Others reported that social class differences in health are strongly related to self esteem, sense of coherence, level of distress, and other measures of psychological well-being and coping resources (Matthews, 1989; Anson et al, 1993b; Macintyre, 1994).

Our findings from rural HeBei strongly support hypotheses suggested by the "soft" version of the materialist / structural approach. As demonstrated in Chapter 6, mental health was consistently associated with all three measures of social class. Moreover, marginality on the community level had significant psychological costs for its people. Residents of villages in peripheral parts of the county reported poorer mental health than their counterparts in villages close to the county center.

Finally, we turn to the cultural/behavioral explanation. Health behavior, both that which fostered health and that which endangered it, was unevenly distributed among the social classes. In rural HeBei, we observed such patterns with regard to smoking, though not alcohol consumption or seeking medical help. Better educated persons were less likely to smoke, but consumed alcohol more often and sought medical help with less frequency. The pattern of association between substance consumption and age, however, especially the decline in consumption after mid-life, could be the result of the harm done by such behavior to health, causing premature death among the men involved. But it is also possible that men of this age no longer needed to establish their social status by overt behaviors that culturally symbolized independence and maturity. Women at this stage of the life-cycle were more likely than younger women to adopt such behaviors, to signify their independence from traditional social controls.

Summary

Each of the previous chapters has been devoted to a specific aspect of health and health care. In this chapter, the findings of our research in rural HeBei, secondary sources, and previous studies in the PRC have been discussed in light of the three aims presented in the introduction to the book. Lessons for policy makers in developing as well as in industrial countries have been suggested.

We started by presenting the changes in the ideology of the welfare state that took place in industrial societies, particularly in Western Europe, during the 1980s, a time of reform for health care systems throughout the world. No such ideological change occurred in the PRC, despite the transition to a market economy. The dismantling of the collective health scheme and mass privatization of the rural health services were a by-product of the implementation of 'the system of household responsibility', rather than of a change in basic ideology or a decline in ideological commitment to health, education, and welfare for all.

We discussed the ways in which the PRC has coped with the universal need to contain costs. The measures taken were in line with the ideological commitment to maintain access to affordable care for all, without compromising the quality of the care. These measures have many characteristics in common with the health care reforms implemented by Western European countries: the combination of public and private care delivery, managed competition, and price control. However, they seem unlikely to achieve the goal of cost containment and may produce inequality in access to care.

Public involvement in health and health delivery, another factor which propelled the need for health reforms in the West, was one of the unique features that have underscored the admirable achievements of China in improving the health of the population since 1949. This mass mobilization has declined in the past two decades, but we suggest that this fall derives more from the changing nature of public health needs and less from the decline in public willingness to contribute its time to collective health action. We have proposed possible ways to revive mass mobilization to cope with the high prevalence of risky health behavior, road and work safety.

The provision of primary care has been discussed in terms of recent criticism by social scientists concerned with the consequences of the privatization of social services for access to health care and professional behavior. As suggested by this line of argument, we found evidence that market forces are likely to increase inequity. The adequate distribution of primary care services in rural China, embedded in the ideology of the CCP, was achieved by deliberate state intervention. Privatization, however, does not seem to have increased inequality in the accessibility and affordability of health care. What appear to be paradoxical findings can be explained by the social context in which the doctor-patient encounter takes place.

Sociological analyses of the social power of the profession of medicine in Western societies have backed the claim that this is largely based on monopoly by the profession of knowledge and technology, on professional organization, and on the discrepancy in status between providers and lay persons. We have discussed the ways in which the characteristics of the village doctors corresponded to those of their Western counterparts. Though the professional training of village doctors is very different from the vocational training of doctors in the West, inequality of knowledge between providers and consumers does exist in rural China. Social distance, however is considerably smaller than in the West. Village doctors are not organized in professional associations that secure their status and monopoly over the provision of health care. Licensing was initiated by the state, stimulated by the state's responsibility for the health of its citizens, rather than by collective political action of a cohesive professional group aimed at protecting its own interests.

The current cultural perception of health defines acute conditions that bring about a precipitate decline in performance in regular social roles as the main reason for seeking medical help. We have discussed possible explanations for this phenomenon, but whatever the explanation, the relative neglect of chronic conditions presents a public health problem. Untreated and uncontrolled chronic conditions increase the risk for cardiovascular and cerebrovascular mortality and health educators should attend to this issue.

We have also discussed the cultural meaning of the consumption of substances currently viewed as harmful to health. The consumption of saturated fat and the use of tobacco and alcohol emerged as symbols of prosperity and maturity. Thus, health education and traditional mechanisms of social control will be unable to limit this behavior as long as the positive cultural meaning attached to them persists.

As might be expected both from the findings of previous studies of the fee-for-service care system and from the social proximity of village doctors and their patients, village doctors were sensitive to their patients' beliefs, attitudes, and preferences. Their medical practice also considered the structural constraints faced by their patients and the coping resources at their possession.

Although the PRC formally abolished all class systems, fully egalitarian access to social goods, including health, has not been achieved. Health status varies by the three indicators most commonly used to determine social class and health inequalities in industrial and post-industrial societies: level of education, income and, though to a much lesser degree, occupation. We have discussed the findings from rural HeBei in light of the four explanations for class health gradients in Western countries. According to our reading of the data, there is no evidence for the selection argument, neither in it's "hard" nor in its "soft" versions. The "soft" versions of the cultural/behavioral hypotheses gained some support. Our data lend the strongest support to the materialist/structural explanation of class health inequalities in its "soft" formulation, which emphasizes the role of the psychological consequences of disadvantaged class position in bringing about health inequalities.

Bibliography

Anderson, B. and Silver, B. D. (1995). Ethnic differences in fertility and sex ratios at birth in China: Evidence from Xinjiang. *Population Studies*, 49, pp. 211-226.

Annandale, E. (1998). *The Sociology of Health and Medicine*. Malden MA: Blackwell Publishers, Inc.

Annandale, E. (1998). *The Sociology of Health and Medicine*. Cambridge: Polity Press.

Annandale, E. (1999). Working on the front line: Risk culture and nursing in the new NHS. *Sociological Review*, 44, pp. 416-451.

Annandale, E. and Hunt, K. (eds) (1999). *Gender Inequalities in Health*. Buckingham: Open University Press.

Anson, J. (1998). Development towns in Israel: Proletarian periphery or surplus populations? Paper presented in the International Conference on Urban Development: A Challenge for Frontier Regions, 4–7 April, Beer-Sheva, Israel.

Anson, O. (1989). Marital status and women's health revisited: The importance of a proximate adult. *Journal of Marriage and the Family*, 51, pp. 185-194.

Anson, O. (1999). Professionalism and the Israeli Patient's Right Law. *Medical Law International*, 4, pp. 59-68.

Anson O. (2000). Health and Ethnicity in the Brussels Region. *Inter-university Papers in Demography*, IPD-WP 2000-3.

Anson, O. and Haanappel, F. W. (1999). 'Remnants of feudalism'? Women's health and their utilization of health services in rural China. *Women & Health*, 30, pp. 105-123.

Anson, O. and Sun, S. (2002). Gender and health in rural China: Evidence from HeBei Province. *Social Science & Medicine*, 55, pp. 1039-1054.

Anson O., Levinson A. and Bonneh D. (1998). Gender and health on the kibbutz. In Peplau, L. A. (ed) *Gender, Culture and Ethnicity*. Mayfield Publishing Company: Pittsburgh, reprint from *Sex Roles*, 22, pp. 213-232 (1990).

Anson, O., Paran, E., Neumann, L. and Chernichovsky, D. (1993a). Gender differences in health perceptions and their predictors. *Social Science & Medicine*, 36, pp. 419-427.

Anson O., Paran E., Neumann L. and Chernichovsky D. (1993b). Psychological state and health experiences: Gender and social class. *International Journal of Health Sciences*, 4, pp. 143-149.

Anson, O., Sun, S., Zhang, W. and Haanappel, F. W. (2003). *The Village Doctor in Different Ownership Clinics in China's Countryside*. Amsterdam: Royal Tropical Institute.

Antonovsky, A. (1979). *Stress, Coping, and Health*. San Francisco: Jossey-Bass.

Arber, S. and Thomas, H. (2001). From women's health to a gender analysis of health. In W. C. Cockerham (ed), *The Blackwell Companion to Medical Sociology*, pp. 94-113, Malden, MA: Blackwell Publishers.

Avgar, A. (1997). Women's health in Israel: A feminist perspective. *Social Work in Health Care*, 25, pp. 45-62.

Banister, J. (1994). Implications and quality of China's 1990 census data, in *1990 Population Census of China: Proceedings of International Seminar*, pp. 208-238, China Publishing House.

Banister, J. (1997). Perspectives on China's mortality trends, in *International Population Conference, Beijing*, 1997. Vol. 3, pp. 1335-1351, Liege: International Union for the Scientific Study of Population.

Banister, J. (1998). Population, public health and the environment in China. *The China Quarterly*, 156, pp. 986-1015.

Banister, J., Gao, J. and Rao, K. (2000). Survival and health in rapidly developing China. Paper presented at the Annual Meeting of the Population Association of America, Los Angeles, March 2000.

Bates, P. W. (1994). The role of legislation in health services development (with particular reference to China and Australia). *Medicine and Law*, 13, pp. 433-49.

Beaver, P. D., Hou, L. and Wang, X. (1995). Rural Chinese women: Two faces of economic reforms. *Modern China*, 21, pp. 205-232.

Benjamin, D. and Brandt, B. (1995). Markets, discrimination, and the economic contribution of women in China: Historical evidence. *Economic Development and Cultural Change*, 44, pp. 63-104.

Bernandez, T. (1984). Prevalent disorders of women: Attempts toward a different understanding and treatment. In C. T. Mowbray, S. Lanir, and M. Hulce (eds), *Women and Mental Health: A New Directions for Change*. New York: The Haworth Press.

Berrios, X., Koponen, T., Huiguang, T., Khaltaev, N., Puska, P. and Nissinen, A. (1997). Distribution and prevalence of major risk factors of noncommunicable diseases in selected countries: the WHO Inter-Health Programme. *Bulletin of the World Health Organization*, 75, pp. 99-108.

Bhat, R. (1993). The private/public mix in health care in India. *Health Policy and Planning*, 8, pp. 43-56.

Bietlot, M., Demarest, S., Tafforeau, J. and Van Oyen, H. (2000). *La Santé en Belgique, ses Communautès et ses Règions: Rèsultat de L'Enquête de Santé par Interview, 1997*. Brussels: Institute Scientifique de la Santé Publique.

Bird, C. E. and Pieker, P. P. (1999). Gender Matters: an Integrated Model for Understanding Men's and Women's Health. *Social Science & Medicine*, 48, pp. 745-755.

Bledsoe, C.H., Ewbank, D.C. and Isiugo-Abanhe, U.C. (1988). The effect of child fostering on feeding practices and access to health services in rural Sierra Leone. *Social Science & Medicine*, 27, pp. 627-636.

Bogg, L. (1998). Family planning in China: Out of control? *American Journal of Public Health*, 88, pp. 649-651.

Browning, H. L. and Fiendt, W. (1969). Selectivity of migrants to a metropolis in a developing country: A Mexican case study. *Demography*, 6, pp. 347-357.

Cahan, I. J. (2001). Continuing medical education. An effective tool or faulty fantasy? *Maryland Medicine*, 2, pp. 14-16.

Cao, G. and Zhong, B. (1990). Study of the evolution and development of rural health system in China. *Primary Health care in China*, 7, pp. 5-10 (Chinese).

Carmel S., Anson O. and Levin M. (1990). Emergency department utilization by two subcultures in the same geographical region. *Social Science & Medicine*, 31, pp. 557-564.

Carpenter, M. (2000). Reinforcing the pillars: Rethinking gender, social divisions, and health, in E. Annalndale and K. Hunt, *Gender Inequalities in Health*, pp. 36-63, Buckingham: Open University Press.

Carrin, G., Ron, A., Wang, S. C., et al.(1996). *The Reform of the Rural Cooperatives System in the People Republic of China*. Geneva: World Health Organization.

Chang, Y., Zhai, W., Li, W., Ge, K., Jin, D. and de Onis, M. (1994). Nutritional status of preschool children in poor rural areas of China. *Bulletin of World Health Organization*, 72, pp. 105-112.

Chen, M. S. (2001). Transformation of health care in the People's Republic of China, in W. C. Cockerham (ed). *The Blackwell Companion to Medical Sociology*, p 456-482, Malden, MA: Blackwell Publishers.

Chen, Z. P. (1998). Big advances in IDD elimination: The examples of China and Peru. *IDD Newsletter*, 14(4).

Chen, Z. P. (1999). Summary of regional coordinator progress report in China. *IDD Newsletter*, 15(3).

Chen, Z. P. (2000). China – the Third National Monitoring Survey applying the ICCIDD/ WHO/UNICEF criteria. *IDD Newsletter*, 16(2).

Chen, S. T. and Hamid, N. P. (1996). A Chinese symptom checklist: Preliminary data concerning reliability and validity. *Journal of Social Behavior and Personality*, 11, pp. 241-252.

Chen, J., Bloom, G. and Wilkes, A. (1997). The impact of China's health care reforms on county hospitals. *World Hospitals and Health Services*, 33, pp. 19-22.

Chen, L., Zheng N., et al. (1992). An investigation analysis of conditions in village clinics in Fujian Province. *Primary Health care in China*, 7, pp. 28-30 (Chinese).

Chen, M. Z., Xu, G. and Shi, Y.Q. (1995). Medicine in China, in S.K. Majumdar, L.M. Rosenfeld, D.B. Nash and A.M. Audet (eds). *Medicine and Health Care into the Twenty-First Century*, pp. 518-531, PA, USA: Pennsylvania Academy of Sciences.

Chen, P., Yu, E. S. H., Zhang, M., Liu, W. T., Hill, R. and Katzman, R. (1995). ADL dependence and medical conditions in Chinese older persons: A population-based survey in Shanghai, China. *JAGS*, 43, pp. 378-383.

Chen, X. M., Hu, T. W. and Lin, Z. (1993). The rise and the fall of the cooperative medical system in rural China. *International Journal of Health Services*, 23, pp. 731-742.

Chernichovsky, D. (1995). Health sector reforms in industrialized economy: The emerging paradigm. *The Milbank Fund Quarterly*, 73, pp. 339-372.

Chernichovsky, D. (1995). What can developing economies learn from health system reforms of developed economies? *Health Policy*, 32, pp. 79-91.

Chernichovsky, D. and Shirom, A. (1996). Equity in the Israeli health care system, in Y. Kop (ed) *Resources Allocation for Social Services*, pp. 157-182, Jerusalem: The Social Policy Research Center. (Hebrew).

China YearBook, 1998, 1999. Beijing: China Statistical Publishing House.

China Population Yearbook. (1997). Beijing: Economic Management Press.

China All-Women Federation (1993). *Women Status Survey in 1990*. Beijing: Women's Press House (Chinese).

Chinese Medical News. (2001a). Five hospitals in Wuhan to be punished for receiving large illegal drug discount. *Chinese Medical News*, 108.

Chinese Medical News. (2001b). Nationwide drug price fall initiates. *Chinese Medical News*, 111.

Chitsulo, L., Engels, D., Montesor, A. and Savioli, L. (2000). The global status of schistosomiasis and its control. *Acta Tropica*, 77, pp. 41-51.

Cho, S. Il., Li, Q., Yang, J., et al. (1999). Drinking water source and spontaneous abortion: A cross-sectional study in a rural Chinese population. *International Journal of Occupational and Environmental Health*, 5, pp. 164-169.

Choe, M. K., Hao, H. and Wang, F. (1995). Effects of gender, birth order, and other correlates on childhood mortality in China. *Social Biology*, 42, pp. 50-64.

Choi, K. H., Zheng, X., Zhou, ., Chen, W. and Mandel, J. (1999). Treatment delay and reliance on private physicians among patients with sexually transmitted diseases in China. *International Journal of STD and AIDS*, 10, pp. 309-315.

Clayton, S., Yang, H., Guan, J., Lin, Z. and Wang, R. (1993). Hepatitis B control in China: Knowledge and practice among village doctors. *American Journal of Public Health*, 83, pp. 1685-88.

Cockerham, W. C. (2001). Medical sociology and sociological theory, in W. C. Cockerham (ed), *The Blackwell Companion to Medical Sociology*, pp. 3-22, Malden, MA: Blackwell Publishers.

Connor, R. A., Hillson, S. D. and Krawelski, J. E. (1995). Competition, professional synergism, and the geographical distribution of rural physicians. *Medical Care*, 33, pp. 1067-1078.

Cooney, R. S. and Li, J. (1994). Household registration types and compliance with the "one child" policy in China, 1979-1989. *Demography*, 31, pp. 21-32.

Cooney, R. S., Wei, J. and Powers, M. G. (1991). The one child certificate in Hebei province, China: Acceptance and consequences, 1979-1988. *Population Research and Policy Review*, 10, pp. 137-155.

Curran, P. J., Muthrn, B. O. and Harford, T. C. (1998). The influence of changes in marital status on developmental trajectories of alcohol use in young adults. *Journal of Studies on Alcohol*, 59, pp. 648-658.

Davies, C. (1996). The sociology of professions and the profession of gender. *Sociology*, 30, pp. 661-678.

De Cock, K. M. and Weiss, H. (2000). The global epidemiology of HIV/AIDS. *Tropical Medicine and International Health*, 5, pp. A3-A9.

De Geyndt, W., Zhao, X. and Liu, S. (1992). *From Barefoot Doctor to Village Doctor in Rural China*. World Bank Technical Report No. 187, Asia Technical Department series, Washington D.C.: The World Bank.

Derber, C., Schwartz, W. and Margrass, Y. (1990). *Power in the Highest Degree: Professionals and the Rise of New Mandarin Order*. Oxford: Oxford University Press.

Dezhi, Y. (1992). Changes in health care financing and health status: The case of China in the 1980s. *UNICEF Economic Policy*, Series 34.

Dong, H., Bogg, L., Wang, K., Rehnberg, C. and Diwan, V. (1999a). A description of outpatient drug use in rural China: Evidence of differences due to insurance coverage. *International Journal of Health Planning and Management*, 14, pp. 41-5.

Dong, H., Bogg, L., Rehnberg, C. and Diwan, V. (1999b). Drug policy in China: Pharmaceutical distribution in rural areas. *Social Studies & Medicine*, 48, pp. 777-786.

Dong, H., Bogg, L., Rehnberg, C. and Diwan, V. (1999c). Association between health insurance and antibiotic prescribing in four counties in rural China. *Health Policy*, 48, pp. 29-54.

Economy and Statistical Yearbook of HeBei, 1994. Beijing: China Statistical Publishing House.

Edwards, G. Anderson, P., Babor, T. F., et al. (1994). *Alcohol Policy and the Public Good*. Oxford: Oxford Medical Publications.

Entwisle, B., Henderson, G. E., Short, S. E., et al. 1995. Gender and Family Businesses in Rural China. *American Sociological Review*, 60, pp. 36-57.

Freidson, E. (1986). *Professional Power*. London: Univ. of Chicago Press.

Freidson, E. (1994). *Professionalism Reborn*. Cambridge: Polity Press.

Gautam, K. (1993). Health challenges for China. Paper presented at the International Seminar on Health Reforms under Socialist Market Economy, Beijing, June 1993.

Gershen, B. J. (2001a). Continuing medical education. *Maryland Medicine*, 2, pp. 8-9.

Gershen, B. J. (2001b). Reading the literature. *Maryland Medicine*, 2, pp. 10-12.

Gian, Y. (1991). Collective ownership is a necessary way for the development of village clinics: An investigation report of reorganization of village clinics in Xu Xi city. *Primary Health care in China*, 3, pp. 17-18 (Chinese).

Gijsbers van Wijk, C. M. T., Kolk, A. M., van den Bosch, W. J. H. M. and van den Hoogen, H. J. M. (1992). Male and Female Morbidity in General Practice: the Nature of Sex Differences. *Social science & Medicine*, 35, pp. 665-678.

Gijsbers van Wijk, C. M. T., Kolk, A. M., van den Bosch, W. J. H. M. and van den Hoogen, H. J. M. (1995). Male and female health problems in general practice: The differential impact of social position and social roles. *Social Science & Medicine*, 40, pp. 597-611.

Gissler, M., J., Louhiala, M. R. and Hemmimki, E. (1999). Boys Have More Health Problems in Childhood than Girls: Follow-up of the 1987 Finish Birth Cohort. *Acta Paediatrica*, 88, pp. 310-314.

Goldstein, A., White, M. and Goldstein, S. (1997). Migration, fertility, and state policy in Hubei Province, China. *Demography*, 34, pp. 481-491.

Gong, Y., Wilks, A. and Bloom, G. (1997). Health human resources development in rural China. *Health Policy and Planning*, 12, pp. 320-328.

Greenhalgh, S., Zhu, C. and Li, N. (1994). Restraining population growth in three Chinese villages, 1988-1993. *Population and Development Review*, 20, pp. 365-395.

Gross, R. and Anson, O. (2002). The Reforms in the Israeli Health Care System, in A. Twaddle (ed), *Comparative Medical Care Reform*, pp. 273-303, Westport CT: Greenwood Press.

Gu, X., Bloom, G., Tang, S., Zhu, Y., Zhou, S. and Chen, X. (1993). Financing health care in rural China: preliminary report of a nationwide study. *Social Science & Medicine*, 36, pp. 385-91.

Guidotti, T. L. and Levister, E. C. (1995). Occupational health in China: 'Rising with force and power'. *Occupational Medicine*, 45, pp. 117-124.

Hao, W. (1995). *Alcohol Policy and the Public Good*: a Chinese view. *Addiction*, 90, pp. 1448-150.

Hao, W., Young, D., Xiao, S., Li, L. and Zhang, Y. (1999). Alcohol consumption and alcohol-related problems: Chinese experience from six area samples, 1994. *Addiction*, 94, pp. 1467-1476.

Hardon, A. (1992). Why are injections so popular? *World Health*, 3-4, pp. 18-19.

Henderson G., Jin S., Akin J., Li X., Wang J., Ma H., He Y., Zhang X., Chang Y., Ge K. (1995). Distribution of medical insurance in China. *Social Science & Medicine*, 41, pp. 1119-1130.

Herzog, H. (1994). *Realistic Women*. Jerusalem: The Institute for Jerusalem Studies (Hebrew).

Hesketh, T. and Zhu, W. X. (1997). Health in China: From Mao to market economy. *British Medical Journal*, 314, pp. 1543-1545.

Hesketh, T. and Zhu, W. X. (1997a). Maternal and child health in China. *British Medical Journal*, 314, pp. 1989-1900.

Hesketh, T. and Zhu, W. X. (1997b). The one child family policy: The good, the bad, and the ugly. *British Medical Journal*, 314, pp. 1685-1587.

Hillier, S. and Shen, J. (1996). Health care systems in transition:People's Republic of China. Part I: An overview of China's health care system. *Journal of Public Health Medicine*, 18, pp. 258-265.

Ho, L. S. (1995). Market reforms and China's health care system. *Social Science & Medicine*, 41, pp. 1065-1072.

Hoeman, S. P., Ku, Y. L. and Ohl, D. R. (1996). Health beliefs and early detection among Chinese women. *Western Journal of Nursing Research*, 18, pp. 518-533.

Holroyd, E., Katie, F. K. L., Chun, L. S. and Ha, S. W. (1997). "Doing the month": An explanation of postpartum practices in Chinese women. *Health Care for Women International*, 18, pp. 301-313.

Horsburgh, C. R. (1996). Economic reform and health - lessons from China. *The New England Journal of Medicine*, 335, pp. 429-430.

Hsiao, W. C. L. (1995). The Chinese health care system: Lessons for other nations. *Social Science & Medicine*, 41, pp. 1047–1055.

Huang, S. M. (1988). Transforming China's collective health care system: A village study. *Social Science & Medicine*, 27, pp. 879-888.

Hughes, E. C. (1958). *Men and Their Work*. Glencoe, Il: Free Press.

Hunter, J. M. and Arbona, S. I. (1995). The tooth as a marker of developing world quality of life: A field study in Guatemala. *Social Science & Medicine*, 41, pp. 1217-1240.

ICCIDD (1999). World health organization review. *IDD Newsletter*, 15(2).

Idler, E. L. and Benyamini, Y. (1997). Self rated health and mortality: A review of twenty-seven community studies. *Journal of Health ans Social Behavior*, 38, pp. 21-37.

Ineichen, B. (1998). Influences on the care of demented elderly people in the People's Republic of China. *International Journal of Geriatric Psychiatry*, 13, pp. 122-126.

Ismail, A. I., Tanzer, J. M. and Dingel, J. L. (1997). Current trends in sugar consumption in developing countries. *Community Dental and Oral Epidemiology*, 25, pp. 438-443.

Izuhara, M. (2000). Changing family tradition: Housing choices and constraints for older people in Japan. *Housing Studies*, 15, pp. 89-110.

Jamison, D. T., Evans, J. R., King, T., et al.(1984). *China: The Health Sector*. Washington DC: The World Bank.

Jernigan, H. and Jernigan, M. (1992). *Aging in Chinese Society: A Holistic Approach to the Experience of Aging in Taiwan and Singapore*. New York: The Haworh Pastoral Press.

Jiang, C., Driscoll, P., Woodford, M., et al. (1996). Trauma care in China: Challenge and development. *Injury*, 27, pp. 471-475.

Jiang, L. (1995). Changing kinship structure and its implication for old-age support in urban and rural China. *Population Studies*, 49, pp. 127-145.

Johnson, K. A. (1985). *Women, the Family and Peasant Revolution in China*. Chicago: University of Chicago Press.

Kan, X. (1990). Village health worker in China: Reappraising the current situation. *Health Policy and Planning*, 5, pp. 40-48.

Katz, R. and Peres, Y. (1995). Marital crisis and therapy in their social context. *Contemporary Family Therapy*, 17, pp. 395-412.

Kessler R. C., Mickelson K. D. and Williams D. R. (1999). The prevalence, distribution, and mental health correlates of percieved discrimination in United States. *Journal of Health and Social Behavior*, 40, pp. 208-230.

Kressin, N., Spiro, A, Bossè, R., Gracia, R. and Kasis, L. (1996). Assessing oral health-related quality o life. *Medical Crae*, 34, pp. 416-427.

Kroenke, K. and Spitzer, R. I. (1998). Gender Differences in the Reporting of Physical and Somatoform Symptoms. *Psychosomatic Medicine*, 60, pp. 150-155.

Lahelma, E. (2001). Health and social stratification, in W. C. Cockerham (ed), *The Blackwell Companion to Medical Sociology*, pp 64-93, Malden, MA: Blackwell Publishers.

Lai, D. and Hsi, B. P. (1996). Soil-transmitted helminthiases in China: A special statistical analysis. *Southeast Asia Journal of Tropical Medicine ans Public Health*, 27, pp. 754-759.

Lai, G. (1995). Work and family roles and psychological well-being in urban China. *Journal of Health and Social Behavior*, 36, pp. 11-37.

Landale, N. S., Oropesa, R. S., and Gorman, B. K. (2000). Migration and infant death: Assimilation or selective migration among Puerto Ricans? *American Sociological Review*, 65, pp. 889-909.

Larsen, U. (1990). An assessment of the one-child policy in China from 1980 to 1985. *European Journal of Population*, 6, pp. 257-284.

Larson, M. S. (1977). *The Rise of Professionalism*. Berkeley: University of California Press.

Lawson, J. S. and Lin, V. (1994). Health status differentials in the People's Republic of China. *American Journal of Public Health*, 84, pp. 737-41.

Lee, S. and Lee, A. M. (1999). Disordered eating in three communities of China: A comparative study of female high school students in Hong Kong, Shenzhen, and rural Hunan. *International Journal of Eating Disorders*, 27, pp. 317-327.

Lee, Y. J. and Xiao, Z. (1998). Children's support for elderly parents in urban and rural China: Results from a national survey. *Journal of Cross-Cultural Gerontology*, 13, pp. 39-62.

Lennart, B., Dong, H., Wang, K., Cai, W. and Vidon, D. (1996). The costs pf coverrage: Rural health insurance in China. *Health Policy and Planning*, 11, pp. 238-252.

Leung, J. C. B. (1997). Family support for the elderly in China: Issues and challenges. *Journal of Aging & Social Policy*, 9, pp. 87-101.

Li, B. (1993). Thoughts on the construction of the Three-Tiers medical prevention network in the countryside. *Primary Health Care in China*, 7, pp. 22-23 (Chinese).

Li, J. (1995). China's one-child policy: How and how well has it worked? A case study of HeBei Province, 1979–1988. *Population and Development Review*, 21, pp. 563-585.

Li, W. L. (1998). Aging and welfare policies in China. *Sociological Focus*, 31, pp. 31-43.

Li, G. H. and Baker, S.P. (1991). A comparison of injury death rates in China and the United States. *American Journal of Public Health*, 81, pp. 605-609.

Li, G. H. and Baker, S. P. (1997). Injuries to bicyclists in Wuhan, People's Republic of China. *American Journal of Public Health*, 87, pp. 1049-1052.

Li, H. and Tracy, M. B. (1999). Family support, financial needs, and health care needs of rural elderly in China: A field study. *Journal of Cross Cultural Gerontology*, 14, pp. 357-371.

Li, J. and Cooney, R. S. (1993). Son preference and the one child policy in China: 1979–1988. *Population Research and Policy Review*, 12, pp. 277-296.

Li, J. and Fielding, R. (1995). The measurement of current perceived health among Chinese people in Guangzhu and Hong Kong, southern China. *Quality of Life Research*, 4, pp. 271-278.

Li, X., Fang, X., Stanton, B., Feigelman, S., snd Dong, Q. (1996). The rate and pattern of alcohol consumption among Chinese adolescents. *Journal of Adolescent Health*, 19, pp. 353-361.

Li, Z., Shang, L., Lian, Z., Li, D. and Su, Y. (1999). Control strategies of malaria in Henan Province, China. *Southeast Asian Journal of Tropical Medicine and Public Health*, 30, pp. 240-242.

Liu, G., Liu, X. and Meng, Q. (1994). Privatization of the medical market in socialist China: A historical approach. *Health Policy*, 27, pp. 157-174.

Liu, X., Liang, J. and Gu, S. (1995). Flows of social support and health status among older persons in China. *Social Science & Medicine*, 41, pp. 1175-1184.

Liu, X., Xu, L. and Wang, S. (1996). Reforming China's 50 000 township hospitals - effectiveness, challanges and opportunities. *Health Policy*, 38, pp. 13-29.

Liu, Y., Hsiao, W. C. and Eggleston, K. (1999). Equity in health and health care: The Chinese experience. *Social Science & Medicine*, 49, pp. 1349-1356.

Liu, Z. Y., He, X. Z. and Chapman, R. S. (1991). Smoking and other risk factors for lung cancer in Xuanwei, China. *Int'l Journal of Epidemiology*, 20, pp. 26-31.

Lutz, W. and Cao, G. Y. (2000). China's unfolding educational revolution. *Popnet*, 33, pp. 5-8.

MacCormack, C.P. (1988). Health and the social power of women. *Social Science & Medicine*, 26, pp. 677-684.

Macintyre, S. (1994). Understanding the social patterning of health: The contribution of the social sciences. *Journal of Public Health Medicine*, 10, pp. 231-233.

Macintyre, S. (1997). The Black Report and beyond: What are the issues? *Social Science & Medicine*, 44, pp. 723-745.

Matos-Ferreira, A. (2001). Continuing medical education and continuing professional development: A credit system for monitoring and promoting excellence. *BJU International*, 87, pp. 1-12.

Matthews, K. (1989). Are sociodemographic variables markers for psychosocial determinants of health? *Health Psychology*, 8, pp. 641-648.

McDonald, L. (1997). The invisible poor: Canada's retired widows. *Canadian Journal of Aging*, 16, pp. 553-583.

McGreevey, W. (1995a). Eight steps to health care financing reform, 1996-2001. Mission report, World Bank: Washington DC.

McGreevey, W. (1995b). China health care finance study, 1995, *Office Memorandum*, The World Bank: Washington DC.

McKinlay, J. B. (1981 [1974]). A case of refocussing upstream: The political economy of illness, in P. Conrad and K. R. (eds) *The Sociology of Health and Illness*, pp. 613-633, St. Martin's Press, New York.

McLaughlin, D. K. and Jensen, L. (1995). Becoming poor: The experiences of elders. *Rural Sociology*, 60, pp. 202-223.

Medjuck, S., O'Brian, M. and Tozer, C. 1992. 'From Private Responsibility to Public Policy: Women and Cost of Caring to Elderly Kin', *Atlantis: A Women's Studies Journal* 17, pp. 44-58.

Meng, X. and Miller, P. (1995). Occupational segregation and its impact on gender wage discrimination in China's rural industrial sector. *Oxford Economic Papers*, 47, pp. 136-155.

Meyer, M. H. and Pavalko, E. K. 1996. Family, Work, and Access to Health Insurance among Mature Women. *Journal of Health and Social Behavior*, 37, pp. 311-326.

Ming, T., He, Q. and Huang, H. Y. (1995). Living Arrangements of Elderly Women and Men in Chinese Cities. *Sociological Spectrum*, 15, pp. 491-510.

Ministry of Public Health (1993). Background paper for International Seminar on Health Reforms under Socialist Market Economy, Beijing, June 1993. The Department of Planning and Finance.

Ministry of Public Health (1984). *Chinese Yearbook of Health*, pp. 17-19, People's Health Press: Beijing.

Morgan, L. A. (2000). The continuing gender gap in later life economic security. *Journal of Aging and Social Policy*, 11, pp. 157-165.

Murray, C. J. L. and Lopez, A. 1997. Mortality by cause for eight regions of the world: Global Burden of Disease Study. *Lancet*, 349, pp. 1269-1276.

Nirel, N., Rosen, B., Gross, R., Berg, G. and Yuval, D. (1996). *Immigrants from the Former USSRin the Health Care System*. Jerusalem: JDC-Brookdaile Institute.

Niu, T., Chen, C., Ni, J., Wang, B., Fang, Z., Shao, H. and Xu, X. (2000). Nicotine dependence and its familial aggregation in China. *International Journal of Epidemiology*, 29, pp. 248-252.

Normile, D. (2000). China awakens to fight projected AIDS crisis. *Science*, 288, pp. 2312-2313.

Omran, A. R. (1971). The epidemiological transition: A theory of the epidemiology of population change. *The Milbank Memorial Fund Quarterly*, 64, pp. 355-391.

Pandav, C. S. (1994). The economic benefits of the elimination of IDD. In B. S. Hetzel and C. S. Pandav (eds) *S.O.S. for a Billion: The Conquest of Iodine Deficiency Disorders*. Delhi: Oxford University Press.

Paran, E., Anson, O. and Neumann, L. (1998). The effects of replacing Beta-Blockers with

ACE Inhibitor on the quality of life of hypertensive patients. In *Yearbook of Drug Therapy*, reprint from *The American Journal of Hypertension*, 9, pp. 1206-1213, 1996.

Pearson, V. (1995). Goods on which one loses: Women and mental health in China. *Social Science & Medicine*, 41, pp. 1159-1173.

Pearson, V. (1996). Women and health in China: Anatomy, destiny, and politics. *Journal of Social Policy*, 25, pp. 529-543.

Peng, X. (1987). Demographic consequences of the Great Leap Forward in China's provinces. *Population and Development Review*, 13, pp. 639-670.

Popkin, B. M., Paeratakul, S., Ge, K. and Zhai, F. (1995). Body weight patterns among the Chinese: Results from the 1989 and 1991 China Health and Nutrition Survey. *American Journal of Public Health*, 85, pp. 690-694.

Potter, S. H. and Potter, J. M. (1990). *China's Pesants: The Anthropology of a Revolution*. Cambridge: Cambridge University Press.

Pritchard, C. (1996). Suicide in the People's Republic of China categorized by age and gender: Evidence of the influence of culture on suicide. *Acta Psychiatria Scandinavia*, 93, pp. 3620-367.

Qu, J. B., Zhang, Z. W., Shimbo, S., Liu, Z. M., Wang, L. Q. (2000). Nutrient intake of adult women in Jillin Province, China, with special reference to urban-rural differences in nutrition in the Chinese continent. *European Journal of Clinical Nutrition*, 54, pp. 741-748.

Qu, J. B., Zhang, Z. W., Xu, G. F., Song, L. H., Wang, J. J., et al. (1997). Urban-rural comparison of nutrient intake by adult women in Shandong Province, China. *Tobuku Journal of Experimental Medicine*, 183, pp. 21-36.

Quah, S. R. (1985). Self-medication in Singapore. *Singapore Medical Journal*, 26, pp. 123-126.

Quah, S. R. (1993). Ethnicity, health behavior, and modernization: The case of Singapore, in P. Conard and E. B. Gallagher (eds) *Health and Health Care in Developing Countries: Sociological Perspectives*, pp. 78-107, Philadelphia: Temple University Press.

Quah, S. R. (2001). Health and culture, in W. C. Cockerham (ed), *The Blackwell Companion to Medical Sociology*, pp. 94-113, Malden, MA: Blackwell Publishers.

Ren, X. S. (1994). Infant and child survival in Shaanxi, China. *Social Science & Medicine*, 38, pp. 609-621.

Ren, X. S. (1995). Sex differences in infant and child mortality in China. *Social Science & Medicine*, 40, pp. 1259-1269.

Ren, X. S. (1996). Regional variation in infant survival in China. *Social Biology*, 43, pp. 1-19.

Rigdon, S. M. (1996). Abortion law and practice in China: An overview with comparisons to the United States. *Social Science & Medicine*, 42, pp. 543-560.

Riley, N. (1996). China's "Missing Girls": Prospects and Policy. *Population Today*, 2, pp. 4-5.

Riley, N. and Gardner, R. W. (1997). China's population: A review of the literature. Commissioned paper for the IUSSP International Conference, Beijing (October 1997).

Riska, E. (2001). Health professions and occupations, in W. C. Cockerham (ed), *The Blackwell Companion to Medical Sociology*, pp. 144-158, Malden, MA: Blackwell Publishers.

Roberts, I. (1995). China takes to the roads. *British Medical Journal*, 310, pp. 1311-1313.

Ross, C. (2000). Neighborhood disadvantage and adult depression. *Journal of Health and*

Social Behavior, 41, pp. 177-187.
Sachs, J. and Woo, T. (1996). China's transition experience, reexamined. *Transition*, 7, pp. 1-6.
Schultz, T. P. and Zeng, Y. (1995). Fertility in rural China: Effects of local family planning and health programs. *Journal of Population Economics*, 8, pp. 329-359.
Schumacher, E. F. (1973). *Small is Beautiful: A Study of Economic as if People Mattered.* London: Blond and Briggs.
Secondi, G. (1997). Private monetary transfers in rural China: Are families altruistic? *The Journal of Developmental Studies*, 33, pp. 487-511.
Shackford, S. (1995). The evolution of modern trauma care. *Surgical Clinics of North America*, 75, pp. 147-156.
Shek, T. L. D. (1995). Gender differences in marital quality and well being in Chinese married adults. *Sex Roles*, 32, pp. 699-715.
Shen, T., Habicht, J. P. and Chang, Y. (1996). Effect of economic reforms on child growth in urban and rural reas of China. *The New England Journal of Medicine*, 335, pp. 400-406.
Shen, X., Rosen, J. F., Guo, D. and Wu, S. (1996). Childhood lead poisoning in China. *The Science of the Total Environment*, 181, pp. 101-109.
Shi, L. (1993). Health care in China: A rural-urban comparison after the socio-economic reforms. *Bulletin of the World Health Organization*, 71, pp. 723-36.
Shi, L. (1996). Access to care in post-economic reform rural China: Results from a 1994 cross-sectional survey. *Journal of Public Health Policy*, 17, pp. 347-361.
Shimbo, S., Zhang, Z. W., Gao, W. P., et al. (1998). Prevalnce of hepatitis B and C infection markers among adult women in urban and rural areas in Shaanxi Province, China. *Southeast Asian Journal of Tropical Medicine and Public Health*, 29, pp. 263-268.
Shuval, J. T. (1992). *Social dimensions of Health: The case of Israel.* Westpoint, CN: Praeger.
Shuval, J. T. (1995). Elitism and professional control in a saturated market: Immigrant physicians in Israel. *Sociology of Health and Illness*, 17, pp. 550-565.
Shuval, J. T. and Anson, O. (2000). *Social Structure and Health in Israel*. Jerusalem: Magnes, The Hebrew University Press (Hebrew).
Siegrist, J. (2001). Work stress and health, in W. C. Cockerham (ed), *The Blackwell Companion to Medical Sociology*, pp. 114-125, Malden, MA: Blackwell Publishers.
Sleigh, A., Jackson, S., Li, X. and Huang, K. (1998a). Eradication of schistosomiasis in Guangxi, China. Part 1: Setting strategies, operations, and outcomes, 1953-1992. *Bulletin of the World Health Organization*, 76, pp. 359-370.
Sleigh, A., Jackson, S., Li, X. and Huang, K. (1998b). Eradication of schistosomiasis in Guangxi, China. Part 2: Political economy; management strategy and costs, 1953-1992. *Bulletin of the World Health Organization*, 76, pp. 497-508.
Sleigh, A., Jackson, S., Li, X. and Huang, K. (1998c). Eradication of schistosomiasis in Guangxi, China. Part 3: Community diagnosis of the worst affected areas and maintenance strategies for the future. *Bulletin of the World Health Organization*, 76, pp. 581-590.
Smith, C. J. (1993). (Over)eating success: The health consequences of the restoration of capitalism in rural China. *Social Science & Medicine*, 37, pp. 761-70.
Smith, C. J. (1993). (Over)eating process: The health consequences of the restoration of capitalism in rural China. *Social Science & Medicine*, 37, pp. 761-770.
Starr, P. (1982). *The Social Transformation of American Medicine*. New York: Basic Books.

State of Israel. (1998). *Health Israel*. Jerusalem: Ministry of Health.

Stevens, F. (2001). The convergence and divergence of modern health care systems. In W. C. Cockerham (ed), *The Blackwell Companion to Medical Sociology*, pp. 159-176, Malden, MA: Blackwell Publishers.

Sun, Y. (1992). A report of sampling investigation of rural health services in HeBei Province. *Administration of Rural Health Organization in China*, 7, pp. 20-25 (Chinese).

Sun, F., Wu, Z., Qian, Y., Cao, H., Xue, H., et al. (1998). Epidemiology of human intestinal nematode infections in Wujiang and Pizhou counties, Jiangsu Province, China. *Southeast Asian Journal of Tropical Medicine and Public Health*, 29, pp. 605-610.

Szreter, S. (1999). Rapid economic growth and 'the four Ds' of disruption, deprivation, disease and death: Public health lessons from the nineteen-century Britain for twenty-first-century China? *Tropical Medicine and International Health*, 4, pp. 146-152.

Tang, S. L., Bloom, G., Feng, X. S., et al. (1994). *Financing Health Services in China: Adapting to the Economic Reforms*. Research Report 26, Brighton: Institute of Development Studies.

Tao, R.C., Huang, Z.D., Wu, X.G. et al. (1989). CHD and its risk factors in the People's Republic of China. *International Journal of Epidemiology*, 18, pp. S159-63.

The World Bank (2000). *World Development Indicators*. Washington DC: The World Bank.

Thomas, N. H. and Aiping, M. (2000). Fertility and population policy in two counties in China 1980-1991. *Journal of Biosocial Science*, 32, pp. 125-140.

Tipping, G. and Segall, M. (1995). *Health Care Seeking Behaviour in Developing Countries*. London: Institute of Developing Studies, University of Sussex.

Turner, S. T. (1997). *Medical Power and Social Knowledge*. London: Sage Publications.

Turner, R. J. and Lloyd, D. A. (1999). The stress process and the social distribution of depression. *Journal of Health and Social Behavior*, 40, pp. 374-404.

Twaddle, A. (2002). *Comparative Medical Care Reform*, Westport CT: Greenwood Press.

Uchino, B. N., Cacioppo, J. T. and Kiecolt-Glaser, J. K. (1996). The relationship between social support and physiological processes: A review with emphasis on underlying mechanisms and implications for health. *Psychological Bulletin*, 119, pp. 488-531.

Umberson, D. (1992). Gender, marital status ans social control of health behavior. *Social Science & Medicine*, 34, pp. 907-917.

Umland, B., Waterman, R., Wiese, W., Duban, S., Mennin, S. and Kaufman, A. (1992). Learning from a rural physician program in China. *Academic Medicine*, 67, pp. 307-309.

Verbrugge, L. M. (1985). Gender and Health: an Update on Hypotheses and Evidence. *Journal of Health and Social Behavior*, 26, pp. 156-182.

Verbrugge, L. M. (1989). The twain meet: Empirical explanations of sex differences in health and mortality. *Journal of Health and Social Behavior*, 30, pp. 282-304.

Waldron, I. (1983). Sex Differences in Human Morality: the Role of Genetic Factors. *Social science & Medicine*, 17, pp. 321-333.

Waldron, I. (1993). Recent Trends in Sex Mortality Ratios for Adults in Developed Countries. *Social Science & Medicine*, 36, pp. 451-462.

Wang, M. M. (1995). Family and culture among Han Chinese in Xi-Cun. *Anthropology and Ethnology Studies*, 13, pp. 6-11 (in Chinese).

Wang, C., Burris, M. A. and Ping X. Y. (1996). Chinese village women as visual anthropologists: A participatory approach to reaching policymakers. *Social Science & Medicine*, 42, pp. 1391-1400.

Wang, C. C., Vittinghoff, E., Hua, L. S., Yun, W. H. and Rong, Z. M. (1998). Reducing pregnancy and induced abortion rates in China: Family planning with husband participation. *American Journal of Public Health*, 88, pp. 646-648.

Wang, J., Harris, M., Amos, B., Li, M., Wang, X., Zhang, J. and Chen, J. (1997). A ten year review of the iodine deficiency disorders program of the People Republic of China. *Journal of Public Health Policy*, 18, pp. 219-241.

Wang, M. M. and Xia, Z. L. (1994). Analysis on the responsibility of family care for the elderly in China. *China Demographic Service*, 4, pp. 37-43 (in Chinese).

Wang, Y., Popkin, B. and Zhai, F. (1998). The nutritional status and dietary pattern of Chinese adolescents, 1991 and 1993. *European Journal of Clinical Nutrition*, 52, pp. 908-912.

Ware, E. J., Kosinsky, M. A. and Keller, S. D. (1996). A 12-item Short Form health survey. *Medical Care*, 34, pp. 220-233.

Watkins, D., Dong, Q. and Xia, Y. (1997). Age and gender differences in the self esteem of Chinese children. *The Journal of Social Psychology*, 137, pp. 374-379.

Weber, M. (1978 [1922]). *Economy and Society*. Berkeley: University of California Press.

Weisha, L. (1998). Rural clans in Hubei Province of China: The pattern of moving through marriage and poverty. Paper presented in the International Sociological Association (ISA) conference, Montreal, August, 1998.

Wen, X. (1993). Effect of son preference and population policy on sex ratios at birth in two provinces in China. *Journal of Biosocial Sciences*, 25, pp. 509-521.

Wen, H. and Yang, W. G. (1997). Public health importance of cystic echinococcosis in China. *Acta Tropica*, 67, pp. 133-145.

White, T. (1990). Postrevolutionary mobilization in China: The One Child policy revisited. *World Politics*, 43, pp. 53-76.

White, T. (1994). Tow kinds of production: The evolution of China's family planning policy in the 1980. *Population and Development Review*, 20, pp. 137-158.

Wilenski, P. (1976). *The Delivery of Health Services in the People's Republic of China*. Canberra, Ottawa: Australian National University Press.

Wilkinson, R. (1992). Income distribution and life expectancy. *British Medical Journal*, 304, pp. 165-168.

Wolf, M. (1985). *Revolution Postponed*. Stanford: Stanford University Press.

Wong, V. C. W. and Chiu, S. W. S. (1998). Health-care reforms in the People's Republic of China. *Journal of Management in Medicine*, 12, pp. 270-286.

A World Bank Country Study. (1992). China: Long-term Issues and Options in the Health Transition. The World Bank, Washington DC.

World Health Organization. (1994). Indicators for assessing iodine deficiency disorders and their control through iodization. *WHO/NUT*, 94:36.

World Health Organization. (1995). The state of world health, 1995. *Journal of Public Health Policy*, 16, pp. 440-451.

World Health Organization. (1997). *Health for All Data Base*. Regional Office, Geneva.

World Health Organization. (2000). *World Health Report of 1999*. Geneva: WHO.

Wu, C., Maurer, C., Wang, Y., Xue, S. and Davis, D. L. (1999). Water pollution and human health in China. *Environmental Health Perspectives*, 107, pp. 251-256.

Wu, Z., Qi, G., Zeng, Y. and Detels, R. (1999). Knowledge of HIV/AIDS among health care workers in China. *AIDS Education and Prevention*, 11, pp. 353-363.

Xiang, M., Ran, M. and Li, S. (1994). A controlled evaluation of psychoeducational family intervention in a rural Chinese community. *British Journal of Psychiatry*, 165, pp. 544-8.

Xu, J. and Liu, H. (1997). Border malaria in Yunnan, China. *Southeast Asian Journal of Tropical Medicine and Public Health*, 28, pp. 456-459.

Xu, B., Rimpela, A., Jarvelin, M. R. and Nieminen, M. (1994). Sex Differences of Infant and Child Mortality in China. *Scandinavian Journal of Social Medicine*, 4, pp. 242-248.

Xu, Z., Yu, D., Jing, L. and Xu, X. (2000). Air pollution and daily mortality in Shenyang, China. *Archives of Environmental Health*, 55, pp. 115-120.

Xu, X., Yang, J., Chen, C., Wang, B., Jin, Y., Fang, Z., Wang, X. and Weiss, S. T. (1999). Familial aggregation of pulmonary function in a rural Chinese community. *American Journal of Respiratory Care and Critical Care Medicine*, 160, pp. 1928-1933.

Xue, Y. C., Min, M. J., Zhi, H. D., et al. (1994). Timing and vulnerability of the brain to iodine deficiency in endemic cretinism. *New England Journal of Medicine*, 331, pp. 1739-1743.

Yang, P.L., Lin, V. and Lawson, J. (1991). Health policy reform in the People's Republic of China. *Int'l Journal of Health Services*, 21, pp. 481-91.

Yearbook of Sanitarian Statistic. (1998). Beijing: China Statistical Publishing House.

Yip, W. P., Wang, H. and Liu, Y. (1998). Determinants of patient choice of medical provider: A case study in rural China. *Health Policy and Planning*, 13, pp. 311-322.

Young, M.E. (1989). Impact of the rural reform on financing rural health services in China. *Health Policy*, 11, pp. 27-42.

Young, H. et al. (1998).Ways and Ration of service reimbursement under CMS. *Chinese Journal of Rural Health Services Management*, 18, pp. 44-51 (Chinese).

Yu, D. (1992). Changes in health care financing and health status: The case of China in the 1980s. *Economic Policy Series*, No. 34, Unicef.

Yu, P. (1996). Family planning program and women's status in China, in *The Population Situation in China*, pp. 16-22, Beijing: China population Association.

Yu, M. Y. and Sarri, R. (1997). Women's health status and gender inequality in China. *Social Science & Medicine*, 54, pp. 1885-1898.

Yu, J. J., Glynn, T. J., Pechacek, M. W. and Manley, M. W. (1995). The role of physicians in combating the growing health crisis of tobacco-induced death and disease in the People's Republic of China. *Promotion and Education*, II, pp. 23-25.

Yu, Z., Song, G., Guo, Z., Zheng, G., Tian, H., et al. (1999). Changes in blood pressure, Body Mass Index, and salt consumption in a Chinese population. *Preventive Medicine*, 29, pp. 165-172.

Yuen, P.P. (1992). Private medicine in socialist China: A survey of the private medical market in Guangzhou. *Int'l J of Health Planning and Management*, 7, pp. 211-221.

Zeng, Y. (1996). A demographic profile of marriage and family in China, in *The Population Situation in China*, pp. 23-29, Beijing: Chian Population Association, State Family Planning Commission of China.

Zeng, Y., Vaupel, J. and Wang, Z. (1993). Marrauge and fertility in China: 1950-1989. *Genus*, 49, pp. 17-34.

Zhan, H. J. (1996). Chinese femininity and social control: Gender-role socialization and the state. *Journal of Historical Sociology*, 9, pp. 269-289.

Zhan, S. K., Tang, S. L., Guo, Y. D. and Bloom, G. (1998). Drug prescribing in rural health facilities in China: Implications for service quality and costs. *Tropical Doctor*, 28, pp. 42-48.

Zhang, J. (1996). Suicides in Beijing, China, 1992-1993. *Suicide and Life Threatening Behavior*, 26, pp. 175-80.

Zhang, Y. W. (1998). *Xileito Village Survey*. Beijing: Knowledge Press (Chinese).

Zhang, A. Y. and Yu, L. C. (1998). Life satisfaction among Chinese elderly in Beijing. *Journal of Cross-Cultural Gerontology*, 13, pp. 109-125.

Zhang, J., Yu, J., Zhang, R. Z., et al.(1998). Costs of polio immunization days in China: Implications for mass immunization campaign strategies. *International Journal of Health Planning and Management*, 13, pp. 15-25.

Zhang, J., Yu, J., Linkins, R.W, et al.(1997). Effect of target age of supplemental immunization campaigns on poliomyelitis occurrence in China. *The Journal of Infectious Diseases*, 175, pp. S210-S214.

Zhao, Z. (1998). Demographic conditions, microsimulation, and family support for the elderly: Past, present, and future in China, in P. Herold and R. Smith (eds), *The Locus of Care: Families, Communities, and Provision of Welfare Since Antiquity*, pp. 259-279, London: Routledge.

Zhao, Z. (2000). Coresidential patterns in historical China: A simulation study. *Population and Development*, 26, pp. 263-295.

Zhou, S. (1992). Scholarly views of rural health insurance system. *Primary Health care in China*, 3, pp. 1-5 (Chinese).

Zhou, Y. (2000). *Will China's Current Population policy Change Its Kinship System?* NUPRI Research Paper Series No. 70, Tokyo: Nihon Univ Press.

Zhou, X. and Hou, L. (1999). Children of the Cultural Revolution: The state and the life course in the People Republic of China. *American Sociological Review*, 64, pp. 12-36.

Zhu, N. S., Ling, Z.H., Shen, J., Lane, J.M. and Hu, S. L. (1989). Factors associated with the decline of the cooperative medical system and barefoot doctor in rural China. *Bulletin of the World Health Organization*, 67, pp. 431-41.

Zhu, Y., Chen, D. and Tang, Y. (1993). The forming and the development of health market in rural districts. *Primary Health Care in China*, 12, pp. 4-6 (Chinese).

Index